A HISTORY OF THE NATIONAL ACADEMY OF MEDICINE

50 YEARS OF TRANSFORMATIONAL LEADERSHIP

Editors
Evelynn Hammonds
Howard Markel
David Rosner
Rosemary Stevens

Authors
Laura Harbold DeStefano
Andrea Schultz
Edward Berkowitz

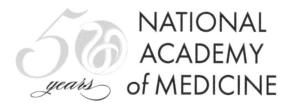

NATIONAL ACADEMY of MEDICINE

THE NATIONAL ACADEMIES PRESS
Washington, DC
www.nap.edu

THE NATIONAL ACADEMIES PRESS   **500 Fifth Street, NW**   **Washington, DC 20001**

International Standard Book Number-13: 978-0-309-69353-0
International Standard Book Number-10: 0-309-69353-5
Digital Object Identifier: https://doi.org/10.17226/26708
Library of Congress Catalog Number: 2022945951

This publication is available from the National Academies Press, 500 Fifth Street, NW, Keck 360, Washington, DC 20001; (800) 624-6242 or (202) 334-3313; http://www.nap.edu.

Cover image credits (left to right, row by row): National Library of Medicine; Science Photo Library (SPL); iStock; Shutterstock; Unsplash (photo by Mick Haupt); Centers for Disease Control and Prevention (CDC)/CDC Connects (photo by Rebecca Myers); Unsplash (photo by National Cancer Institute); Library of Congress; White House Archives; iStock; iStock; SC National Guard on Flickr; iStock; iStock; National Institutes of Health; Cleveland Clinic; CDC (photo by Rana Asghar); National Academy of Medicine (NAM); Dick Swanson/The LIFE Images Collection/Getty Images; Piyaset, iStock; Don Detmer; iStock; iStock; SPL; CDC (photo by Courtney Wheeler); NAM; SPL; CDC (photo by Debra Cartagena).

Suggested citation: Hammonds, E., H. Markel, D. Rosner, and R. Stevens, editors; Harbold DeStefano, L., A. Schultz, and E. Berkowitz, authors. *A History of the National Academy of Medicine: 50 Years of Transformational Leadership*. Washington, DC: The National Academies Press. https://doi.org/10.17226/26708.

ABOUT THE NATIONAL ACADEMY OF MEDICINE

The **National Academy of Medicine** is one of three Academies constituting the National Academies of Sciences, Engineering, and Medicine (the National Academies). The National Academies provide independent, objective analysis and advice to the nation and conduct other activities to solve complex problems and inform public policy decisions. The National Academies also encourage education and research, recognize outstanding contributions to knowledge, and increase public understanding in matters of science, engineering, and medicine.

The **National Academy of Sciences** was established in 1863 by an Act of Congress, signed by President Lincoln, as a private, nongovernmental institution to advise the nation on issues related to science and technology. Members are elected by their peers for outstanding contributions to research. Dr. Marcia McNutt is president.

The **National Academy of Engineering** was established in 1964 under the charter of the National Academy of Sciences to bring the practices of engineering to advising the nation. Members are elected by their peers for extraordinary contributions to engineering. Dr. John L. Anderson is president.

The **National Academy of Medicine** (formerly the Institute of Medicine) was established in 1970 under the charter of the National Academy of Sciences to advise the nation on issues of health, health care, and biomedical science and technology. Members are elected by their peers for distinguished contributions to medicine and health. Dr. Victor J. Dzau is president.

Learn more about the National Academy of Medicine at NAM.edu.

Acknowledgments

The National Academy of Medicine extends its gratitude to the following individuals for their valuable contributions to the research, writing, review, and production of this volume:

Alina Baciu
Clyde Behney
Libby Beri
Madeleine Deye
Donna Duncan
Victor Dzau
Harvey Fineberg
Kenneth Fulton
James Hinchman
Radhika Hira
Morgan Kanarek
Seth LaShier
Alan Leshner
Rachel Marcus

Rose Marie Martinez
J. Michael McGinnis
Sharyl Nass
Jenna Ogilvie
Steve Olson
Julie Pavlin
Samantha Phillips
Andrew Pope
Olivia Ramirez
Kenneth Shine
Samuel Thier
Ann Yaktine
Tadataka Yamada
Keith Yamamoto

Glossary

Action Collaborative: A program type of the National Academy of Medicine (NAM) that brings multi-sectoral stakeholders together on a term-limited basis to catalyze action around shared priorities.

Consensus Report (or Consensus Study): An evidence-based report containing findings, conclusions, and recommendations authored by an expert committee appointed by the National Academies of Sciences, Engineering, and Medicine (the National Academies).

Convening Activity: A one-time event (e.g., a public workshop) or standing mechanism (e.g., a roundtable) to convene stakeholders to discuss or advance specific issues or fields.

Council (or Councilor): A governing and oversight body to which Academy members are elected on a term-limited basis. Members of the Councils of the National Academy of Sciences (NAS), National Academy of Engineering (NAE), and the NAM are referred to as Councilors.

Division Committee: An advisory body, to which volunteers are appointed on a term-limited basis, that informs the work of the Health and Medicine Division (HMD) and other program divisions of the National Academies.

Forum (or Roundtable): A standing mechanism to convene stakeholders from a defined field and advance issues of common interest.

Health and Medicine Division (HMD): A program division of the National Academies that was created in 2015 after the Institute of Medicine (IOM) became the NAM.

Home Secretary: An officer elected from among the NAM (or the NAS or the NAE) membership to oversee member elections, interest groups, and other activities related to member engagement.

Institute of Medicine (IOM): The precursor organization to the NAM, which was known under the IOM name from 1970 until 2015.

International Secretary: An officer elected from among the NAM (or the NAS or the NAE) membership to lead and advise on international affairs. This position was called Foreign Secretary until 2021, when the name was changed to International Secretary.

Member of the IOM/NAM: An individual elected to the IOM (later the NAM) on the basis of exceptional achievement and commitment to service within the National Academies.

National Academies of Sciences, Engineering, and Medicine: The name of the organization made up of the NAS, the NAE, the NAM, and programmatic units including the HMD. The organization began using this name in 2015.

National Academy of Engineering (NAE): An independent, evidence-based advisor on matters of engineering and an honorific membership organization for exceptional leaders in engineering fields (founded in 1964).

National Academy of Medicine (NAM): An independent, evidence-based advisor on matters of biomedical science, medicine, and health and an honorific membership organization for exceptional leaders in these fields. Founded in 1970, the NAM was known as the IOM until 2015.

National Academy of Sciences (NAS): An independent, evidence-based advisor on matters of science and technology and an honorific membership organization for exceptional leaders in these fields (founded in 1863).

National Research Council (NRC): The operational arm of the NAS and the NAE, which houses programmatic units that carry out consensus studies, convenings, and other activities. The NRC name was no longer used publicly after 2015.

Contents

FOREWORD   xi

PREFACE   xv

PART I   INSTITUTIONAL HISTORY   1

1   THE FOUNDING OF THE INSTITUTE OF MEDICINE   3
The Need for Independent Advice in Health and Medicine, 4
Establishment of the National Academy of Sciences' Board on Medicine and
    Public Health, 7
Proposal for a National Academy of Medicine, 10
Establishment of the Institute of Medicine, 11
Conclusion, 13

**2   A COMMITMENT TO SERVICE: MEMBERS AND LEADERS OF THE INSTITUTE OF MEDICINE
AND THE NATIONAL ACADEMY OF MEDICINE**   15
Volunteerism, 15
Multidisciplinarity, 16
Achievement, 18
Presidents of the Institute of Medicine and the National Academy
    of Medicine, 22
Institute of Medicine and National Academy of Medicine Staff Leaders, 36
Building the Leadership Pipeline and Recognizing Excellence, 39
Conclusion, 40

3   THE CREATION OF THE NATIONAL ACADEMY OF MEDICINE   43
    History of Campaigns to Establish the National Academy of Medicine, 44
    Success of the 2013–2015 Campaign, 47
    Organizational Transitions, 50
    The National Academy of Medicine's Program Takes Shape, 52
    Conclusion, 54
    Chapter 3 Appendix Figures, 55

PART II IMPACT   61

4   BIOMEDICAL SCIENCE   63
    The Human Genome: From Sequencing to Editing, 65
    Vaccine Safety and Efficacy, 68
    The Science of Childhood and Adolescent Development, 73
    Facilitating Progress in Cancer Research, 77
    Scientific Advisor to the U.S. Government, 83
    Building Capacity of International Science Academies, 99
    Conclusion, 100

5   U.S. HEALTH CARE AND POLICY   101
    Building a Culture of Health Care Quality, 102
    A Value and Science-Driven Health System, 111
    Health Disparities and Health Equity, 115
    The Health Care Workforce and Informal Caregivers, 120
    Complex and Serious Health Conditions, 125
    Health Care Reform and Uninsurance, 132
    Conclusion, 136

6   ADVANCING THE HEALTH OF THE PUBLIC IN THE UNITED STATES AND GLOBALLY   139
    Defining and Shaping Public Health, 139
    Responding to Public Health Pandemics and Epidemics, 141
    Responding to Chronic Conditions, 154
    Environmental Health, 171
    Protecting Health in an Interconnected World, 174
    Conclusion, 183

PART III A NEW ERA: THE EARLY YEARS OF THE NATIONAL ACADEMY
         OF MEDICINE   185

7   RESPONDING TO NATIONAL AND GLOBAL CRISES, 2015–2021   187
    Identifying, Addressing, and Inspiring Action in Response to Critical Issues
    (Strategic Goal 1), 187
    Diversifying and Activating Members and Engaging Emerging Leaders
    (Strategic Goal 2), 201
    Building Leadership Capacity Across Diverse Disciplines (Strategic Goal 3), 203
    Conclusion, 207

8   CONCLUSION   209

EPILOGUE **213**

BIBLIOGRAPHY **215**

EDITOR AND AUTHOR BIOGRAPHIES **239**

Foreword

"The tragedy of life is often not in our failure, but rather in our complacency; not in our doing too much, but rather in our doing too little; not in our living above our ability, but rather in our living below our capacities."

—Benjamin Mays, U.S. Civil Rights Leader

I was elected as a member of the Institute of Medicine (IOM), now the National Academy of Medicine (NAM), in 1998. It was the highest honor of my career.

I was born in Shanghai, grew up in Hong Kong, and traveled to Montréal to earn my undergraduate and medical degrees at McGill University. I moved to New York for my postdoctoral training and have lived in the United States ever since—since 1990, as a proud U.S. citizen. As an immigrant, my adopted country has given me many remarkable opportunities. It is a privilege and a joy to give back by serving the mission of the NAM—*to improve health for all by advancing science, accelerating health equity, and providing independent, authoritative, and trusted advice nationally and globally.*

In 2014, I was appointed as the final president of the IOM and, 6 years later, elected for a second term as the first president of the newly reconstituted NAM. Although it meant spending less time with my family in North Carolina and taking a leave of absence from my role at Duke University, taking the job was a no-brainer. It is not hyperbole to say that no other organization can match the impact of the IOM/NAM.

As you will read in the chapters ahead, it was the IOM that launched the patient safety movement in U.S. health care, laid the foundation for mapping the human genome, galvanized the public health response to the AIDS epidemic, and upheld the safety of vaccines—among other impacts too numerous to list in science, medicine, and population health. IOM/NAM members are luminaries in their fields, more than 75 Nobel Prize winners among them at the time of this writing. Approximately 25 percent represent professions outside the traditional health sciences, in a nod to the inter-disciplinarity of health. I marvel at how many members give freely of their time and expertise each year to support the work of the NAM and advance the common good.

This volume details the long path to reconstitute the IOM as the NAM, an organizational transformation that had been debated almost without pause since the IOM's founding in 1970.

When I took the helm of the IOM in 2014, the latest campaign to form an Academy, begun by my predecessor, Harvey V. Fineberg, was nearing its successful conclusion.

The establishment of the NAM, finalized in 2015, was the culmination of decades of work by IOM leaders to achieve organizational parity with the National Academy of Sciences (NAS) and the National Academy of Engineering (NAE). As an Academy, the NAM had an equal role in the governance of the overarching organization, which was rebranded alongside the NAM as the National Academies of Sciences, Engineering, and Medicine (the National Academies). The move signaled a commitment to greater integration and efficiency in an age in which society's greatest challenges require an increasingly interdisciplinary toolkit.

Indeed, the creation of the NAM was cause for celebration. But the transition was difficult in many ways. The IOM brand was beloved among members and staff and trusted by sponsors, policy makers, and researchers in the United States and abroad. The reorganization required the IOM's legacy boards, roundtables, and forums—and the majority of its staff—to be rehoused in a new National Academies' Health and Medicine Division (HMD). The NAM, left with just a few programs, had to chart a new course.

It has been hard work, but I am deeply proud to say that we have succeeded. In the few short years since its creation, the NAM has established a dynamic portfolio of programs that leverage its new independence as an Academy while remaining deeply rooted in the rigorous science that propelled the IOM's influence for 45 years.

In fact, it is my belief that the NAM has extended the impact of the organization well beyond what the IOM's founders ever imagined. As I write, we are at a pivotal moment in history. No less than three existential crises threaten the health of humanity and the environment that sustains us: pandemics, climate change, and structural racism. The new Academy has evolved and innovated to meet these challenges head on. We do not wait until we are called on to act. Instead, we move proactively to catalyze collective action among the diverse stakeholders who hold the levers for change. Together with colleagues throughout the National Academies and partners across the world, we are pioneering solutions for the most urgent challenges of the future. A quote from the German poet Johann Wolfgang von Goethe, which appeared in the front matter of IOM reports for many years, still says it best: *"Knowing is not enough; we must apply. Willing is not enough; we must do."*

In early 2020, the NAM—and the health and medical community worldwide—was put to the test when SARS-CoV-2, the virus that causes COVID-19, became the most dangerous pandemic in a century. We put the Academy's existing programmatic priorities on hold in order to focus fully on fighting the pandemic. Alongside the HMD and other National Academies units, the NAM provided crucial scientific expertise to the government and members of the public as the crisis unfolded, on topics ranging from how COVID-19 is transmitted to the efficacy of face coverings and physical distancing, to the efficacy of testing and need for crisis standards of care. We also called for a national strategy to protect clinician well-being during the pandemic, as stressors such as lack of personal protective equipment and life-saving supplies sharply increased the strain on an already burdened workforce.

As COVID-19 vaccines drew closer to approval in fall 2020, the National Institutes of Health and the Centers for Disease Control and Prevention (CDC) turned to the NAM and the National Academies to guide the equitable allocation of an initially limited supply. We produced a consensus report in just over 3 months that helped to inform the CDC's recommendations as well as many state-level plans for allocation. By the end of 2021, more than 60 percent of the U.S. population had been fully vaccinated against COVID-19 (Pariseault, 2021). However, the pandemic continues to evolve and challenge us. The emergence of highly contagious variants has stretched the U.S.

health care system to the breaking point. Meanwhile, populations around the world still struggle to access vaccines—a tragic inequity that threatens the health of people everywhere.

Throughout the pandemic, NAM members have been crucial leaders driving solutions in their own spheres—several as heads of government agencies and task forces, many more as scientists, clinicians, educators, and advocates. Alongside myself and the presidents of the NAS and the NAE, members spoke out against the dangerous politicization of science during the pandemic, as well as the temporary breakdown of the U.S. relationship with the World Health Organization, a critical partner in combatting COVID-19 globally. The NAM's response to COVID-19 will continue as long as the virus continues to infect individuals anywhere across the globe.

Among many lessons, COVID-19 has taught us that quick, collective action among the scientific and medical communities is possible—and powerful. We must turn that passion and purpose toward other major challenges, both new and enduring, that threaten human health. In that spirit, I am proud that the NAM has committed to confronting structural racism and the impacts of climate change on health and equity.

There is much to be learned from looking back at what we have accomplished—and, crucially, at how we have accomplished it. The IOM/NAM continues to be impactful because of its commitment to science, evidence, and independence, as well as the dedication of countless members, volunteers, and staff who work tirelessly on behalf of its mission. This unique formula allows us to cut across geographic, political, and disciplinary divides and unite leaders around common goals—particularly in times of crisis, as recent events have demonstrated.

But we cannot and will not rest on our laurels. As rapid developments in science, technology, and communication transform the social landscape and climate change, infectious disease, and inequities fuel new threats to health, the unique contributions of the IOM/NAM are just as vital, if not more so, than 50 years ago. Decision makers at every level—within governments, organizations, communities, and households—need evidence-based solutions that support equitable good health. More than that, they need decisive leadership and innovative strategies to anticipate the formidable challenges of the future and ensure that everyone benefits from exponential gains in knowledge.

The NAM, alongside the HMD and drawing on the deep interdisciplinary expertise of the broader National Academies, stands ready to provide this crucial leadership. As we look ahead to the next half-century as an Academy, our legacy will be one of action.

—**Victor J. Dzau, MD**
President
National Academy of Medicine

December 2021

Preface

This volume was originally intended to be published in 2020 to mark the occasion of the 50th anniversary of the founding of the Institute of Medicine (IOM). The COVID-19 pandemic slowed its completion, and, as the chapters that follow detail, led to lasting changes across the organization. The final volume describes events within and outside the organization through the end of 2021. The National Academy of Medicine's (NAM's) response to major events in 2022, such as Russia's invasion of Ukraine, racially motivated and other mass shootings in the United States, and the U.S. Supreme Court's decision to overturn *Roe v. Wade,* are covered in the Epilogue.

This volume is organized into three parts. Part I, "Institutional History," describes the circumstances that led to the IOM's founding, the members and leaders who built and sustained the organization, and the process by which the NAM and the Health and Medicine Division were formed. Part II, "Impact," details a selection of the IOM/NAM's most influential contributions to biomedical science, U.S. health care, and population health. Finally, Part III, "A New Era: The Early Years of the National Academy of Medicine," describes how the NAM navigated unprecedented national and global crises between 2015 and 2021 and developed an innovative programmatic approach that led to changes across the National Academies of Sciences, Engineering, and Medicine.

Part I

Institutional History

The following chapters describe the founding of the Institute of Medicine (IOM) in 1970, its journey toward establishment as a trusted and influential advisor on health and medicine, and institutional steps toward becoming the National Academy of Medicine (NAM) in 2015. This part also includes descriptions of the roles of IOM/NAM presidents, members, and staff leaders, as well as the NAM's response to national and global challenges in its first years as an Academy alongside the National Academy of Sciences and the National Academy of Engineering.

1

The Founding of the Institute of Medicine[1]

In 2011, *The New York Times* described the Institute of Medicine (IOM) as one of "the nation's most esteemed and authoritative advisors on issues of health and medicine" (Harris, 2011) with the power "to transform medical thinking around the world" (Ince, 2015, p. 15). Such a ringing endorsement may have come as a surprise to the charter members of the IOM in 1970, although it was a perfect match for their ambition.

The roots of the organization can be traced to the 1960s, when highly politicized debates over the prospect of national health insurance in the United States revealed the need for an unbiased, evidence-based source of advice to guide health policy and its implementation. The IOM, which began as the Board on Medicine and Public Health within the National Academy of Sciences (NAS), set out to meet that need. The IOM's association with the prestigious NAS, as well as an influential public statement it made on the safety of heart transplantation (described later in this chapter), garnered almost immediate visibility for the fledgling organization. Yet, it faced formidable challenges in establishing its infrastructure and governance in its early years.

Nevertheless, elements of the organization *The New York Times* would later deem capable of changing the world were already evident. From the beginning, the IOM's founding leaders and members determined that it would be a working organization, rather than solely honorific, and be dedicated to solving pressing health and medical challenges. Because such challenges required a multidisciplinary approach, the IOM established a requirement that one-quarter of its members should represent disciplines outside medicine and the biomedical sciences. The IOM's early leaders also demonstrated a keen understanding of the influence of social factors on health, as well as a commitment to an active agenda that serves the needs of the public. These elements continue to be critical to the mission and approach of the organization, which was reconstituted as the National Academy of Medicine (NAM) in 2015.[2]

---

[1] Except where otherwise noted, historical facts presented in this chapter are drawn from a 1998 history of the Institute of Medicine authored by Edward Berkowitz (IOM, 1998a).

[2] At the same time the IOM was reconstituted as the NAM, a new Health and Medicine Division (HMD) was created within the National Research Council. All of the IOM's boards and many of its convening activities were moved to HMD. See Chapter 3 for more on the 2015 reorganization.

THE NEED FOR INDEPENDENT ADVICE IN HEALTH AND MEDICINE

In 1964, Irvine Page (see Figure 1-1), a prominent physician who would later become a founding member of the IOM, wrote an editorial in the journal *Modern Medicine* titled "Needed—A National Academy of Medicine." At the time, the notion of national health insurance preoccupied health policy makers, but faced opposition from private physicians who feared it would stifle their businesses. The future of the National Institutes of Health (NIH) was also the subject of spirited debate, as politicians advocated for the funding of pet issues and scientists contended that priorities should be set by experts in accordance with the most critical needs in health and medicine.

For Page, a leading expert on hypertension and heart disease at Cleveland Clinic, such disputes illustrated the need for a national organization that could speak with independent, nonpartisan authority on questions of health policy. In his 1964 editorial, Page argued that government required the advice of a group of physicians who were "truly representative of excellence in all branches of medicine" and who could provide "decisions of wisdom" (Page, 1964).

The American Medical Association and Academic Medicine

The largest medical association at the time, the American Medical Association (AMA), was a grassroots organization founded in 1847 to represent the interests of practicing physicians across the nation. Its goals included professionalizing the practice of medicine and instilling science as the foundation of medical education and practice. In 1883, the AMA established the *Journal of the American Medical Association* (*JAMA*) as a vehicle to distribute peer-reviewed research and encourage the practice of evidence-based medicine among its members. The AMA was a broadbased organization that brought all medical specialties inside its tent. However, because of its demo-

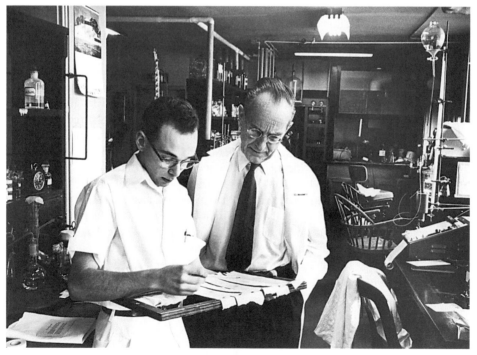

FIGURE 1-1 Irvine Page (at right) is pictured in laboratory in the 1960s.
SOURCE: Cleveland Clinic (CC BY 4.0).

cratic structure, the AMA's policy positions reflected the influence of the majority of its physician members, who worked in private practice settings.

Page and his colleagues had a different perspective. Doctors on the faculty of medical schools often had teaching, clinical, and research responsibilities. External funding was crucial to their endeavors. As tertiary care settings receiving patients with the most critical medical problems, medical schools relied on specialists in a wide range of fields. At some academic institutions, physicians were paid on a salaried basis, in contrast to doctors working in private practice, or relied on grants from the NIH and private foundations. Academic physicians and medical researchers, in Page's estimation, had fundamentally different concerns than did doctors engaged in general practice in their communities.

Many private doctors opposed the passage of Medicare, for example, believing it was in effect the first step toward the socialization of medicine. They worried in particular about the possibility that government would set prices and enforce national standards that violated the norms of local medical practice. Reflecting these concerns, the AMA, beginning in the late 1930s and the 1940s, had become the leading opponent of proposals for national health insurance, frequently testifying on the subject before Congress. Despite efforts by the Truman administration (1945–1953) and liberal members of Congress, proposals had failed in every congressional session after 1949. Medical researchers and academic physicians such as Page, on the other hand, had a much more collaborative relationship with the federal government (e.g., through work with the NIH), and therefore less apprehension about federally funded health care (Chapin, 2015).

It was in this context that Page and other prominent academic physicians began to explore the idea of an "academy of medicine," an organization that could represent the views of the academic medical community and balance the influence of the AMA.

Health Policy Priorities of the 1960s

The future of the NIH was at the center of Page's concerns. The agency enjoyed a wide base of political support; throughout the 1950s, Congress had consistently allocated more money for the NIH than the Eisenhower administration requested. However, some believed it was a fragile organization of relatively recent vintage that could be easily misdirected.[3] The NIH had extensive programs of intramural and extramural research, with work being done across the nation in medical schools as well as the sprawling Bethesda headquarters. It was commonplace for politicians to try to secure funding for their local institutions and for members of Congress to urge that research into a disease of particular interest to them be brought to the forefront of the NIH's priorities.

Page and others wanted to protect the NIH from what they considered to be harmful political influences. They advocated for policies to ensure that the NIH's funding decisions reflected an expert understanding of the most critical research needs in health and medicine—not the political flavor of the week. They insisted, for example, that grant proposals submitted to the NIH undergo peer review by leading medical experts, rather than government officials. (In 2020, this issue would come full circle as the presidents of the NAS, the NAM, and the NAE spoke out against the political review of scientific proposals under the Trump administration; see Chapter 7.)

President John F. Kennedy (1961–1963), unlike his predecessor President Dwight D. Eisenhower (1953–1961), supported a socially progressive agenda with significant implications for the practice of medicine. Medicare, long a subject of contention, finally gained traction during the Kennedy administration and was ultimately signed into law in 1965. It was clear that the legislation would fundamentally alter the relationship between the medical profession and the federal govern-

---

[3] The NIH was established in 1949 with the creation of the National Institute of Mental Health.

ment. Page believed that government needed the best possible independent advice to implement this complicated new program and that such advice should come from leaders of academic medicine.

Other elements of Kennedy's political agenda had relevance to Page's effort. Federal aid to education (including aid to medical schools) continued to be a hotly contested issue. By expanding existing medical schools and creating new ones, the federal government could insure against an anticipated doctor shortage that might cripple the nation and put it at a disadvantage in the Cold War. The Civil Rights Act of 1964 also had broad ramifications for health care, bringing about the desegregation of health facilities and setting the stage for efforts to build a more diverse clinical workforce. In this period of complex and sweeping change, Page believed that an independent medical advisory organization would serve the nation well.

Irvine Page Convenes Founding Members of the Institute of Medicine

In a March 1965 follow-up editorial, Page argued for an academy of medicine that, unlike the AMA, would not be a grassroots organization lobbying for change from the bottom up. Instead, he envisioned an academy that would draw its membership from the "upper, relatively thin layer of the best medical and scientific talent" and would adapt continuously as medical science evolved (Page, 1965). The academy would be a "working organization" positioned at the forefront of medical research and science. However, the "upper layer" described by Page did not necessarily reflect the makeup of U.S. society or the challenges faced by its diverse population. As the photo of Page's group (see Figure 1-2) illustrates, leaders of the medical field in the 1960s and 1970s were almost overwhelmingly White and male. Yet, the civil rights and women's movements in the era of the IOM's founding demanded equity and access to positions of influence for women, Black people and other people of color. This tension endured for decades, even as the IOM issued reports that highlighted the crisis of racial and other health disparities. Diversification of the IOM/NAM membership across dimensions of demographics and expertise remained both a challenge and a priority for the organization in 2020, when the NAM launched a membership diversity task force (Dzau, 2020).

On January 17, 1967, with the help of a $6,000 grant from the Cleveland Foundation, Page convened a group of 16 leading physicians and scientists in Cleveland, Ohio, to refine his idea of

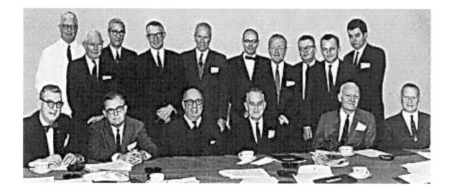

FIGURE 1-2 Irvine H. Page's group to discuss the formation of a National Academy of Medicine met for the first time on January 17, 1967, at the Cleveland Foundation.
SOURCE: Institute of Medicine. 1998. *To Improve Human Health: A History of the Institute of Medicine*. Washington, DC: The National Academies Press. https://doi.org/10.17226/6382.

an academy of medicine. The attendees were well connected in political and philanthropic networks. Nearly all of them worked in medical schools or for the NIH; the group included the NIH's then current director, James Shannon, an influential malaria researcher who had advised the U.S. Secretary of War on tropical diseases during World War II (NASEM, 1967a; NIH, n.d.a). Other attendees included Ivan Bennett, Deputy Director of the Office of Science and Technology Policy under President Lyndon B. Johnson (1963–1969). Colin MacLeod, a scientist who discovered the hereditary properties of DNA, served as Vice President for Medical Affairs at The Commonwealth Fund, an important source of support for public health and medical research. Shannon and McLeod were also elected members of the NAS.

The NAS enjoyed a strong reputation as an unbiased, independent advisor to the nation on complex scientific and technical questions, as it had for more than a century. Its membership included physicians such as Shannon who worked in academic medical centers and made outstanding scientific contributions. However, the large majority of the NAS's membership hailed from fields such as physics, biology, or mathematics.

Before Page's group met for a second time in March 1967, Shannon and Bennett arranged a meeting in Washington, DC, with Frederick Seitz, a prominent physicist who was then president of the NAS. Seitz was receptive to the Cleveland group's ideas. He offered to move its meetings to the NAS headquarters in Washington, DC, and establish a Board on Medicine and Public Health under the auspices of the academy. The board would not only contemplate the formation of an academy of medicine, perhaps as an offshoot of the NAS, but would also meet with foundations and government agencies to discuss issues of concern, including urban health challenges and the complexities of national health insurance. Members of the Cleveland group agreed to the move (NASEM, 1967b).

ESTABLISHMENT OF THE NATIONAL ACADEMY OF SCIENCES' BOARD ON MEDICINE AND PUBLIC HEALTH

In June 1967, the NAS Council approved the creation of a Board on Medicine and Public Health charged to "formulate recommendations on matters of policy related to medicine and public health" (IOM, 1998a, p. 10). Seitz indicated that the Board could "possibly lead to the formation of a National Academy of Medicine somewhat analogous to the NAE [National Academy of Engineering]" (IOM, 1998a, p. 10). The NAE had been established in 1964 under the charter of the NAS to honor eminent engineers and tap engineering expertise for the nation's most important scientific projects (NAE, n.d.). During this time of transition for the Cleveland group, Page continued to advocate for the creation of an academy of medicine that would not be a purely honorific organization like the NAS. However, on June 2, 1967, Page suffered a heart attack. Although he remained active in the discussions of the Board on Medicine and Public Health, he no longer took the lead.

As an NAS activity, the new Board on Medicine and Public Health (ultimately shortened to the Board on Medicine) required an NAS member as its leader. Seitz made the appointment, setting a precedent for NAS involvement in IOM leadership decisions that would remain until the IOM's reconstitution as an independent academy in 2015. Seitz chose Walsh McDermott, a professor at Cornell Medical School known for his contributions to the development of antibiotics and anti-tuberculosis drugs, to serve as the board's first chair (see Figure 1-3). McDermott had served as the head of the Division of Infectious Diseases at New York Hospital, where he performed important clinical trials on penicillin, streptomycin, and the other "wonder drugs" of the era. In the 1950s, he shifted his focus to the task of bringing medical treatment to underserved populations, and organized a successful effort to treat tuberculosis among members of the Navajo Nation living in Arizona and New Mexico. He had served as a member of the NIH's National Advisory Health Council as well New York City's Board of Health.

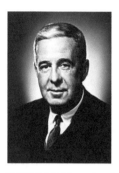

FIGURE 1-3 Portrait of Walsh McDermott.
SOURCE: National Library of Medicine (http://resource.nlm.nih.gov/101422334).

Under the banner of the Great Society in the 1960s,[4] the federal government attempted to confront large-scale societal challenges facing the nation, including poverty and health disparities, physician shortages related to the Vietnam War and the implementation of Medicare, ensuring access to affordable health care, and the need to increase government support for medical research. Culturally, there was a sense of optimism that progress was possible on all of these fronts in an increasingly prosperous America with a developing commitment to civil rights. McDermott's strong interest in public health was a contributing factor in developing the portfolio of the Board on Medicine, and subsequently the IOM. Even more so than Page, McDermott envisioned an organization of working members who were actively engaged by the most pressing medical and health concerns for society.

Together, McDermott and Seitz selected the original members of the Board on Medicine, with Page, Bennett, and MacLeod among them (see Box 1-1). The membership also included non-physicians deliberately selected for the expertise they could bring to social problems. Adam Yarmolinsky, for example, was a lawyer with experience in the Kennedy and Johnson administrations who had helped to organize the Johnson administration's war on poverty. Yarmolinsky became an active member of the IOM, eventually writing the organization's charter bylaws and serving on its governing council. Rashi Fein, another non-physician member, had served on the staff of President Kennedy's Council of Economic Advisors, making him an expert on what would soon become the field of health economics.

Representation of a wide range of medical specialties and social expertise became an explicit objective of the board—a criterion that would extend to membership in the IOM and NAM. Lucile Leone, a nurse who had led the U.S. Cadet Nurse Corps during World War II, was a charter member of the board and the only woman in the group (Thurber, 2000). Just two of the Board's original 21 members were African American (see Figure 1-4). Samuel Nabrit, a marine biologist and the first African American to receive a PhD from Brown University, was a member of President Johnson's Atomic Energy Commission (Brown University, n.d.). Alonzo Yerby, a physician who served as the first African American Commissioner of Hospitals in New York City, had helped the Johnson

---

BOX 1-1
Members of the Board on Medicine, June 1969

Walsh McDermott, MD, *Chair*	Joseph Murtaugh
Ivan L. Bennett, Jr., MD	Samuel M. Nabrit, PhD
Charles G. Child III, MD	Irvine H. Page, MD
Julius H. Comroe, Jr., MD	Henry W. Riecken, PhD
John Dunlop, PhD	Walter A. Rosenblith, IngRad
Rashi Fein, PhD	Eugene Stead, Jr., MD
Robert J. Glaser, MD	Dwight L. Wilbur, MD
Lucile P. Leone, MA	Bryan Williams, MD
Irving M. London, MD	Adam Yarmolinsky, LLB
Colin M. MacLeod, MD	Alonzo S. Yerby, MD

---

[4] The "Great Society" refers to a series of socially progressive policies and initiatives under the Johnson administration. See https://www.washingtonpost.com/wp-srv/special/national/great-society-at-50 (accessed September 7, 2022).

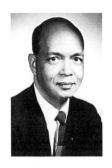 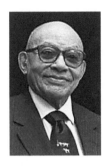 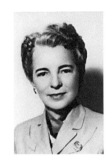

FIGURE 1-4 The first African American and female members of the IOM. From left to right: Alonzo Yerby, Samuel Nabrit, and Lucile Leone.
SOURCES: Center for the History of Medicine. 2020. "Alonzo Yerby," OnView: Digital Collections & Exhibits, https://collections.countway.harvard.edu/onview/items/show/6197 (accessed July 8, 2022); NASEM. n.d. "Samuel M. Nabrit." http://www.cpnas.org/aahp/biographies/samuel-m-nabrit.html (accessed July 8, 2022); Smithsonian Institution. 2011. "Lucile Petry Leone (1902–1999)." Acc. 90-105—Science Service, Records, 1920s–1970s, Smithsonian Institution Archives. https://www.flickr.com/photos/smithsonian/5494539024 (accessed July 8, 2022).

administration to draft Medicare and Medicaid legislation (Harvard T.H. Chan School of Public Health, n.d.). Diversification of the IOM/NAM membership (across race/ethnicity, age, gender, and geography) would be an ongoing challenge for the IOM/NAM (discussed further in Chapter 7).

The Board on Medicine held its first formal meeting on November 15, 1967. Its formation garnered national attention, including a front-page story in *The New York Times* titled "Medical Board Set Up to Speed Benefits of Research to Public." Walsh McDermott was quoted in the article, describing the board as a "good balanced mix of people who could be counted on for dispassionate and expert judgments about a broad range of problems" (Clark, 1967). From its earliest days, the organization's determination to engage the nation's current concerns resonated with the public.

The Board on Medicine Issues Its First Public Statement

In December 1967, less than 1 month after the first meeting of the Board on Medicine, news broke that Christiaan Barnard, a South African surgeon, had completed the world's first heart transplant (see Figure 1-5). Interest in the procedure skyrocketed among Americans, who welcomed a bit of good news at a moment when the United States appeared to be losing the Vietnam War and race riots had broken out in many cities. Although many viewed heart transplants as a medical miracle in the company of penicillin or polio vaccinations, the Board on Medicine responded more warily. Outcomes data for the heart transplants were lacking, and operations were proceeding in an ad hoc manner across the United States. Members of the board understood that a successful transplant depended as much on immunology—the question of whether the body would reject the donor heart—as it did on the skill of the surgeon. The board concluded that there was insufficient scientific evidence to support the widespread adoption of heart transplants.

On February 28, 1968, the Board on Medicine issued a public statement titled "Cardiac Transplantation in Man," in which it argued that heart transplants should not yet "be regarded as an accepted form of therapy, even as a heroic one" (Board on Medicine, 1968). Rather, the statement read, heart transplants should be viewed as scientific experiments for which reliable results were still pending, and should only be conducted by institutions "in which the total array of scientific expertise necessary for the proper conduct of the whole experiment (can) be brought to bear on every case" (Board on Medicine, 1968). This expertise included an experienced surgical team, a

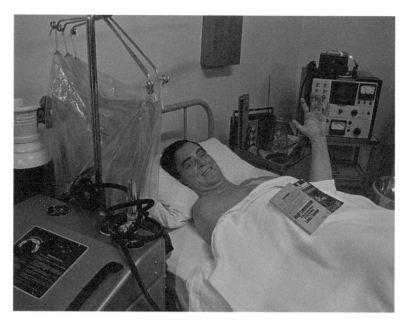

FIGURE 1-5 Fifty-three-year-old South African Louis Washkansky recovers after receiving the world's first heart transplant in 1967. Washkansky died of pneumonia 18 days after the surgery.
SOURCE: Mallix, Heart of Cape Town Museum (CC BY-NC-ND 2.0).

supporting team of immunologists, and meticulous efforts to record the long-term outcomes of transplant patients.

The Board on Medicine's statement was covered by almost every major U.S. newspaper. An article in *The New York Times* noted that five of the six people who had received heart transplants in recent weeks had died. The article quoted McDermott as saying that, while the statement was intended to inform the medical community, "the issues are of such importance to the lay public as well that it is hoped they will take notice" (Clark, 1968). But not all of the attention was favorable. Francis Moore, a prominent Harvard surgeon, questioned the board's expertise in heart transplants, claiming in a letter to McDermott that it would "have been prudent ... to seek some consultation from those who have been intimately concerned with these problems for almost twenty years" (IOM, 1998a, p. 19). McDermott countered that the statement exemplified the board's mission of acting as a "disinterested group." The Board on Medicine, he wrote, "sought to be helpful on the more important issues as they arise considering both medicine itself and its relationship to our society." For McDermott, the statement exemplified the board's utility (IOM, 1998a, p. 19).

Publicity from the heart transplant statement, along with the board's well-connected membership and association with the prestigious NAS, paved the way for preliminary funding discussions with foundations. MacLeod and fellow board member Robert J. Glaser fostered a relationship between the board and the Commonwealth Fund, ultimately securing $150,000 in support. The Commonwealth Fund, in turn, arranged a meeting between the board and five other large foundations. The Rockefeller Foundation, the Milbank Memorial Fund, the Carnegie Foundation, and the Association for the Aid of Crippled Children also became early funders of the Board on Medicine.

PROPOSAL FOR A NATIONAL ACADEMY OF MEDICINE

In July 1968, McDermott asked a committee of Board on Medicine members to prepare a report evaluating the prospect of creating an academy of medicine. After about 8 months of deliberation, the committee reached consensus and recommended the creation of an academy that would remain affiliated with the NAS but would initiate its own studies and activities. This decision represented a compromise between McDermott, who sought the continuation of the Board on Medicine, and Page, who favored an independent academy. On March 12, 1969, the full Board on Medicine accepted the committee's recommendation.

NAS leadership, however, greeted the proposal with skepticism. The NAS, which largely served as an honorific membership organization, had an operational arm called the National Research Council (NRC), which was tasked with responding to requests from the federal government for studies and advice on scientific policy. The NRC had a Division of Medical Sciences, which had advised the Surgeons General of the Navy and Army on medical research and medical care during World War II (NAS, 1947). When McDermott met with the Executive Committee of the NAS Council at the end of March 1969, the members expressed concern that an independent academy of medicine might create competition with the NRC and fragment the organization.

The debate highlighted issues that would become fundamental to the mission of the IOM and eventually the NAM. For example, the board's stated commitment to examining and responding to important social challenges, such as health disparities and the social determinants of health, did not fit neatly into the scientific method. Some NAS members believed that such topics should not fall under the purview of the Academy. Supporters of this view contended that the role of the NAS should be to honor achievement and promote academic discussion, rather than take positions in what they viewed as social concerns with political undercurrents and implications.

A five-person delegation[5] from the Board on Medicine met with the full NAS Council on June 7, 1969. When the group presented the board's proposal, NAS Councilors cemented the Executive Committee's doubts about an academy that could initiate its own studies. Such an arrangement, they felt, ran counter to the organization, operation, and tradition of the NAS, which relied on the NRC to conduct studies (and then only at the request of the federal government). Ultimately, however, the Council deferred a decision on the proposal.

Around this time, the NAS underwent a leadership transition that would influence the debate over an academy of medicine. Philip Handler, Chair of the Department of Biochemistry at Duke University, succeeded Seitz as NAS President on July 1, 1969. Determined to provide strong leadership and uphold the NAS's high scientific standards, Handler was less sympathetic to the idea of an academy of medicine than his predecessor. He made it clear that he did not support the establishment of an academy during his tenure, preferring instead to expand the NAS's Medical Sciences Section and the NRC's Division of Medical Sciences. In a letter to the NAS Council, Handler voiced his concern that proponents of an academy of medicine wanted to "undertake a type of lobbying activity which is not in keeping with the history of the Academy" (IOM, 1998a, p. 31). Finally, on July 19, 1969, the Executive Committee of the NAS Council formally rejected the idea of an academy of medicine, although it expressed support for the board's stated goals.

ESTABLISHMENT OF THE INSTITUTE OF MEDICINE

The floundering of the Board on Medicine's proposal to create an academy of medicine under the NAS charter reinvigorated Page's campaign to create a fully independent organization. Some members of the board urged McDermott to inform Handler that they would proceed with the formation of an academy, even if it meant disengaging entirely from the NAS. Both McDermott and Handler hoped to avoid this outcome, however, and worked for nearly 1 year to engineer a

---

[5] The delegation consisted of McDermott, Adam Yarmolinsky, James Shannon (the retired head of the NIH who served as a consultant to the Board), Robert Glaser, and Irving London, who chaired the Department of Medicine at the Albert Einstein College of Medicine and had chaired the subcommittee to consider the formation of an academy of medicine.

compromise. By May 1970, members of the Board on Medicine had come to agreement around the notion of an *institute* of medicine that—although lacking the stature of an academy and reporting to the NAS Council—would nevertheless have the freedom to set its own agenda and conduct studies with the support of an independent staff.

Yarmolinsky took the lead in drafting a charter for the new Institute of Medicine. The IOM would aim for an initial membership of approximately 100, with plans to grow to 250. Members of the IOM, like their counterparts in the NAS and the NAE, would be people of merit and achievement. In a continuation of the multidisciplinary focus that defined the Board on Medicine, at least 25 percent of the IOM's members would come from fields outside medicine and the biomedical sciences. "The problems posed in provision of health services are so large, complex and important as to require, for their solution, the concern and competences not only of medicine but also of other disciplines and professions," the charter read (IOM, 1998a, p. 40).

On June 5, 1970, McDermott presented the IOM's proposed charter to the NAS Council. The following day, the NAS Council authorized Handler "to take the necessary steps to create an Institute of Medicine." On June 10, the NAS made a formal announcement that it would establish an Institute of Medicine "to address the larger problems of medicine and health care" (IOM, 1998, p. 39).

With approval in place, the Board on Medicine began its metamorphosis into the IOM. The new institute would operate under multiple organizational restraints because of its relationship to the NAS. For example, the NAS Council retained the right to review IOM publications using NRC procedures and to add or remove individuals nominated for IOM membership. In effect, the NAS Council would assume responsibility for quality control and high-level oversight of the IOM.

Members of the Board on Medicine orchestrated the organizational transition. One early decision touched on the institute's leadership structure. The typical institute, such as those found in universities, had a director who reported to the university president. According to this model, the IOM director would report to the NAS president. Members of the Board on Medicine found such an arrangement unacceptable, because it would not reflect the IOM's independent authority to initiate and conduct studies, and proposed that a president rather than a director lead the institute.

The NAS Council acquiesced to the notion of an IOM president, and Handler appointed Glaser, then dean of the Stanford University School of Medicine, to act in the role. The IOM officially launched its operations on December 21, 1970.

The Institute of Medicine Selects Its First Members

The IOM's first task was to delineate the terms of membership and select its first members. As a starting point, members of the Board on Medicine were grandfathered into the IOM and reconstituted as its Executive Committee (see Box 1-2). A membership subcommittee then set about identifying a list of nominees to expand the IOM membership to its initial target of 100 eminent leaders. The 1971 inaugural class was nominated by the membership subcommittee, approved by the IOM Executive Committee and the NAS president, and invited to join the organization. In addition, members of the NAS's Medical Sciences Section automatically received invitations. In subsequent years, new classes of IOM members would be elected by the existing membership.

In June 1971, 77 new members of the IOM were announced. Among them, Glaser identified at least 19 different fields, including administration, basic sciences, engineering, community medicine, dentistry, nursing, and nutrition. Notably, the inaugural class also included two future IOM presidents: Donald Fredrickson, then general director of the National Heart Institute, and David A. Hamburg, then a psychiatrist at Stanford University.

BOX 1-2
Charter Members of the Institute of Medicine

Paul B. Beeson, MD	Walsh McDermott, MD
Ivan L. Bennett, Jr., MD	Carl V. Moore, MD
Charles G. Child III, MD	Samuel M. Nabrit, PhD
Julius H. Comroe, Jr., MD	Irvine H. Page, MD
Jerome W. Conn, MD	Henry W. Riecken, PhD
Rashi Fein, PhD	Walter A. Rosenblith, IngRad
Robert J. Glaser, MD	Ernest W. Saward, MD
Robert A. Good, MD, PhD	James A. Shannon, MD, PhD
Leon O. Jacobson, MD	Thomas H. Weller, MD
Henry G. Kunkel, MD	Dwight L. Wilbur, MD
Lucile P. Leone, MA	Bryan Williams, MD
Irving M. London, MD	W. Barry Wood, Jr., MD
Colin M. MacLeod, MD	Adam Yarmolinsky, LLB
Maclyn McCarty, MD	Alonzo S. Yerby, MD

CONCLUSION

Despite its long and occasionally contentious path to creation, the IOM found a fruitful home within the NAS complex, where it would remain for the next 45 years. In the story of its founding are themes that would color its journey for the next five decades. The organization's emphasis on a multidisciplinary, action-oriented membership would endure, with IOM (and later NAM) members regularly posting higher rates of volunteerism in studies and advisory activities than their peers in the NAS and the NAE. The statement on heart transplants, too, with its "outsider" perspective, began to define the IOM and the NAM's unique value as an advisor to government and the public. The organization would soon develop a firm reputation for independence and objectivity, even and especially when its recommendations were unpopular or controversial. Finally, the debate over creating an academy of medicine was far from settled. The IOM would continue to both benefit from the NAS's influence and chafe under its restrictions. In the ensuing decades, IOM leadership would fail repeatedly to advance the notion of an academy of medicine, until finally finding success in 2015 (see Chapter 3).

2

A Commitment to Service:
Members and Leaders of the Institute of Medicine
and the National Academy of Medicine[1]

T he bylaws of the Institute of Medicine (IOM), which became those of the National Academy of Medicine (NAM) in 2015, specified that, in part, "membership in the Academy shall be based upon … skills and resources likely to contribute to achieving the Academy's mission; and willingness to be an active participant in the Academy."[2] This provision originated in conversations led by charter member Irvine Page years before the founding of the IOM, in which Page was adamant that the organization should exist not only to honor professional excellence in health, medicine, and biomedical sciences, but also to serve society and improve the health of the public.

VOLUNTEERISM

Volunteerism became established as a tenet of IOM (and later NAM) membership from the moment the organization opened its doors in 1970. IOM/NAM members volunteered their expertise to support the programmatic work of not only the IOM/NAM, but also other program divisions within the National Academies of Sciences, Engineering, and Medicine (the National Academies) (e.g., the Division on Earth and Life Studies and the Division of Behavioral and Social Sciences and Education). Many IOM/NAM members were also members of the National Academy of Sciences (NAS) and/or the National Academy of Engineering (NAE) and participated in activities of those organizations. Member service took the form of serving as chairs or members of consensus study committees; advising programmatic boards, roundtables, forums, or workshop planning committees; reviewing reports and publications; and more. Such participation was strictly without financial remuneration.

Members also volunteered for roles in the governance of the organization, including service on its Council.[3] The Council, chaired by the IOM/NAM president, met several times per year and had

---

[1] Except where otherwise noted, historical facts presented in this chapter are drawn from a 1998 history of the Institute of Medicine authored by Edward Berkowitz (IOM, 1998a).

[2] National Academy of Medicine Articles of Organization, Article II: Membership, Section 3.

[3] In 2021, the NAM Council comprised three officers (President, Home Secretary, and International Secretary) and 15 at-large Council members, all elected by the NAM membership.

oversight of organizational policies, procedures, funds, and activities. In addition to the president, the IOM/NAM's governing officers included the Home Secretary and International Secretary.[4] The Home Secretary was responsible for the conduct of membership affairs (chiefly, member elections), while the International Secretary served as the organization's chief liaison and representative in global affairs.

In 2000 the organization established three annual member awards to recognize outstanding volunteer service (see Box 2-1). The Walsh McDermott Medal, named in honor of the Chair of the Board on Medicine and charter member of the IOM (see Chapter 1), recognized members for distinguished service over an extended period of time. The David Rall Medal was named for an IOM member who served as Foreign Secretary from 1994 to 1998. Rall was the Director of the National Institute of Environmental Health Studies (1971–1990) and the National Toxicology Program (1978–1990). The award in his name honored members who demonstrated particularly distinguished leadership as chair of a study committee or other activity. Finally, the Adam Yarmolinksy Medal, named for the lawyer who was lead author of the IOM's charter and bylaws (see Chapter 1), recognized service by members representing a discipline outside the health and medical sciences.

MULTIDISCIPLINARITY

The Yarmolinsky Medal highlighted the importance of "nontraditional" perspectives in the IOM's work. As noted in Chapter 1, the IOM (later the NAM) bylaws specified that "no more than three-quarters of the members shall be drawn from the fields of health and medicine."[5] This requirement reflected an understanding of the role of social, political, economic, and environmental

---

BOX 2-1
Recipients of Member Service Awards, 2000–2021

Walsh McDermott Medal: Mary Ellen Avery, MD; Julius Richmond, MD; Enriqueta Bond, PhD; Leon Eisenberg, MD; Floyd Bloom, MD; Ada Sue Hinshaw, PhD, RN; Elena Nightingale, MD, PhD; Jack Barchas, MD; Gilbert Omenn, MD, PhD; Don Detmer, MD; David Challoner, MD; Robert Wallace, MD; Haile Debas, MD; Donald Berwick, MD; Dan Blazer, MD, PhD, JP; Alan Leshner, PhD; Lynn Goldman, MD, MS, MPH; Barbara McNeil, MD, PhD; Elaine Larson, PhD, RN; Cato Laurencin, MD, PhD; David Relman, MD; Christine Cassel, MD

David Rall Medal: Stuart Bondurant, MD; Dorothy Rice, ScD; Joshua Lederberg, PhD; Daniel Federman, MD; Marie McCormick, MD, ScD; Torsten Wiesel, MD; Fitzhugh Mullan, MD; William Richardson, PhD; Sheila Burke, RN, MPA; Bernard Guyer, MD, MPH; Nancy Adler, PhD; Virginia Stallings, MD; Linda Rosenstock, MD, MPH; Ellen Wright Clayton, JD, MD; Richard Johnston, Jr., MD; Jonathan Samet, MD, MS; Donna Shalala, PhD; Richard Hynes, PhD; Hedvig Hricak, MD, PhD; David Savitz, PhD; David Eaton, PhD; Mary Wakefield, PhD, RN

Adam Yarmolinksy Medal: Rashi Fein, PhD; Walter McNerney, MHA; Richard Bonnie, JD; Paul Rogers, JD; Lawrence S. Lewin, MBA; Henry Riecken, PhD; Lawrence Gostin, JD; Karen Davis, PhD; David Mechanic, PhD; Joseph Newhouse, PhD; Gail Warden, MHA; R. Alta Charo, JD; Susan Scrimshaw, PhD; Mary Woolley, MA; Ruth Faden, PhD, MPH; Nicholas Peppas, ScD; Gail Wilensky, PhD; Sara Rosenbaum, JD

---

[4] The IOM/NAM President, Home Secretary, and International Secretary were the only governance positions that received financial remuneration. The President (a full-time role) received a salary, while the secretaries (part-time roles) received stipends. Prior to 2020, the International Secretary position was known as Foreign Secretary.

[5] National Academy of Medicine Articles of Organization, Article II: Membership, Section 1.

factors on human health and acknowledged that solutions to national and global health challenges would require broad and diverse viewpoints.

In addition to this basic qualification, the IOM developed disciplinary "sections" to organize its membership. Election policies were designed to ensure proportionate representation in each of these sections. Each section had an elected chair and vice chair, who facilitated communication among members and shared relevant volunteer opportunities across the National Academies. The IOM also developed interest groups to allow members from across sections to convene and discuss issues of cross-cutting importance. Member sections and interest groups continued after the establishment of the NAM in 2015 (see Boxes 2-2 and 2-3).

BOX 2-2
NAM Member Sections, 2021

- SECTION 1: Physical, Mathematical, Computer, Information, Engineering Sciences
- SECTION 2: Biochemistry, Cellular and Developmental Biology, Medical Microbiology and Immunology, and Genetics
- SECTION 3: Neurosciences, Physiology, and Pharmacology
- SECTION 4: Internal Medicine, Pathology, and Dermatology
- SECTION 5: Pediatrics and Obstetrics/Gynecology
- SECTION 6: Surgery, Surgical Subspecialties (excluding ophthalmology), Anesthesiology, Radiology, Nuclear Medicine, Radiation Oncology, and Ophthalmology
- SECTION 7: Psychiatry and Neurology
- SECTION 8: Family Medicine, Emergency Medicine, Physical Medicine, and Rehabilitation
- SECTION 9: Public Health, Biostatistics, and Epidemiology
- SECTION 10: Dentistry, Nutrition, Nursing, Allied Health Professions, Pharmacy, and Veterinary Medicine
- SECTION 11: Social Sciences, Humanities, and Law
- SECTION 12: Administration of Health Services, Education, and Research

---

BOX 2-3
NAM Member Interest Groups, 2021

- Health Policy and Health Care Systems
- Global Health, Infectious Diseases, and Microbiology
- Neuroscience, Behavior, Brain Function, and Disorders
- Maternal and Child Health and Human Development
- Health of Populations and Health Disparities
- Education of the Health Care and Science Workforce
- Biology of Aging and Geriatrics
- Nutrition, Diabetes, and Obesity
- Cancer, Stem Cell Biology, and Transplantation
- Human Rights, Professional Ethics, and the Value of Medicine
- Rehabilitation and Human Function
- Primary Care
- Health Technology
- Climate Change

ACHIEVEMENT

In a 2008 address to members, then-IOM President Harvey V. Fineberg remarked that the organization's impact depended in part on "the credibility that is earned by virtue of [members'] stature."[6] The "primary criterion" of IOM/NAM membership, alongside active engagement both within and outside the organization, was "distinguished professional achievement in a field related to medicine and health" (NAM, n.d.l). A new class of IOM/NAM members was elected annually by the existing membership. In 2021, the new class was composed of 90 members from the United States and 10 international members. The total membership numbered approximately 2,400 (NAM, n.d.l).

Since its founding in 1970, the IOM/NAM membership has included highly accomplished and influential leaders, including heads of federal agencies; Surgeons General and members of Congress; presidents and chief executive officers of foundations, universities, businesses, and health systems; and scientists, inventors, educators, and clinicians of all kinds. Internationally, the membership has included leaders of peer scientific academies, ministers of health, and heads of global multilateral organizations. More than 75 IOM/NAM members had been awarded Nobel Prizes in Physiology/Medicine, Chemistry, Peace, Physics, or Economics by 2021 (see Tables 2-1 through 2-3). In a 2019 survey of NAM members, Eva Feldman, a pioneer in stem cell implantation therapy for amyotrophic lateral sclerosis (ALS, or Lou Gehrig's disease), described NAM membership as "an unparalleled opportunity to meet and interact with colleagues who are pushing the boundaries of scientific and medical innovation with a common goal: to understand and treat disease and promote health worldwide."[7]

Presidential Citation for Exemplary Leadership

On October 19, 2020, at the 50th annual meeting of the NAM, then-President Victor J. Dzau presented the Academy's first-ever Presidential Citation for Exemplary Leadership to NAM member Anthony S. Fauci, Director of the National Institute of Allergy and Infectious Diseases (NIAID) (see Figure 2-1). When the meeting occurred, the COVID-19 pandemic was in its eighth month, and the United States had seen nearly 8 million cases and more than 220,000 deaths (STAT, n.d.). As NIAID director, Fauci had become the nation's de facto spokesperson for scientific information about the virus and a strong proponent of preventive public health measures. He was unequivocal about the danger of the pandemic, yet projected a sense of optimism that the virus could be controlled through measures such as physical distancing and face coverings—and ultimately, through a soon-to-be-developed vaccine. The presidential citation, presented on behalf of the NAM Council, recognized Fauci's present contributions as well as his long career of federal service, which spanned six presidential administrations. The citation also recognized Fauci's scientific contributions to the fields of human immunoregulation and the prevention and treatment of HIV/AIDS (NAM, 2020h) (see Box 2-4).

Upon accepting the award, Fauci remarked, "We are going through a time that is disturbingly anti-science in certain segments of our society.... We really need a group of scientists and physicians and health care providers to really stick together in our principles ... we need to be the steadfast vocal defenders of the scientific process" (Fauci, 2020). Illustrating his point, on the same day Dzau presented the citation to Fauci, U.S. President Donald J. Trump, who had downplayed the gravity of the virus and spoken against physical distancing measures that prevented large public gatherings and resulted in the closing of businesses, was quoted as saying "People are tired of COVID.... People are tired of hearing Fauci and these idiots, all these idiots who got it wrong" (Stolberg et al., 2020). By the end of Trump's term, U.S. COVID-19 cases had neared 24 million

---

[6] IOM/NAM Records.
[7] Internal survey of NAM members, summer 2019.

BOX 2-4
The NAM Awards First-Ever Presidential Citation for
Exemplary Leadership to Anthony S. Fauci

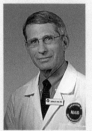 On October 19, 2020, during the 50th Annual Meeting of the National Academy of Medicine (NAM), NAM President Victor J. Dzau presented the Academy's inaugural Presidential Citation for Exemplary Leadership to Anthony S. Fauci, director of the National Institute of Allergy and Infectious Diseases (NIAID). The citation read:

In recognition of extraordinary service and outstanding contributions to biomedical science, health care, and public health in the United States, in particular: Pioneering advances in the field of human immunoregulation and life-saving therapies for rare immune disorders; Seminal research and groundbreaking leadership in prevention and treatment of HIV/AIDS, impacting countless lives now and in the future; Enduring, visionary guidance to the field of biomedical research globally and nationally; Unprecedented public service as director of the National Institute of Allergy and Infectious Diseases for nearly four decades; Distinguished service as a trusted advisor to six U.S. presidents during public health crises including HIV/AIDS, SARS, anthrax, influenza, and Ebola; and Firm and steady leadership during the COVID-19 pandemic, offering an unwavering, trusted voice to the nation and world on behalf of science-based policy and public health.

SOURCE: National Academy of Medicine. 2020. NAM Awards First Ever Presidential Citation for Exemplary Leadership to Anthony Fauci. https://nam.edu/nam-awards-first-ever-presidential-citation-for-exemplary-leadership-to-anthony-fauci (accessed December 23, 2020).
PHOTO SOURCE: NIAID (CC BY 2.0 via Wikimedia Commons).

---

and deaths had reached more than 400,000 (STAT, n.d.). President Joseph Biden (2021–) asked Fauci to serve as his chief medical advisor and continue in his role at NIAID (Evelyn, 2020).

TABLE 2-1 Nobel Prizes in Physiology or Medicine Awarded to IOM/NAM Members

IOM/NAM Member(s)	Year	Achievement
Frederick Chapman Robbins and Thomas Huckle Weller	1954	Discovery of the ability of poliomyelitis viruses to grow in cultures of various types of tissue
Joshua Lederberg	1958	Discoveries concerning genetic recombination and the organization of the genetic material of bacteria
Marshall W. Nirenberg	1968	Interpretation of the genetic code and its function in protein synthesis
Salvador E. Luria	1969	Discoveries concerning the replication mechanism and the genetic structure of viruses
Julius Axelrod	1970	Discoveries concerning the humoral transmitters in the nerve terminals and the mechanism for their storage, release, and inactivation
George E. Palade	1974	Discoveries concerning the structural and functional organization of the cell
David Baltimore and Howard Martin Temin	1975	Discoveries concerning the interaction between tumor viruses and the genetic material of the cell
Baruch S. Blumberg	1976	Discoveries concerning new mechanisms for the origin and dissemination of infectious diseases
Allan M. Cormack	1979	Development of computer assisted tomography
Baruj Benacerraf	1980	Discoveries concerning genetically determined structures on the cell surface that regulate immunological reactions

continued

TABLE 2-1 Continued

IOM/NAM Member(s)	Year	Achievement
Torsten N. Wiesel	1981	Discoveries concerning information processing in the visual system
Sune K. Bergström, Bengt I. Samuelsson, and John R. Vane	1982	Discoveries concerning prostaglandins and related biologically active substances
Michael S. Brown and Joseph L. Goldstein	1985	Discoveries concerning the regulation of cholesterol metabolism
Gertrude B. Elion	1988	Discoveries of important principles for drug treatment
J. Michael Bishop and Harold E. Varmus	1989	Discovery of the cellular origin of retroviral oncogenes
Joseph E. Murray	1990	Discoveries concerning organ and cell transplantation in the treatment of human disease
Phillip A. Sharp	1993	Discovery of "split genes"
Alfred G. Gilman	1994	Discovery of G-proteins and the role of these proteins in signal transduction in cells
Peter C. Doherty	1996	Discoveries concerning the specificity of the cell-mediated immune defense
Stanley B. Prusiner	1997	Discovery of prions—a new biological principle of infection
Louis J. Ignarro and Ferid Murad	1998	Discoveries concerning nitric oxide as a signaling molecule in the cardiovascular system
Günter Blobel	1999	Discovery that proteins have intrinsic signals that govern their transport and localization in the cell
Arvid Carlsson, Paul Greengard, and Eric R. Kandel	2000	Discoveries concerning signal transduction in the nervous system
Sydney Brenner and H. Robert Horvitz	2002	Discoveries concerning genetic regulation of organ development and programmed cell death
Linda B. Buck	2004	Discoveries of odorant receptors and the organization of the olfactory system
Barry J. Marshall	2005	Discovery of the bacterium *Helicobacter pylori* and its role in gastritis and peptic ulcer disease
Andrew Z. Fire	2006	Discovery of RNA interference—gene silencing by double-stranded RNA
Mario R. Capecchi and Oliver Smithies	2007	Discoveries of principles for introducing specific gene modifications in mice by the use of embryonic stem cells
Françoise Barré-Sinoussi	2008	Discovery of human immunodeficiency virus
Harald zur Hausen	2008	Discovery of human papilloma viruses causing cervical cancer
Elizabeth H. Blackburn and Carol W. Greider	2009	Discovery of how chromosomes are protected by telomeres and the enzyme telomerase
Bruce A. Beutler	2011	Discoveries concerning the activation of innate immunity
Ralph M. Steinman	2011	Discovery of the dendritic cell and its role in adaptive immunity
John B. Gurdon and Shinya Yamanaka	2012	Discovery that mature cells can be reprogrammed to become pluripotent
James E. Rothman, Randy W. Schekman, and Thomas C. Südhof	2013	Discoveries of machinery regulating vesicle traffic, a major transport system in our cells

TABLE 2-1 Continued

IOM/NAM Member(s)	Year	Achievement
Edvard I. Moser and May-Britt Moser	2014	Discoveries of cells that constitute a positioning system in the brain
James P. Allison	2018	Discovery of cancer therapy by inhibition of negative immune regulation
William G. Kaelin, Jr., and Gregg L. Semenza	2019	Discoveries of how cells sense and adapt to oxygen availability
Harvey J. Alter	2020	Discoveries that led to the identification of a novel virus, hepatitis C virus
David Julius	2021	Discoveries of receptors for temperature and touch

NOTE: In some cases, the prize was shared or split with individuals not listed in this table.
SOURCE: The Nobel Prize. https://nobelprize.org.

TABLE 2-2 Nobel Prizes in Chemistry Awarded to IOM/NAM Members

IOM/NAM Member(s)	Year	Achievement
Paul Berg	1980	Fundamental studies of the biochemistry of nucleic acids, with particular regard to recombinant-DNA
Thomas R. Cech	1989	Discovery of catalytic properties of RNA
E. J. Corey	1990	Development of the theory and methodology of organic synthesis
Richard R. Ernst	1991	Contributions to the development of the methodology of high-resolution nuclear magnetic resonance (NMR) spectroscopy
Mario J. Molina and F. Sherwood Rowland	1995	Work in atmospheric chemistry, particularly concerning the formation and decomposition of ozone
Peter Agre	2003	Discovery of water channels
Aaron Ciechanover	2004	Discovery of ubiquitin-mediated protein degradation
Martin Chalfie and Roger Y. Tsien	2008	Discovery and development of the green fluorescent protein (GFP)
Brian K. Kobilka and Robert J. Lefkowitz	2012	Studies of G-protein-coupled receptors
Paul Modrich and Aziz Sancar	2015	Mechanistic studies of DNA repair
Frances H. Arnold	2018	Directed evolution of enzymes
Jennifer A. Doudna	2020	Development of a method for genome editing

NOTE: In some cases, the prize was shared or split with individuals not listed in this table.
SOURCE: The Nobel Prize. https://nobelprize.org.

TABLE 2-3 Nobel Prizes in Economics, Peace, and Physics Awarded to IOM/NAM Members

IOM/NAM Member(s)	Year	Achievement
Nobel Prize in Economics		
Kenneth J. Arrow	1972	Pioneering contributions to general economic equilibrium theory and welfare theory
Thomas C. Schelling	2005	For having enhanced our understanding of conflict and cooperation through game-theory analysis
Nobel Peace Prize		
Bernard Lown	1985	Accepted the prize on behalf of the International Physicians for the Prevention of Nuclear War
Denis Mukwege	2018	Efforts to end the use of sexual violence as a weapon of war and armed conflict
Nobel Prize in Physics		
Robert Hofstadter	1961	Pioneering studies of electron scattering in atomic nuclei and for his thereby achieved discoveries concerning the structure of the nucleons

NOTE: In some cases, the prize was shared or split with individuals not listed in this table.
SOURCE: The Nobel Prize. https://nobelprize.org.

PRESIDENTS OF THE INSTITUTE OF MEDICINE AND THE NATIONAL ACADEMY OF MEDICINE

After the IOM's leadership structure was carefully negotiated by Yarmolinksy and colleagues in 1970 (see Chapter 1), the IOM/NAM presidency became a prestigious and influential position capable of drawing prominent IOM/NAM members away from established careers for a 6-year term in Washington, DC.[8] The president served as the full-time chief executive officer of the organization as well as the vice chair of the National Research Council (NRC). Each president put his own stamp on the IOM/NAM, taking the organization in new operational and programmatic directions. Eight presidents and two acting presidents had led the IOM and NAM by 2021 (see Box 2-5), all of whom were men and all but one of whom were White.

BOX 2-5
Presidents of the Institute of Medicine and the National Academy of Medicine

Robert J. Glaser, MD (1970–1971)*
John R. Hogness, MD (1971–1974)
Donald Fredrickson, MD (1974–1975)
David A. Hamburg, MD (1975–1980)
Frederick Chapman Robbins, MD (1980–1985)
Samuel O. Thier, MD (1985–1991)
Stuart Bondurant, MD (1991–1992)*
Kenneth I. Shine, MD (1992–2002)
Harvey V. Fineberg, MD, PhD (2002–2014)
Victor J. Dzau, MD (2014–Present)

---

* Acting President.

---

[8] The IOM/NAM presidential term was 5 years prior to Harvey Fineberg's term (2002–2014).

John R. Hogness (Term: 1971–1974)

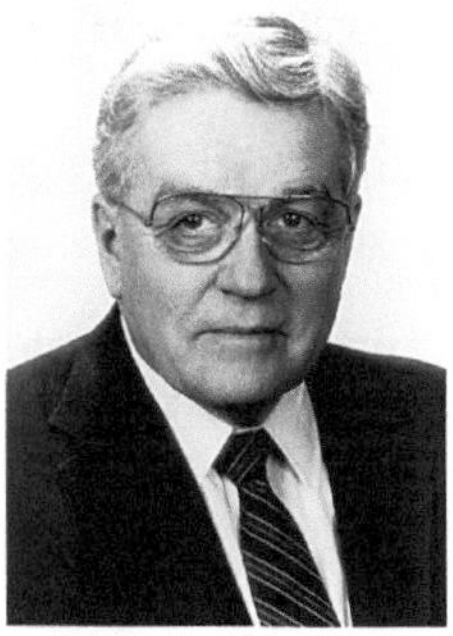

FIGURE 2-1 John Hogness.
SOURCE: University of Washington.

On March 30, 1971, approximately 3 months after the IOM's founding, the IOM and NAS[9] announced that John R. Hogness would become the first IOM president (see Figure 2-1). "With the appointment of Dr. Hogness, the Institute of Medicine becomes a reality," said NAS President Philip Handler (IOM, 1998a, p. 55). In July, Hogness succeeded Robert J. Glaser, a charter IOM member who had served as acting president and overseen the selection of the first IOM members, as well as the presidential search process.

A 48-year-old physician and former dean of the medical school at the University of Washington, Hogness enthusiastically assumed the challenging task of building the IOM's infrastructure and programs. He was inspired by the IOM's mission to provide rigorous, evidence-based advice, describing the presidency as "one of the most important jobs in the health field." Hogness declared that the IOM "alone in the health field will speak ... without an axe to grind" (IOM, 1998a, p. 57). He believed strongly that the IOM should stay out of politics and be guided only by scientific evidence—and that the organization's value was rooted in its independence.

Hogness set about establishing the IOM's basic governing structure, beginning with the appointment of its first executive director, Roger Bulger. He also appointed the first members of the IOM Council and established Executive, Program, and Finance Committees within it. In 1972, to give the IOM's programmatic portfolio coherence, the Program Committee issued a set of general guidelines for studies in an effort to identify projects that would fulfill the IOM leadership's vision for the organization. The guidelines encouraged the IOM to recognize "a fundamental unity to health policy issues" instead of approaching them piecemeal (IOM, 1998a, p. 76). Accordingly, the Program Committee suggested that the IOM build capacity to initiate its own studies, rather than awaiting requests from the government.

Lack of capital proved a significant obstacle. As Hogness recalled, "the financial support of the Institute of Medicine was, to put it mildly, a bit shaky at first" (IOM, 1998a, p. 76). With a goal of raising $700,000 to support the IOM's general operations, Hogness began to cultivate relationships with private foundations that had an interest in health and medicine. Among these was the Robert Wood Johnson Foundation (RWJF), which had not yet opened its doors when Hogness approached its soon-to-be president, fellow IOM member David Rogers, in 1971. Hogness's argument proved persuasive, and RWJF ultimately issued a grant of $750,000 to be spent over 3 years, noting in a statement its confidence that the IOM would "make a contribution of the first importance to the outcome of the difficult and decisive policy decisions confronting the nation's health enterprise" (IOM, 1998a, p. 77). RWJF's contribution allowed the IOM to more than double its staff and marked the beginning of an enduring relationship between the two organizations.

Four other major foundations soon joined RWJF in supporting the IOM's early infrastructure. The W.K. Kellogg Foundation and the Richard King Mellon Foundation each provided $100,000 per year for 3 years. The Commonwealth Fund, where Glaser was a vice president and trustee, offered $200,000 per year for 3 years; and the Andrew Mellon Foundation agreed to $750,000.

Hogness announced his intention to resign from the IOM presidency in spring 1973 after being recruited to serve as president of the University of Washington. He had accomplished a great deal in a very short time, having established the IOM's operating structure, built strong ties with the

---

[9] As described in Chapter 1, the NAS played a role in IOM governance until the creation of the NAM in 2015.

federal government and private foundations, and begun cultivating an endowment that would give the IOM freedom to pursue its own priorities. Following his tenure at the University of Washington, Hogness became president and chief executive of the Association for Academic Health Centers. He passed away in 2007 at the age of 85 (Altman, 2007).

Donald Fredrickson (Term: 1974–1975)

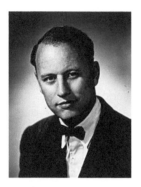

Donald Fredrickson, a senior official in the National Heart and Lung Institute, succeeded Hogness as president in 1974 but spent less than 1 year in the role before departing to become Director of the National Institutes of Health (NIH). Fredrickson had been selected as part of the IOM's 1971 inaugural class and quickly become engaged in its activities.

Addressing IOM members during his presidency, Fredrickson spoke of bridging the worlds of science and policy, arguing that the IOM had an obligation to "lend the scientific method to the direction of a whole social movement." He noted, as Hogness had, that the IOM's success rested upon the "essence, not merely the appearance, of nonpartisan objectivity" (IOM, 1998a, p. 85).

FIGURE 2-2 Donald Fredrickson SOURCE: National Library of Medicine.

However, Fredrickson had little time to shape the organization. He departed in June 1975 before a successor could be appointed. During the interim, Julius Richmond, then Vice-Chair of the IOM Council, and Bulger provided leadership and day-to-day management for the organization and its staff.

David A. Hamburg (Term: 1975–1980)

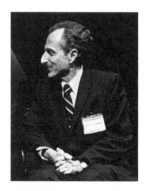

David Hamburg, an academic psychiatrist who specialized in the behavioral components of health, took office as IOM president in fall 1975 (see Figure 2-3). Born in 1925, he had spent his childhood and completed his education in Indiana, where his grandfather arranged refuge for about 50 of Hamburg's relatives who fled Eastern Europe as the Nazis took power ahead of World War II. Witnessing the Holocaust instilled in Hamburg a lifelong global sensibility, commitment to human rights, and interest in the psychological underpinnings of behavior, particularly violence (Roberts, 2019).

FIGURE 2-3 David Hamburg at the 1975 Annual Meeting of the Institute of Medicine. SOURCE: National Library of Medicine. Reproduced with the permission of Paul Conklin and courtesy of the Institute of Medicine. https://profiles.nlm. nih.gov/101584939X198.

The same year he was recruited as IOM President, Hamburg, then Chair of the Department of Psychiatry at Stanford University, was enmeshed in a global hostage crisis involving several of his students who were kidnapped by militants in the Democratic Republic of the Congo (Roberts, 2019). The experience, he said, sharpened his motivation to unravel the "policy issues that brought about that hatred and violence and ignorance and disease and severe poverty" (Carnegie Council, 2009).

Hamburg delivered inaugural remarks to IOM members at the 1975 Annual Meeting. Like Hogness and Fredrickson, he praised the organization's impartiality, remarking that it had "no over-riding doctrine, no party line, no cow too sacred to be examined" (IOM, 1998a, p. 97). He did, however, see potential liabilities and missed opportunities that prevented the IOM from maximizing its influence. He therefore initiated a thorough review of IOM activities during his first year in office. After extensive conversations with staff, members, and funders, Hamburg decided it would be important for the IOM to build a national, even global, perspective, rather than a narrow focus on Washington, DC–centric health policy minutiae. He also concluded that the IOM needed to respond more quickly to requests in order to make a more timely impact on current policy debates.

Building on the work of Hogness's Program Committee, Hamburg set out to "map out the terrain" and organize the IOM into five major policy areas: (1) health services, including national health insurance; (2) health sciences policy; (3) the prevention of disease; (4) education for the health professions; and (5) mental health (IOM, 1998a, p. 104). In March 1977, Hamburg announced the creation of six IOM operating divisions, each with its own staff director and advisory board composed of member and non-member experts. Elena Nightingale, an MD-PhD Holocaust survivor who became a long-serving member of the IOM staff and was elected as a member in 1985, founded and headed the Division of Health Promotion and Disease Prevention. Other inaugural divisions included the Division of Health Care Services, the Division of Health Manpower and Resources Development, the Division of Health Sciences Research, the Division of International Health, and the Division on Legal, Ethical, and Educational Aspects of Health. Later called "boards," these divisions provided a structure for the IOM that, with variation over time that reflected current health concerns and funding streams, remained in place until the creation of the NAM in 2015 (IOM, 1998a).

Other changes to the IOM's operating structure in the Hamburg era included the appointment of Karl Yordy as executive officer, following Bulger's departure to become Chancellor of the University of Massachusetts and Dean of its medical school. Bulger would be elected as an IOM member in 1977. Hamburg also created two new senior staff positions in program development and finance and operations. The new structure accomplished three major goals for Hamburg and the IOM Council: it increased the participation of members, expanded the role of staff, and more clearly demonstrated the IOM's breadth and capacity to funders and collaborators.

During Hamburg's tenure, shared interests with President Jimmy Carter's (1977–1981) administration—such as mental health, cost containment, health care as a component of foreign aid, and the relationship between health and behavior—facilitated a solid working relationship between the IOM and the federal government. In 1979 alone, the IOM reviewed the planning process for the Department of Health, Education, and Welfare[10]; reported on food safety policy and the safety of sleeping pills for the Food and Drug Administration; evaluated the research agenda of the National Institute on Alcohol Abuse and Alcoholism; and reported on health in Egypt for the Agency for International Development.

After only 3 years in office, Hamburg informed the IOM Council that he would not pursue a second 5-year term as IOM president, noting that McDermott and the IOM founding fathers were wise to encourage fresh leadership at regular intervals. In his remaining time, he said, he would focus on establishing "valuable, long-term directions for the Institute" (IOM, 1998a, p. 128). Despite the IOM's close collaboration with the government during the Carter years, Hamburg warned that if the IOM wished to fulfill its potential, it needed to find unrestricted, nongovernmental support and an infusion of new ideas and new people in key positions.

Hamburg left office 1 month before Ronald Reagan (1981–1989) was elected president. NAS President Philip Handler thanked Hamburg for his service in a personal letter, noting that, "Under your leadership, the Institute of Medicine has been brought to maturity. It has earned a place in the Washington scene and become the instrument to which we aspired when it was first created" (IOM,

---

[10] The Department of Health, Education, and Welfare later became the Department of Health and Human Services.

1998a, p. 139). Hamburg went on to serve as president of the Carnegie Corporation and president of the American Association for the Advancement of Science. He passed away in 2019 at the age of 93 (Roberts, 2019).

Frederick Robbins (Term: 1980–1985)

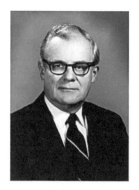

FIGURE 2-4 Frederick Robbins. SOURCE: National Academy of Sciences. 2006. *Biographical Memoirs: Volume 88*. Washington, DC: The National Academies Press. https://doi.org/10.17226/11807.

Frederick Robbins, a scientist who had earned a Nobel Prize for his work in isolating the polio virus, also limited his service to a 5-year term before retiring in 1985 (see Figure 2-4). Robbins's term was marked by challenges that included internal turmoil at the NAS and the Reagan administration's efforts to downsize the federal government, including the NIH.

Robbins was appointed as the IOM's fourth president in the fall of 1980. At age 63, he was older than previous presidents and brought experience from a full and illustrious career in medical research. Arriving at the IOM after leaving his position as dean of the Case Western Reserve University School of Medicine, Robbins remarked that he was "not going to revolutionize things" (IOM, 1998a, p. 138). Instead, he wanted to maintain the program that Hamburg had built. However, this proved difficult in the atmosphere of the times.

Continuing financial shortfalls had led NAS leaders to recommend that the IOM be disbanded and its program of studies be subsumed by the NRC. The matter escalated into a controversy that occupied much of Robbins's term and marked a crucial turning point in the organization's struggle to move beyond its start-up phase to a new era of growth and stability.

Before leaving the IOM in 1980, Hamburg had created a taskforce to evaluate the organization's structure and relationship to the NAS. The taskforce, which completed its work during Robbins's presidency, was chaired by Washington University in St. Louis Chancellor William H. Danforth. The Danforth report recommended that the Division of Medical Sciences (DMS) be moved from the NRC to the IOM. In the fall of 1981, Robbins confided to the NAS's new President Frank Press that he felt there was a "significant and disturbing problem of overlap in the interests of the IOM" and the DMS (IOM, 1998a, p. 147).

Meanwhile, NAS Vice President James Ebert undertook a parallel assessment. Ebert's 1982 report proposed that the NRC be divided into six major units, including one devoted to human health and medicine that would encompass some functions of the DMS and some functions of the IOM. Demonstrating support for the IOM, Ebert recommended that this new unit be housed in the IOM and overseen by the IOM Council. However, the NAS Council opposed the proposal, and the recommended merger never took place.

In 1984, the IOM's role again came under scrutiny, this time at the behest of its sponsors. Robert Ebert, president of the Milbank Memorial Fund, proposed a study of the IOM at the impetus of a group of private foundations that had supported its work, including the Commonwealth Fund and RWJF. The foundations' leaders wanted to assess how well the IOM was fulfilling its mission and determine whether it deserved continuing philanthropic support.

A nine-person committee chaired by Robert Sproull, a distinguished physicist and president of the University of Rochester, undertook the evaluation. Robbins testified before the committee in June 1984, arguing that the IOM's primary challenge was the lack of an endowment. He estimated that it would take $20 million to generate enough income to replace the funds that were provided by the foundations.

The Sproull committee's report, released in November 1984, called for "a strengthening of the IOM that amounts to a rebirth" (IOM, 1998a, p. 168). Reopening the debate of more than a decade before, the committee recommended the creation of an academy of medicine to take the place of the IOM in the NAS structure. In a departure from the original vision of the IOM's founders, the committee also recommended that the studies undertaken by the IOM be moved to the NRC.[11]

For many on the IOM Council, such a move would dissolve the founders' vision for a proactive, working organization. They preferred to preserve the designation of "institute" rather than "academy," especially if it meant preventing the transfer of the IOM's studies to the NRC. However, it was the NAS Council that would decide whether to adopt the Sproull committee's recommendations.

At a climactic NAS Council meeting in February 1985, Robbins expressed his views on the future of the IOM. He was disappointed by the Sproull committee's report, stating that it contained "drastic recommendations for change" and indicated "a true lack of support for the concept of the IOM" (IOM, 1998a, p. 171). As Robbins' term was nearing its end, the NAS Council decided to delay making a final decision on the Sproull report until the arrival of his successor. This deferral amounted to a reprieve for the IOM—the current structure would hold for the time being.

Robbins's term was consumed by the need to repeatedly defend the IOM's structure, even its very existence. Despite his vigorous efforts, the matter was not resolved by the end of his tenure. As a result, his successor faced the formidable task of bolstering the IOM's position in the NAS, restoring morale, and—perhaps most difficult of all—raising enough money to keep the IOM solvent. The outlook for the fiscal year 1986 indicated a quarter-million-dollar shortfall in the IOM budget.

Robbins returned to Case Western Reserve University after leaving the IOM. The technique he and his colleagues developed to grow the polio virus in a lab continued to be used by vaccine researchers worldwide. In 2003, the year Robbins passed away at the age of 86, the technique was used to identify the virus that causes severe acute respiratory syndrome (SARS) (Altman, 2003).

Samuel Thier (Term: 1985–1991)

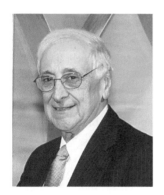

FIGURE 2-5 Samuel Thier in 2015.
SOURCE: National Academy of Medicine.

At the September 23, 1985, meeting of the IOM Council, NAS President Frank Press announced that Samuel Thier, a prominent kidney scientist who was then head of the Internal Medicine Department at Yale University, would become the next president of the IOM (see Figure 2-5). At the relatively young age of 48, Thier looked to the IOM as the next challenge of his career. Thier, who had been an IOM member since 1978 and had chaired the Board on Health Sciences Policy, presided over what could be considered the "rebirth" of the IOM as an expanded and reinvigorated organization.

Thier brought a new vitality and a reassuring self-confidence to the presidency of the IOM. Although he vowed to make changes, such as speeding up the report process and increasing the IOM's visibility to the federal government, he held to the IOM's original mission and touted the organiza-

---

[11] The prospect of transforming the IOM into an academy of medicine would be debated repeatedly until it became a reality in 2015. See Chapter 3 for a detailed account of the decades-long campaign.

tion's accomplishments. He believed that too much time and energy had been expended trying to determine whether the IOM should focus on health policy or health science—a false dichotomy in his mind. Thier stated that not only could the IOM do both, but it should cover "the entire spectrum of activities within the National Academy of Sciences complex that deal with human health" (IOM, 1998a, p. 181). He regarded the problems identified in the Sproull report as settled matters, and he used the report as leverage within the NAS and the foundation community. Thier believed that the foundations that had subjected the IOM to such in-depth and painful analysis had an obligation to continue to provide support in light of the internal efforts being made to improve the organization and its operations.

Thier took an assertive approach in his interactions with Press, whom he regarded as an important ally, and with the NAS Council. He secured a 2-year grace period to put the IOM's financial affairs in order and requested additional financial support from the NAS to make up for any deficits. Thier then launched an outreach campaign to the major health foundations, starting with RWJF. Although an early supporter of the IOM, RWJF's interest had begun to waver by Thier's tenure, due in part to the slow pace of IOM studies. These doubts had led the foundation to become one of the driving forces behind the Sproull report.

In the fall of 1986, Thier met with a small subcommittee of the RWJF board and succeeded in securing a $5 million contribution to the IOM's endowment. As conditions of the grant, the IOM was required to raise $2 for every $1 it received from the foundation. By March 1987, the IOM was prepared to announce a capital campaign, seeded not only by RWJF but also by sizable grants from The Commonwealth Fund, the Andrew W. Mellon Foundation, the W.K. Kellogg Foundation, and the MacArthur Foundation.

In addition to building the IOM's endowment, which reached nearly $19 million by the end of 1989, Thier expanded the organizational scope of the IOM to include two units that were previously part of the NRC—the exact opposite of the transfers suggested in the Sproull report. On July 1, 1988, the Medical Follow-Up Agency (MFUA) and the Food and Nutrition Board (FNB)—both with histories dating to World War II—became part of the IOM, consolidating more of the NRC's health activities under the purview of the Institute. By then, the IOM had the largest budget within the NAS complex, and the broad external support of the IOM began to quiet the criticisms that had appeared in the Sproull report.

During the Thier years, the IOM also acquired a new degree of flexibility and agility. Thier emphasized the IOM's convening power as an alternative to the more formal consensus study for which the National Academies were known. Although he did not invent the idea of an IOM forum or roundtable, he helped popularize the mechanism and made it a staple of IOM activities. For the IOM, the forum provided a less inhibited venue for open discussion among interested parties than did the traditional study committees, which were bound by conflict-of-interest rules and required sometimes lengthy, closed-door deliberations to come to consensus. Unlike study committees, forums and roundtables did not issue recommendations, and, with the exception of planning sessions, the majority of their work was conducted publicly through workshops and other meetings.

Thier departed the IOM in 1991, during the first year of his second term as IOM president, to become the president of Brandeis University. His fundraising efforts had resulted in a larger, more influential organization. By this time, the IOM had made a decisive turn in its history and was on its way to becoming a nationally recognized force in the health policy world. IOM member Stuart Bondurant, then dean of medicine at the University of North Carolina at Chapel Hill, stepped in as Acting President during the search for Thier's successor.

Kenneth Shine (Term: 1992–2002)

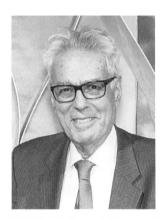

FIGURE 2-6 Kenneth Shine in 2015.
SOURCE: National Academy of Medicine.

Kenneth Shine arrived as the new IOM president in the fall of 1992 (see Figure 2-6). Shine was a Harvard-trained physician and one of the nation's most prominent cardiologists. When asked to consider the IOM presidency following Thier's resignation, Shine was dean of the School of Medicine at the University of California, Los Angeles.

Shine informed the IOM Council that he had accepted the presidency because of the IOM's remarkable membership, the legacy left by Thier, and the chance to respond to health challenges facing the nation—most notably a dysfunctional care system with shrinking resources. He talked about the fragile environment in which science and research were undertaken and the nation's increased interest in health care reform. Shine's goals for his presidency included maintaining a balance between careful, deliberative studies and timeliness; pursuing projects that would have a measurable impact on policy and practice; continuing Thier's fundraising efforts; and exploring projects with regional or state foci.

Shine, who would become the first two-term president of the IOM, led strategic planning processes in 1993 and 1997. The 1993 plan, developed in consultation with the IOM membership and its key governing committees, was designed to help establish a consensus across numerous internal stakeholders around the goals and directions for the IOM. The first step involved structured interviews with IOM staff that featured candid discussions of the IOM's strengths and weaknesses. The second step entailed regional dinners for IOM members held in late 1992 and early 1993 that Shine and Enriqueta Bond, by then the IOM's executive officer, hosted in Irvine, Chicago, and Washington. These consultations led to the development of a mission statement and accompanying goals, objectives, and strategies that the IOM Council approved in November 1993.

Among the plan's key objectives was the creation of a mechanism to identify important issues and priorities that the IOM should consider addressing, regardless of funding availability. The plan suggested the annual selection of a "special initiative" as an area of emphasis that was broad, crossed sectoral lines, and could command the focus of the entire IOM. Identifying areas in which the IOM could break new ground and achieve lasting impact was a key concern. Shine, drawing on conversations with IOM member and RAND Corporation Vice President Robert H. Brook, advanced the quality of health care as the topic of the IOM's first special initiative.

Due to the controversy of the subject, which highlighted the fallibility of clinicians and the system in which they operated, Shine was unable to secure external funding for the initiative's first study. Several potential sponsors he approached questioned why the IOM "would want to frighten the public with this information."[12] Ultimately, Shine used interest from the IOM's endowment and $750,000 in a matching gift supplied by NAS President Bruce Alberts to launch the initiative under the leadership of Staff Director Janet Corrigan.[13] In 1999, the initiative produced one of the IOM's most influential reports, *To Err Is Human: Building a Safer Health System.*[14]

---

[12] Personal communication between Kenneth Shine and Laura H. DeStefano, April 18, 2020.
[13] Ibid.
[14] Ibid. For more on the IOM's Quality Initiative, see Chapter 5.

In 1994, Shine led a new push to change the IOM's name to the National Academy of Medicine. Although the effort ultimately failed, it represented another step toward the creation of an academy, which would be realized in 2015 (see Chapter 3). The IOM's leadership structure became more robust during Shine's tenure, with the creation of two new officer positions within the IOM Council: Home Secretary and Foreign Secretary[15] (see Box 2-6).

In 1997, at the start of Shine's second term, he led the IOM Council in assessing progress and refining the 1993 strategic plan. Along with central goals related to the timely identification and engagement of priority issues, fundraising, membership diversity, and staff enrichment, the plan resulted in the delineation of key focus areas for the IOM to consider in the development of its program: the strength and function of the health care workforce; the implications of scientific breakthroughs (such as genetics and informatics) for the practice of health; health literacy and health communication; health of vulnerable populations; and designing health approaches for an increasingly diverse U.S. society. The IOM would go on to develop a significant body of work in each of these areas.

Shine's presidency was marked by continued growth and stability for the organization as the world entered a new millennium. After completing his second term as IOM president in 2002, Shine served briefly as a scholar at the RAND Corporation before beginning a distinguished tenure as Chancellor ad interim and Executive Vice Chancellor for Health Affairs at the University of Texas.

BOX 2-6
Home and International Secretaries of the Institute of
Medicine and the National Academy of Medicine

The Council Officer positions of Home Secretary and Foreign/International Secretary were formally established by amendment to the IOM bylaws in 2000, although informal operations began earlier. The Home Secretary is responsible for the conduct of membership affairs, including member elections, while the Foreign/International Secretary is responsible for the conduct of international affairs.

Home Secretaries of the IOM/NAM

- Harold J. Fallon, MD (1999–2004; 2013–2014)
- Stephen J. Ryan, MD (2004–2013)
- Jane E. Henney, MD (2014–2020)
- Elena Fuentes-Afflick, MD, MPH (2020–)

International Secretaries of the IOM/NAM

- James Wyngaarden, MD (1990–1994)
- David P. Rall, MD, PhD (1994–1998)
- David R. Challoner, MD (1998–2006)
- Jo Ivey Boufford, MD (2006–2014)
- Margaret A. Hamburg, MD (2014–2020)
- Carlos del Rio, MD (2020–)

---

[15] In 2020, the NAM membership voted to change the name of this position from Foreign Secretary to International Secretary.

Harvey Fineberg (Term: 2002–2014)

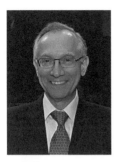

FIGURE 2-7 Harvey Fineberg at the 2012 IOM Annual Meeting. SOURCE: National Academy of Medicine.

Harvey Fineberg took office as the IOM's seventh president in 2002, and, like Shine, served two full terms before leaving his post in June 2014 (see Figure 2-7).[16] Fineberg came to the IOM as a distinguished medical practitioner and academic administrator with a unique blend of medical and public policy expertise.[17] He completed his education at Harvard, where he also spent much of his career. Fineberg served as the Dean of the Harvard School of Public Health before being named Provost of Harvard University in 1997.

As President, Fineberg's calm demeanor, congenial manner, and willingness to share credit endeared him to members and staff. "The IOM has this unique responsibility as the nation's science adviser on matters of health," Fineberg said upon news of his appointment, and described its membership as "an all-star national faculty to work on the most pressing issues of the day." Taking office soon after the September 11, 2001, terrorist attacks, Fineberg also noted that "the tenor of the times made the job all the more appealing. It's a great opportunity for service at a very critical time in the nation's history" (Rakoczy, 2001).

From the beginning of his presidency, Fineberg emphasized measuring and expanding the impact of the IOM and its reports. In this regard, he expanded on work started by Shine. Within a few years of Fineberg's arrival, he announced the creation of the Harvey V. Fineberg Impact Fund as an option to which members could contribute during annual fundraising. The Impact Fund would raise funds to initiate studies "where the need is great, where government may be disinterested or conflicted, where private sources may not be ready yet to provide support." During his 2013 Annual Meeting address, Fineberg stated, "the Impact Fund spells out its own components: I, Initiate, M, Motivate, P, Participate, and ACT" (Fineberg, 2013).

In 2011, the IOM published a schematic, called the Degrees of Impact Thermometer (see Figure 2-8), which defined the types of impact the IOM's activities could have and would be measured against. By the time Fineberg's second term ended, every Council meeting included an impact report. Following the IOM-NAM transition, the Health and Medicine Division (HMD) retired its use of the Impact Thermometer in favor of a new schematic that better captured the outcomes of convening activities such as roundtables, forums, and smaller-scale studies that did not necessarily change policy but were nevertheless of important use to sponsors and participants.[18]

Fineberg, like his predecessors, engaged in strategic planning, which involved developing a "strategic vision" to guide the IOM between 2003 and 2008. The plan envisioned a "vibrant and vital" IOM that provided a public service by "working outside the framework of government to ensure scientifically informed analysis and independent guidance." The portfolio of IOM studies continued to embrace the critical public issues of the day, which by Fineberg's tenure included homeland security and the threat of bioterrorism. With Fineberg's goal to increase impact, the IOM continued the mission begun by his predecessors to center its activities on coherent themes that promoted longer-term visibility and increased the organization's impact on public policy and private medical practice. Themes identified as important at the time included vaccine safety, quality of

---

[16] By the time of Fineberg's presidency, the IOM Council had voted to extend the length of a single presidential term from 5 to 6 years.

[17] Interview between Harvey Fineberg and Edward Berkowitz, October 15, 2018.

[18] Personal correspondence, Clyde Behney to Laura H. DeStefano, April 2020.

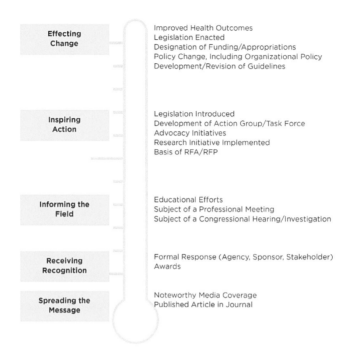

FIGURE 2-8 The Institute of Medicine's Degrees of Impact Thermometer (2014).
SOURCE: National Academy of Medicine.

care, health system redesign, global health, and genomics.[19] Fineberg felt particularly strongly that the IOM needed to reinvigorate its focus on global health. The prospect of eliminating the IOM's Board on Global Health had arisen during Shine's tenure, which Fineberg believed "undervalued the critical importance of global health, even when taking a relatively narrow view of American interests."[20] His focus on the interconnectedness of the health of the globe led to the revitalization of the Board on Global Health and its associated activities, which has published more than 170 reports and proceedings since 1996.

In an effort to sharpen the focus of the IOM, Fineberg, in collaboration with Executive Officer Susanne Stoiber, decided to reduce the number of IOM boards from eight to six and to convert the Board on Neuroscience and Behavioral Health into a convening activity in January 2005. Part of the motivation for this reorganization was to expand and elevate the IOM's standing convening activities (e.g., forums and roundtables), a program mechanism that the IOM had advanced under Thier. Although roundtables and forums did not issue recommendations, Fineberg emphasized that discussions and relationships formed during these activities constituted important contributions to the contemporary health policy agenda in national and international health.

The IOM's "Perspectives" platform arose in 2011 as a mechanism for participants in round-tables and forums to comment on issues of interest. In an early article for the platform, Fineberg wrote, "In the spirit of our mandate to serve as 'advisor to the nation to improve health,' this new venture to share ideas and insights presents an exciting opportunity to use the IOM's unique resource of the nation's leading experts in health and health policy to sharpen national dialogue on today's health challenges" (Fineberg, 2012). "Perspectives" remained with the NAM after the 2015 IOM-NAM reorganization and was reformed as a formal digital periodical called *NAM Perspec-*

---

[19] Institute of Medicine, "Strategic Vision 2003–2008," April 14, 2003, IOM/NAM Records.
[20] Personal correspondence, Harvey Fineberg to Laura H. DeStefano, December 2021.

tives. In 2021, 10 years after its establishment under Fineberg, *NAM Perspectives* became a journal indexed by the National Library of Medicine.

Like Shine's presidency, Fineberg's two terms in office saw continued growth and stability for the IOM. As a major element of his legacy, Fineberg began a process that would finally lead to the IOM's reconstitution as the NAM—an endeavor that had failed several times in the past. The success of the campaign headed by Fineberg lay in its framing as the establishment of a more integrated and efficacious National Academies overall, rather than focusing solely on the future of the IOM (discussed further in Chapter 3). By the time of Fineberg's departure in 2014, the changes were set in motion that will transform the trajectory of the IOM as well as the National Academies.

Fineberg's next role was as president of the Gordon and Betty Moore Foundation. He remained very active in the work of the NAM and the National Academies, notably as chair of a standing committee to advise the government on its response to the COVID-19 pandemic.

Victor J. Dzau (Term: 2014–Present)

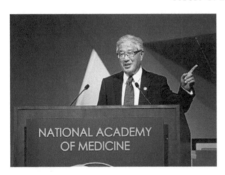

FIGURE 2-9 Victor Dzau at the 2019 NAM Annual Meeting.
SOURCE: National Academy of Medicine.

Victor Dzau became both the final president of the IOM and the first president of the newly formed NAM (see Figure 2-9). By the time Dzau took office in 2014, the IOM-NAM reorganization was already in motion, and he inherited the complex task of negotiating the details with NAS and NAE, communicating the change to membership, securing the approval votes from NAS and IOM members and navigating the transition (see Chapter 3). As the new Academy expanded its operations, Dzau spearheaded an innovative and proactive orientation that represented a significant departure from the IOM's previous approach and ultimately led to changes throughout the National Academies (described below and further in Chapter 7).

Dzau brought a dynamic presence and distinguished clinical, academic, and administrative background to the IOM/NAM. Born in Shanghai, Dzau, an immigrant, was the first non-White president of the IOM, the first of Asian descent, and the first to be born outside the United States. A cardiologist and an active researcher in the field of gene therapy for vascular disease who made significant contributions to the development of ACE inhibitors, Dzau chaired the departments of medicine at Stanford and Brigham and Women's Hospital before becoming the president and chief executive officer of the Duke University Health System and the chancellor in charge of the university's many health activities. Dzau served as a member of the NAM Council for 6 years before being selected as IOM president in 2014.

After the IOM-NAM reorganization, the programs of the IOM including all six boards, which conducted consensus studies and convening activities, were moved into a new Health and Medicine Division within the National Academies. Left with close to a blank slate, Dzau set out to develop the NAM's distinct priorities and programmatic approach. Like his predecessors, Dzau quickly undertook a strategic planning process to position the NAM for success within the National Academies complex and as a proactive, galvanizing leader on the domestic and international stage. The NAM's strategic planning model proved so fruitful that Dzau led the NRC Strategic Plan in 2019–2020 in which fellow leaders of the National Academies adapted the NAM model to map future directions for the NRC. (The particulars of the IOM-NAM reorganization and the NAM's strategic planning process are described in Chapter 3.)

From the start of his presidency, Dzau emphasized innovation—both in terms of the IOM/NAM's program models and the rapid advances in science, technology, and health care to which the organization should respond. In his inaugural president's address to the NAM membership, Dzau expressed his belief that

> these days, a lot of people in health and medicine are hunkered down, operating in siloes that focus narrowly on their own problems. The world needs aspirational and audacious goals to inspire confidence that we can do more, much more, to change the course of health. Many of us believe that major breakthroughs can be achieved through partnerships of the best minds across all sectors, sharing a common vision and goals, working collectively to address big, bold problems, creating the right environment with robust resources and aligning incentives and value. (Dzau, 2015b)

To mobilize resources around such goals, Dzau developed a new "Grand Challenge" program model for the NAM, establishing the Healthy Longevity Global Grand Challenge in 2019 and the Grand Challenge on Climate Change, Human Health, and Equity in 2021.

An unwavering focus on providing leadership in the domestic and global spheres became a hallmark of Dzau's tenure. Early in Dzau's first term, the West African Ebola crisis presented an opportunity for another new program model focused on international leadership. Observing the slow and poorly coordinated international response to the outbreak, Dzau saw a role for the NAM in gathering global experts to collectively assess shortcomings and develop solutions to improve health security. The NAM became the Secretariat for an independent International Commission, overseen by an International Oversight Board, which issued a fast-track report with recommendations in the areas of public health, global and regional coordination, and research and development. The commission's recommendations were embraced by the World Health Organization, the United Nations, and the World Bank. The International Commission model became part of the NAM's new capability portfolio, next used to address human genome editing, healthy longevity, influenza vaccine preparedness, and financing pandemic preparedness.

Throughout his tenure, Dzau also maintained a strong international presence in his personal capacity, serving as a member of the Global Preparedness Monitoring Board and Access to COVID-19 Tools (ACT) Accelerator and the interim board of directors for the Coalition for Epidemic Preparedness Innovations as well as co-chair of a scientific report of the G20 global health summit, among other global engagements (G20, 2021b). He participated in the European Union's Coronavirus Global Response Pledging Conference, which raised 7.5 billion euros to fund the global response to the COVID-19 pandemic (Borger, 2020; European Commission, 2020; European Union and Italian G20 Presidency, 2021).

Dzau believed that NAM should be an academy of action and impact, beyond providing advice. He often quoted the German philosopher Goethe: "Knowing is not enough. We must apply. Willing is not enough. We must do." An innovative programmatic mechanism pioneered successfully under Dzau's leadership was the "Action Collaborative," a standing body that convened multi-sectoral stakeholders to develop collective solutions and actions around shared priorities (see Box 2-7). NAM Action Collaboratives became high-visibility vehicles for collective commitment and action around subjects of broad concern in health and medicine. The NAM's inaugural Action Collaborative on Clinician Well-Being and Resilience achieved national recognition of the problem of clinician burnout and galvanized a new body of research to better understand the crisis and develop effective interventions. By 2022, the NAM had applied its Action Collaborative model to the U.S. opioid epidemic and the intersection of climate change, human health, and equity. The Action Collaborative on Climate and Health took on the bold goal of decarbonizing the entire U.S. health sector (NAM, 2018b, 2021m). The National Academies also adapted the model for an initiative on preventing sexual harassment in academic science, engineering, and medicine.

BOX 2-7
The Action Collaborative Model

The concept of the "Action Collaborative" predated the creation of the NAM, although the model was reshaped and adopted as a core program model by the Academy. The Leadership Consortium, which was founded in 2006 as an IOM program called the Roundtable on Value & Science-Driven Health Care, had established "Innovation Collaboratives" and "Action Collaboratives" as informal subgroups of volunteers within its activities. These subgroups were able to make statements and take action toward self-determined priorities—independent of the IOM, but inspired by their engagement with the IOM and facilitated by its staff. Innovation/Action Collaboratives continued to be used by a range of IOM and later HMD programs, although with policies distinct from Action Collaboratives under the NAM.

Under the NAM, the Action Collaborative became a standalone mechanism to convene and enable key stakeholders with similar responsibilities and shared interests to develop solutions and act collectively to address a specific, multi-faceted, and significant problem and provide stakeholder participants with a collaborative platform on which to build a shared "action agenda" for advancing progress. Members of NAM Action Collaboratives have produced individually authored papers and other resources, hosted public events, and worked directly with policy makers and health leaders to drive change.

Dzau also focused significant efforts on fundraising, securing $10 million from RWJF to launch the Culture of Health Program in 2015, half of which was allocated to the NAM's endowment. RWJF committed another $5 million to the program in 2020. Dzau also mobilized more than $30 million to support an international competition under the Healthy Longevity program. These and other efforts contributed significantly to a $100 million NAM capital campaign launched publicly in 2021.

Dzau believed that Academies should stand up for their foundational values and core beliefs based on science and evidence. He became one of the most publicly outspoken presidents in the history of the organization as policies during the Trump administration threatened to undercut the integrity of science and ran counter to many of the evidence-based recommendations issued by the IOM/NAM. He was quick to respond publicly after the murder of George Floyd at the hands of Minneapolis police officers in 2020, issuing a statement to NAM staff and then publicly that read, in part, "I commit to using our platform to improve the lives of people who experience disproportionate health disparities as a result of socioeconomic inequity, bias, and structural racism" (Dzau, 2020). Dzau was also motivated by, and spoke often of three "existential threats to health and well-being everywhere: COVID-19 and future pandemics, the negative impacts of structural racism, and climate change."

In 2020, Dzau was elected by the NAM membership for a second term as president. The election was the first of its kind for the organization, enabled by governance rules in the new NAM bylaws that empowered members to elect their own president (as opposed to having one appointed by the NAS president, as dictated in the IOM bylaws). Just 8 months into Dzau's historic second term, the global COVID-19 pandemic upended society worldwide. Dzau focused on pivoting the Academy's programs to respond to the crisis, working with NAM members to fill a gulf in federal scientific leadership in the early days of the pandemic, and leading NAM and National Academies staff through a complex transition to remote work. In 2021, as vaccinations rose steadily in the United States, Dzau turned to promoting vaccine equity worldwide. Importantly, Dzau positioned the NAM to respond to other challenges that threatened the health and stability of an increasingly global society, such as climate change and structural racism.

INSTITUTE OF MEDICINE AND NATIONAL ACADEMY OF MEDICINE STAFF LEADERS

Building a staff of the right size and expertise was a consuming early focus of the IOM. When the institute opened its doors in 1970, then-President John Hogness had a single person on staff. He quickly determined the need for a "deputy" to assist him in priority setting and program building, and by 1972 had hired the IOM's first executive officer, Roger Bulger (see Box 2-8). Two other significant hires that Hogness made included Karl Yordy, who would ultimately succeed Bulger as executive officer, as staff director for the IOM's new program committee, and Ruth Hanft as senior research associate. Figure 2-10 shows many of the IOM's staff members on the steps of the NAS Building in 1973.

Hanft, a distinguished researcher with extensive federal service who would be elected as an IOM member in 1978, led the key early studies for the organization (*The Washington Post*, 2011). These studies helped to build a sustainable staffing model for the IOM. In the days of the Board on Medicine (see Chapter 1), the organization relied on temporary consultants. Under Hanft, however, the IOM began increasing the numbers of dedicated, full-time staff. In 1972, Congress directed the IOM to study the costs of education of health professionals. Hanft hired a staff of 20 to collect data on the cost of educating medical students across institutions. However, the IOM's lack of core funding meant that those staff would have to move on when the study concluded—a soft-money problem that posed an ongoing challenge.

Hanft's study also revealed another problem that the IOM needed to solve—the division of labor and the degree of supervision between staff and the volunteer members and external experts who made up study committees. Although members of the committee were named as the formal "authors" of the study, they had limited involvement in the work of data collection, and it was Hanft, not Committee Chair Julius Richmond (who would later become U.S. Surgeon General), who presented the findings of the costs of education study to Congress.

This tension continued into Hamburg's tenure as Hanft concluded an intensive follow-up study, this time with a staff of 45, that examined Medicare's role in funding medical education. Hanft and Study Committee Chair Adam Yarmolinsky disagreed about the appropriate balance of data

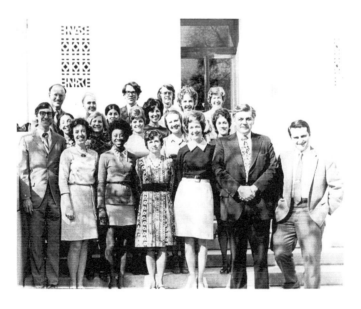

FIGURE 2-10 IOM staff pictured in 1973.
SOURCE: Courtesy of Don Detmer.

and policy recommendations. Hanft, who favored a focus on data, prevailed. The lack of clarity around the respective roles of the IOM's staff and its members was a focus of Hamburg's review of the organization's programmatic structure and approach (described earlier in this chapter). He found that both groups—members and staff—wanted more meaningful involvement in the IOM's work. Ultimately, Hamburg's solution was to create six program divisions (later called boards), each headed by a staff director and advised by a group of members. This practice enabled ongoing, productive collaboration among members and staff.

Hamburg's structure became the foundation for the model that endured until the 2015 IOM-NAM transition and carried through in the structure of the new HMD. In 2021, the HMD had five boards (Food and Nutrition; Global Health; Health Care Services; Health Sciences Policy; Population Health and Public Health Practice) and a sixth (Children, Youth, and Families) shared with the Division of Behavioral and Social Sciences and Education. In addition, there was an Office of Military and Veterans' Health. As during Hamburg's tenure, each board was overseen by a staff director and advised by a group of members of the NAM, the NAS, and the NAE and other experts.

As they had in Hanft's day, both HMD and NAM staff served as directors of individual studies, convening activities, and other projects, applying their own considerable expertise to synthesize the findings and recommendations of expert committees. In addition to the directors, a cadre of research, administrative, and communications staff supported the conduct of projects and the dissemination of recommendations. In 2000, in recognition of the crucial role of its staff in carrying out the work of the organization, the IOM/NAM began conferring annual awards, called Cecil Awards,[21] to recognize superlative staff contributions (see Box 2-9). Upon his retirement in 2021 as Executive Director of the HMD, Clyde Behney received a special Cecil Award in recognition of "40 years of unparalleled service leading and shaping the nation's ability to receive expert and unbiased advice on scientific and technical matters of particular priority and potential in advancing the human condition."

BOX 2-8
Executive Officers of the Institute of Medicine and
the National Academy of Medicine

Roger Bulger, MD (1972–1976)[a]
Karl Yordy, MPA (1976–1981)
Charles Miller, MA (1981–1989)
Enriqueta Bond, PhD (1989–1994)[a]
Karen Hein, MD (1995–1998)
Susanne Stoiber, MPA, MS (1998–2007)
Judith Salerno, MD, MS (2008–2013)[a]
Clyde Behney, MBA (2013–2015)[b]
J. Michael McGinnis, MD, MPP (2015–)[a,b]

---

[a] NAM member.
[b] After the 2015 IOM-NAM transition, Clyde Behney, who had been the interim Leonard D. Schaeffer Executive Officer of the IOM since 2013, became the executive director of the new Health and Medicine Division. J. Michael McGinnis became the Leonard D. Schaeffer Executive Officer of the NAM.

---

[21] The name "Cecil" came from IOM staff's informal name for the serpent in the IOM/NAM's logo. IOM reports bore the following explanation for the logo: "The serpent has been a symbol of long life, healing, and knowledge among almost all cultures and religions since the beginning of recorded history. The serpent adopted as a logotype by the Institute of Medicine is a relief carving from ancient Greece, now held by the Staatliche Museen in Berlin."

BOX 2-9
Recipients of the Institute of Medicine and the National
Academy of Medicine Cecil Staff Award

Established in 2000, the Cecil Award recognized IOM/NAM staff for exceptional contributions to the work of the organization. As of 2020, Cecil Awards are conferred in the categories of individual excellence and excellence of a group or team. A third award for administrative excellence is given in honor of staff member Sandra H. Matthews, who supported three IOM presidents during her tenure (see Figure 2-11). Matthews also served as chair of the National Academies' African American Histories Program, which recognizes the contributions of outstanding African Americans to science, engineering, medicine, and to the nation's welfare. Notably, she invited school-age children from the Washington, DC, area to attend program events and learn more about careers in science and medicine.

Recipients, 2000–2021: Laura Aiuppa, Charlee Alexander, Elle Alexander, Bruce Altevogt, Pamella Atayi, Aurelia Attal-Juncqua, Alina Baciu, Emily Backes, Erin Balogh, Anton Bandy, Jim Banihashemi, Sue Barron, Clyde Behney, Natacha Blain, Katharine Bothner, Katie Bowman, Lisa Brown, Sarah Brown, David Butler, Kyra Cappelucci, Joe Cassells, Rosemary Anne Chalk, Rebecca Chevat, Ivory Clarke (2), Heather Cook, Janet Corrigan, Thelma Cox, Laura H. DeStefano, Donna Duncan, Marilyn Field, Emma Fine, Elizabeth Finkelman, Carolyn Fulco, Amy Geller, Mary Ghitelman, Annalee Espinosa Gonzales, Roger Herdman, Lyla Hernandez, Lois Joellenbeck, Ben Kahn, Morgan Kanarek, Rajbir Kaur, Bridget Kelly, Geraldine Kennedo, Linda Kilroy, Heather Kreidler, Cathy Liverman, Tracy Lustig, Cypress Lynx, Guru Madhavan, Rose Marie Martinez (2), Sandra Matthews, Meg McCoy, Janice Mehler, Marc Meisnere, Linda Meyers, Marie Michnich, Abigail Mitchell, Sharyl Nass, Amanda Nguyen, Lynn Parker, Mary Burr Paxton, Samantha Phillips, Yumi Phillips, Andrew Pope (2), Imani Rickerby, Andrea Schultz, Judith Shamir (2), Dara Shefska, Leslie Sim, Brian Smedley, Stacy Smit, Kirsten Sampson Snyder, Doug Sprunger, Christine Stencel, Janet Stoll, Kathleen Stratton, Jama Surdi, Elizabeth Townsend, Danitza Valdivia, Gary Walker, Toby Warden, Roberta Wedge, Yvonne Wise, Gooloo Wunderlich, Ann Yaktine, Karl Yordy, Mariana Zindel

NOTE: Recipients are presented in alphabetical order.

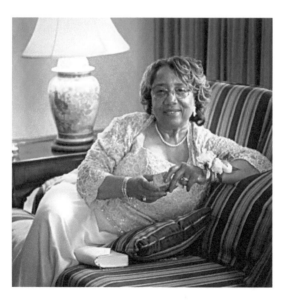

FIGURE 2-11 Longtime IOM staff member Sandra H. Matthews.
SOURCE: Courtesy of the family of Sandra H. Matthews.

BUILDING THE LEADERSHIP PIPELINE AND RECOGNIZING EXCELLENCE

In addition to its members, officers, and staff, the IOM/NAM developed programs to foster the next generation of health and medical leaders and recognize superlative contributions to the field.

Fellowships

The RWJF Health Policy Fellows program, established in 1973, is the IOM/NAM's longest-running program as of 2021. The program began under Hogness's tenure with a $710,000 grant from RWJF to "offset severe shortages of faculty members in the nation's academic medical centers who are specifically qualified for research, teaching, and service in the complex field of health policy." The foundation hoped to take advantage of the IOM's strong connections in Washington to expose health researchers and administrators to the intricacies of policy making, with the ultimate goal of building productive relationships that would encourage a scientific approach to federal health policy and its implementation at the local level. Robert Q. Marston, former director of the NIH, served as the program's first director.

The IOM announced its inaugural six fellows, culled from a list of 43 nominations and 12 finalists, in the spring of 1974. The fellows spent the 1974–1975 academic year in Washington, DC, beginning with an orientation at the IOM and then taking up temporary posts in congressional and executive offices on Capitol Hill. The program continued to followed this model for nearly 50 years, and many of its approximately 300 alumni went on to assume prominent roles in national health policy.

In a notable example, Jo Ivey Boufford, class of 1979–1980, became the first woman to serve as President of New York City Health and Hospitals Corporation in 1985. She then served in the Clinton administration as the principal deputy assistant secretary for health in the Department of Health and Human Services. Elected to membership in the IOM/NAM in 1992, she ultimately served as its Foreign Secretary. Karen Hein, who spent her 1993–1994 fellowship with the Senate Finance Committee, became executive officer of the IOM and president of the William T. Grant Foundation. "The rest of my life started the day I heard I had gotten this fellowship, and there's been no looking back since then," Hein noted.

Following the 2015 IOM-NAM transition, the RWJF Health Policy Fellows and five other fellowship programs became part of the new Academy (see Box 2-10). In 2021, the NAM announced the formation of a new Scholars in Diagnostic Excellence Program in collaboration with the Council of Medical Specialty Societies, sponsored by the Gordon and Betty Moore Foundation. The program was designed to support 10 scholars per year in a "one-year, part-time experience to advance the scholars' diagnostic skills, reduce diagnostic errors that lead to patient harm, and accelerate their career development as national leaders in this field" (NASEM, 2021a).

Awards

Starting in 1986, the IOM began conferring the Gustav O. Lienhard Award for Advancement of Health Care. The award was named in honor of the chairman of the RWJF Board of Trustees from 1971 to 1986. Funded by RWJF and consisting of a medal and $40,000, the award recognizes individuals for outstanding achievement in improving health care services in the United States. In 1992, the IOM added the Rhoda and Bernard Sarnat International Prize in Mental Health, established by the Sarnats out of a desire to improve the science base for and the delivery of mental health services. Accompanied by a medal and $20,000, the award honored individuals or organizations for notable achievements. Like the Lienhard Award, the Sarnat Prize is open to members as well as non-members of the IOM/NAM (see Box 2-11).

BOX 2-10
National Academy of Medicine Fellowship Programs

Robert Wood Johnson Foundation Health Policy Fellowship program (1973–). An opportunity for mid-career professionals to participate in federal policy making and apply new knowledge to their careers.

Distinguished Nurse Scholar-in-Residence program (1992–). An opportunity for nurse leaders to contribute to the development of national health policy.

Food and Drug Administration Tobacco Regulatory Science Fellowships (2012–2021). An opportunity for midcareer professionals to learn about the regulation of tobacco products following the Family Smoking Prevention and Tobacco Control Act.

NAM Fellowships (2005–). Originally established as the IOM Anniversary Fellowships, an opportunity for early- to mid-career professionals to participate in the work of the National Academies of Sciences, Engineering, and Medicine.

Endowed NAM Fellowships

- Norman F. Gant/American Board of Obstetrics and Gynecology Fellowship
- James C. Puffer, MD/American Board of Family Medicine Fellowship
- Gilbert S. Omenn Fellowship
- American Board of Emergency Medicine Fellowship
- Greenwall Fellowship in Bioethics
- NAM Fellowship in Pharmacy
- NAM Fellowship in Osteopathic Medicine

International Fellowships (2017–). An opportunity for global scholars to train in the areas of international health policy and global health leadership. Included the NAM-HKU Fellowship in Global Health Leadership (a collaboration between the NAM and The University of Hong Kong) and the NAM International Health Policy Fellowship, designed for early- to mid-career scholars in the fields of bioethics, medical ethics and law, economics and health policy, and health care.

NAM Scholars in Diagnostic Excellence (2021–). An opportunity for professionals to develop personal proposals to reduce diagnostic errors, as well as to learn, network, and receive mentoring opportunities.

In October 2021, the NAM established a new annual award, the David and Beatrix Hamburg Award for Advances in Biomedical Research and Clinical Medicine. Named for the former IOM president, who passed away in 2019, and his wife, Beatrix, an NAM member who specialized in child and adolescent psychiatry, the award recognized an "exceptional biomedical research discovery, translation, or public health intervention … that has fundamentally enriched the understanding of biology and disease" (NAM, 2021o; see Figure 2-12). The inaugural member of the Hamburg Award, which was accompanied by a $50,000 prize, was scheduled to be announced at the 2022 NAM Annual Meeting.

CONCLUSION

This chapter chronicles the people who carried out the work of the IOM/NAM. Upon acceptance of their election to the Academy, NAM members made a commitment to advance the work of the organization—and thereby further its mission of improving human health. They served and helped to steer the organization in diverse leadership as well as voluntary roles. IOM/NAM staff,

---

BOX 2-11
Recipients of Institute of Medicine and National Academy
of Medicine Awards for Professional Achievement

Gustav O. Lienhard Award for Advancement of Health Care

Recipients, 1986–2020: Julius B. Richmond, MD; Ernest W. Saward, MD; Marie-Louis Ansak; Robert J. Haggerty, MD; Henry K. Silver, MD; Loretta C. Ford, EdD, RN; Robert M. Ball, MA; C. Everett Koop, MD, ScD; Faye G. Abdellah, EdD, ScD, RN; David E. Rogers, MD; Byllye Y. Avery; Lawrence L. Weed, MD; Robert N. Butler, MD; T. Franklin Williams, MD; Lester Breslow, MD, MPH; H. Jack Geiger, MD; Elma L. Holder, MSPH; Philip R. Lee, MD; Ruth Watson Lubic, RN, CNM, EdD; Kathryn E. Barnard, PhD, RN; T. Berry Brazelton, MD; B. Jaye Anno, PhD; Bernard P. Harrison, JD; Kenneth W. Kizer, MD, MPH; Robert H. Brook, MD, ScD; Aaron T. Beck, MD; Howard H. Hiatt, MD; John E. Wennberg, MD, MPH; Thomas E. Starzl, MD, PhD; Joseph A. Califano, Jr., LLB; Jerold F. Lucey, MD; Donald M. Berwick, MD; Steven A. Schroeder, MD; Linda Aiken, PhD, RN; Robert L. Brent, MD, PhD; David Cella, PhD; Diane E. Meier, MD; Stuart Altman, PhD; Patricia Gabow, MD; Anthony Fauci, MD; Risa Lavizzo-Mourey, MD, MBA

Rhoda and Bernard Sarnat International Prize in Mental Health

Recipients, 1992–2020: Daniel X. Freedman, MD; Seymour S. Kety, MD; Myrna Weissman, PhD; Gerald Klerman, MD; Samuel B. Guze, MD; Leon Eisenberg, MD; Herbert Pardes, MD; David Kupfer, MD; Nancy C. Andreasen, MD, PhD; Rosalynn Carter; Michael L. Rutter, MD; Solomon H. Snyder, MD; David Satcher, MD, PhD; Aaron T. Beck, MD; Albert J. Stunkard, MD; Floyd E. Bloom, MD; Jack D. Barchas, MD; Beatrix Hamburg, MD; David Hamburg, MD; Paul R. McHugh, MD; David Mechanic, PhD; Eric J. Nestler, MD, PhD; Charles P. O'Brien, MD, PhD; William E. Bunney, MD; Ellen Frank, PhD; Huda Akil, PhD; Stanley J. Watson, MD, PhD; William T. Carpenter, MD; Vikram Patel, FMedSci; Kay Redfield Jamison, PhD; Kenneth S. Kendler, MD; Steven E. Hyman, MD; Robin Murray, FRS; Catherine Lord, PhD; Matthew State, MD, PhD; Joseph T. Coyle, MD; Kenneth B. Wells, MD, MPH; Daniel Weinberger, MD; Stephen Hinshaw, PhD; Spero M. Manson, PhD

NOTE: Recipients are presented in chronological order.

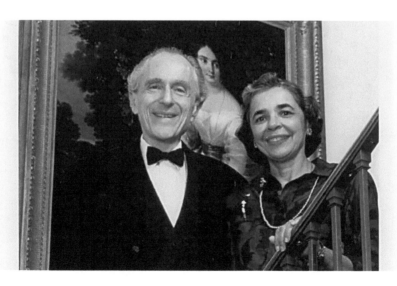

FIGURE 2-12 David and Beatrix Hamburg.
SOURCE: National Academy of Medicine.

too, played a historically significant role. Executive officers served as "deputies" to the presidents and oversaw the organization's staff and operations. Directors of boards and studies, experts in their own right, collaborated with advisory groups and consensus committees made up of members as well as external volunteers to determine programmatic direction and execute studies and convening activities. Finally, the IOM/NAM looked beyond its members and staff to foster excellence and leadership in the field of health through fellowships and awards. The collective expertise and commitment of these many individuals made the organization a powerful force for change throughout its history.

3

The Creation of the National Academy of Medicine[1]

On April 28, 2015, Ralph Cicerone, then the president of the National Academy of Sciences (NAS), announced that "today the membership of the National Academy of Sciences voted to change the name of the Institute of Medicine [IOM] to the National Academy of Medicine [NAM]." The announcement marked the end of a concentrated, 2-year campaign to reconstitute the IOM as the NAM, conferring a new structure and authority parallel to that of the NAS and the National Academy of Engineering (NAE). As described in Chapters 1 and 2, the campaign was by no means the first attempt to transform the IOM into an Academy; indeed, the notion had persisted in some form for nearly five decades.

Cicerone's announcement detailed, in part, the rationale that had fueled the campaign for so long. The addition of the new Academy would bring greater harmony to the work of the broader organization, which was rebranded at the same time as the National Academies of Sciences, Engineering, and Medicine (the National Academies).[2] Continual advances in science, engineering, and medicine over the past 50 years meant that scientific inquiry was increasingly multidisciplinary, Cicerone explained. Solutions to society's most pressing challenges required "knowledge, techniques, and tools from multiple areas of expertise." The reorganization would provide a more unified organizational and governance structure and encourage expanded collaboration across the three Academies. It would create what Cicerone described as "a greater symmetry in the roles, scope of activities, and responsibilities within the organization."[3]

As a result of the reorganization, the NAM gained co-equal status with the NAE in overseeing the joint program of the National Academies, including what had once been separately administered by the IOM. Indeed, achieving these goals meant a near-total reconfiguration of the IOM's programs and profoundly changed the way the organization conducted its work. During the reorganization,

---

[1] Except where otherwise noted, historical facts presented in this chapter are drawn from a 1998 history of the Institute of Medicine authored by Edward Berkowitz (IOM, 1998a).

[2] Concurrent with the IOM/NAM rebranding, the name "National Research Council," which had described the operating arm of the National Academy of Sciences and the National Academy of Engineering until 2015, was supplanted publicly by the "National Academies of Sciences, Engineering, and Medicine."

[3] Ralph J. Cicerone to National Academies staff, April 28, 2015, IOM/NAM Records.

the IOM's activities were divided between the NAM and a new NRC programmatic unit called the Health and Medicine Division (HMD). Ongoing consensus studies and most convening activities (e.g., boards, as well as forums and roundtables, which also housed around 20 Action or Innovation Collaboratives) of the former IOM were moved to HMD, while membership activities, fellowships, awards, and select program activities remained with the NAM (see Chapter 3 Appendix Figures 3A-1 through 3A-4).

As the NAM defined its new purpose and role within the National Academies, it quickly expanded its programmatic portfolio and field leadership activities. Innovative collaborations, international outreach, and novel program models became hallmarks of the NAM's approach during its first 5 years. Chief among its priorities was establishing a productive working relationship with HMD to carry forward the IOM's legacy.

HISTORY OF CAMPAIGNS TO ESTABLISH THE NATIONAL ACADEMY OF MEDICINE

The campaign to create the NAM had been derailed several times in the past, due largely to an inability to agree on its role and scope within the larger institution. The IOM leaders who decided to renew the campaign in 2012 needed to incorporate the lessons of prior attempts that had met resistance and ended in failure. Although conditions and attitudes had changed over time, and the organization seemed to be ready for a new chapter, many past obstacles remained relevant.

The IOM had begun operations in 1970 as part of the NAS, and that affiliation had both advantages and disadvantages for the organization. The NAS's scientific authority and reputation as an impartial adviser extended to the IOM, easing early efforts to mount new studies and establish a presence in Washington, DC. As an institute, rather than an Academy, the IOM was able to initiate its own studies, and it had more leeway to set its own priorities, allowing the organization to pursue an agenda that included social dimensions beyond the limitations of traditional medical research in the 1960s and 1970s. Walsh McDermott, one of the IOM's founders, strongly believed in the IOM's social mission and was a proponent of selecting members from outside the medical sciences. Despite these advantages, the IOM's governance was only semi-autonomous. The IOM was not able to select its own president; rather, it was required to present candidates to the NAS president, who made the ultimate decision. The IOM's association with the NAS also subjected the organization and its decisions to the scrutiny of the governing council of the NAS and the National Research Council (NRC, the operating arm of the National Academy of Sciences and the National Academy of Engineering until 2015), never allowing for complete independence.

The Sproull Report, 1984

The question of an Academy versus an Institute had been one of the central questions around the IOM's founding (see Chapter 1). Fourteen years later, the first formal proposal to reconstitute the IOM as an Academy emerged when a group of foundations, led by Robert Ebert, president of the Milbank Memorial Fund, commissioned a study of the IOM's structure and performance. As described in Chapter 2, a committee headed by physicist Robert Sproull undertook the review.

What became known as the "Sproull report" called for "a strengthening of the IOM that amounts to a rebirth"—in other words, its transformation into a fully autonomous and prestigious academy positioned to lead the nation's response to health and medical challenges. To allow for this expanded leadership capacity, Sproull's committee recommended that the IOM's existing program of consensus studies be moved to an NRC division.

However, many members of the IOM's governing council believed that implementation of the latter recommendation would compromise the founders' design for a proactive, working organization. At its January 1985 meeting, therefore, the Council announced its preference to maintain the IOM's current name and structure. However, the final decision rested with the NAS Council. The following month, then-IOM President Frederick Robbins argued passionately before the NAS Council against implementation of the Sproull recommendations, claiming that the report betrayed "a true lack of support for the concept of the IOM." Robbins was persuasive, to a point; his term as president was soon to conclude, and the NAS Council deferred any decision until the arrival of his successor. However, as described in Chapter 2, Samuel Thier focused on using the Sproull report's expressed support for the IOM to solidify financial and institutional support for the institute in its existing form.

A Second Campaign Fails, 1994–1996

After nearly a decade, the question of transforming the IOM into an Academy arose once again—this time as an internally driven campaign. On July 6, 1994, as the IOM approached its 25th anniversary, then-President Shine wrote to NAS President Bruce Alberts, seeking his advice on asking the NAS Council to approve a name change to the National Academy of Medicine. Shine emphasized that the change would only affect the IOM's name and not its mission or operations. He argued that "Institute of Medicine" created confusion with the National Institutes of Health (NIH), and that the relationship between the NAS and the IOM was not always clear, particularly when the NAE was added to the mix. Shine saw a name change as a way of matching the organization's title to its work and as an appropriate way to celebrate the institute's maturity and influence after 25 years.

Alberts replied positively to the proposal and put the matter before the NAS Council in August 1994, receiving favorable feedback. However, the NAS Council noted that proper procedure would have to be followed to effect the change—a process that would take 2 years when combined with the IOM's own requirements.[4] Approval required a two-thirds majority vote by the NAS membership, because the change would involve an amendment to the NAS charter. The NAS Council would have to approve a charter amendment ballot, with a return deadline of February 1995. Then the Council would present the recommended name change to the NAS members at their regular April 1995 meeting. The NAS membership would vote on the name change in 1996.[5]

Prior to initiating the NAS approval process, IOM members needed to provide their approval of the proposal. A ballot was sent to members in January 1995, accompanied by a letter from Shine that listed the reasons he favored the change. "We are an academy, not an institute," he argued. Institutes carried out research, whereas an academy consisted of a "collection of learned individuals seeking to further art, science, or literature." The term "academy" better described what the IOM did, Shine contended. Counterpart organizations throughout the world typically carried the title of "academy," or, in some countries, royal societies. If the IOM changed its name to the National Academy of Medicine, Shine argued, it would be recognized "almost immediately as to who we are and what we do." Shine emphasized that the name change implied "no other change in the mode of operation, representation, organization or participation of the Institute within the National Academy of Sciences or the National Research Council."[6]

IOM members endorsed the name change with a vote of 380 in favor, 14 opposed, and 3 abstentions. However, by this time, some fissures had started to develop in support for the name change in the broader NAS complex. The NAE argued that, if the new NAM were to be allowed to maintain its independent program of studies, then the NAE should be given the same allowance (rather than its current limitation of carrying out studies through the NRC). Furthermore, at a regional meeting, NAS members expressed concern that they did not know enough about the

---

[4] Kenneth Shine to Bruce Alberts, July 6, 1994, IOM/NAM Records; IOM Council Minutes, October 18, 1994, IOM/NAM Records.

[5] IOM Council Minutes, January 10, 1995, IOM/NAM Records.

[6] Kenneth Shine to IOM Members, January 17, 1995, IOM/NAM Records.

IOM or its operations to vote on the matter. In response to NAS members' concerns, Alberts asked the IOM to prepare material that would make its case. He did not feel he could bring the proposal forward until the NAS membership could be "further educated."[7]

Complicating the situation, the NAE faced internal tensions with the NAS and the NRC. The new NAE president was not nominated through the usual channels but rather ran as a "petition" candidate on a platform opposing the "NAE establishment." When he took office in 1995, he directly criticized and challenged the NAS and the NRC. For example, he felt that the NRC's work was not focused on important topics of the time and that its operations were too heavily influenced by staff members. He wanted the NAS to be able to lobby for the positions it supported—a proposal that was in direct violation of the institution's tax-exempt, nonprofit status. The fraught interactions between the NAS and the NAE at this time overshadowed the discussion of the IOM's name change and dampened some of the support for the change.[8]

Meanwhile, the IOM proceeded with its campaign to educate the NAS membership about the institute and its body of work. The campaign cited 12 reports that illustrated the nature of the IOM's work and its considerable impact, including the report *Preventing Low Birthweight* (IOM, 1985) and the study on *Confronting AIDS: Directions for Public Health, Health Care, and Research* (IOM and NAS, 1986). The IOM also highlighted its convening activities, such as the recently initiated National Roundtable on Health Care Quality. The institute also submitted a statistical analysis of its membership for consideration by NAS members, noting that 17 percent of IOM members also belonged to the NAS and an overwhelming number of the members were either physicians or had doctorates.[9]

On April 2, 1996, Alberts sent NAS members a letter that contained a simple wording change to the NAS Constitution. The change substituted the words "national academy" for "institute" in Section 10, establishing the "National Academy of Medicine ... as a separate membership organization under terms of a charter adopted by the Council of the National Academy of Sciences." The NAS Council recommended that the change be approved by NAS leadership at that annual business meeting and that the membership consider it over the ensuing year, with a final vote at the 1997 business meeting.

To inform the NAS members' decision, the letter from Alberts contained two short statements— one in favor of the name change and the other against. The supporting statement repeated the arguments already presented by Shine and the IOM Council. The statement against the change argued that the name change implied a fundamental shift in "the nature of the organization." The IOM was established not to honor excellence in medicine but rather to respond to challenges for human health. It differed from the NAE, which was an "autonomous organization" and a partner in managing the NRC. Because the proposal did not include amendments to the IOM's operating structure or status within the National Academies, the NAS would remain as the parent body of the National Academy of Medicine and continue to appoint its president. The statement indicated that these differences would lead to an institutional asymmetry that was likely to become a problem in the future.[10]

Some NAS members believed it was important to maintain the distinction between an institute and an academy. Frank Westheimer, a Harvard chemist, maintained that the IOM had a very dif-

---

[7] Kenneth Shine to Colleagues, March 17, 1995, IOM/NAM Records; IOM Council Minutes, April 17–18, 1995, IOM/NAM Records.

[8] IOM Council Minutes, April 17–18, 1995, IOM/NAM Records; IOM Council Minutes, July 18, 1995, IOM/NAM Records.

[9] Kenneth Shine, "Name Change for the Institute of Medicine," Draft Statement, November 21, 1995, IOM/NAM Records.

[10] Bruce Alberts to NAS Members, April 2, 1996, with enclosures "Proposed Change to the Constitution to Change the Name of the Institute of Medicine to the National Academy of Medicine," "Statement Against Changing the Name of the Institute of Medicine to the National Academy of Medicine," "Statement in Favor of Changing the Name of the Institute of Medicine to the National Academy of Medicine," NAS-NRC Archives.

ferent mission from that of the NAS, and that its members were elected on a very different basis. Once the IOM became the NAM, according to Francis Moore, the surgeon-in-chief emeritus at the Peter Bent Brigham Hospital, it would "immediately lose its functional status and become a mere honorary society." Moore also pointed out that the multidisciplinary membership of the IOM, which included nurses, lawyers, pharmacists, and hospital administrators, would be lost in an academy. Neither the NAS nor the NAE had the "broad social contract and the responsibility for improvement of services to the public" of the IOM.[11] Joint IOM/NAS members, many with senior status within the Academies, made what Alberts described as "passionate statements" against the name change. They believed that the IOM was doing so well that nothing needed to change.

Shine rebutted these various arguments, saying that the IOM had already established itself in both an honorific role and a service role. The existing IOM charter prevented it from becoming a purely honorific society, and no amendments to the charter were being proposed with the suggested name change.[12] Therefore, the IOM would continue its operations as it had for the past 25 years.

Although many NAS members objected to the name change, there were some supporters. Maurice Hilleman, Director of the Merck Laboratory for Therapeutic Research, said he would support the name change. The NAS, he explained, had a basic science base and tended to recruit people in basic research who might become Nobel laureates. This practice left little room for the applied aspects of medicine and public health, which he believed also deserved representation in the National Academies.

Ultimately, on April 30, 1996, the NAS members voted against changing the IOM's name to the National Academy of Medicine, and the debate over creating an academy of medicine fell dormant once again. Cicerone attributed the proposal's defeat to the ongoing controversy with the NAE and a prevalent belief that the word "academy" carried a connotation that would fundamentally change the nature of the IOM. Reporting on the outcome, Shine urged his members to "continue our efforts to improve the quality, relevance, and responsiveness of our work.... Who knows what will happen with our name in 21st century?"[13]

In this effort, as in previous efforts to create an Academy, the timing mattered. Internal disputes with the NAE changed the climate in which the vote on the IOM's name change occurred. Another retrospective lesson from this effort was that McDermott's vision for the IOM, one in which the IOM served as an honorific organization also able to initiate its own studies and focus on social aspects of health (in part), had remarkable staying power. The generation that founded the IOM stood by this vision and was reluctant to let it go. Change also came hard to the NAS, which was steeped in tradition and regarded itself as a defender of science. At the time, it was difficult for NAS members to see how the IOM, an organization that put social change on its agenda, could be granted equal footing with the "hard" sciences.

SUCCESS OF THE 2013–2015 CAMPAIGN

Despite this setback, the IOM steadily built its reputation for influence and produced some of its most authoritative work in years following Shine's campaign to change the name of the institute. The issue remained quiet until 2013, when a draft report titled *How to Better Consolidate and Align the Constituent Parts of the National Academies and Strengthen Its Identity* circulated among the NAS, NAE, and IOM Councils. The 2013 draft coincided with the 150th anniversary of the

---

[11] Francis D. Moore to Kenneth Shine, March 22, 1996, IOM/NAM Records.

[12] Kenneth Pitzer to Bruce Alberts, February 5, 1996, NAS-NRC Archives; Maurice Hillerman to Karen Hein, February 9, 1996, IOM/NAM Records; Francis D. Moore to Kenneth Shine, March 22, 1996, IOM/NAM Records; F. H. Westheimer to Peter Ravens, Home Secretary, NAS, April 2, 1996, NAS-NRC Archives.

[13] Kenneth Shine to IOM Members, May 22, 1996, IOM/NAM Records; Bruce Alberts to Kenneth Shine, May 17, 1996, IOM/NAM Records.

NAS, a significant milestone for the organization. Although the NAS represented a stable institution that had maintained the essence of its mission, it had undergone significant changes over the course of its existence. For example, the NRC was added to the organization in 1916, the NAE was established in 1964, and the IOM followed in 1970. A provision implemented in the 1950s made the NAS president the chair of the NRC, ending years of tension between the two organizations. Now, approaching its milestone anniversary, NAS leadership reflected on the Academy's history and organization with greater openness to changes in its structure. The intended goal of the 2013 report was to establish a rebranded "National Academies of Sciences, Engineering, and Medicine," resulting in a unified, more consistent program. If such a change were enacted, the IOM would attain "comparable standing as an academy," and its programmatic work would endure within a new division of the National Academies.[14]

This campaign differed from previous efforts in that, from the beginning, it was presented as a way to rationalize the National Academies' entire structure, rather than as simply a name change for the IOM. It also was framed as a major reorganization of the NAS on the occasion of its 150th anniversary, rather than an IOM-centric request that would benefit a single arm of the institution. The atmosphere across the NAS complex also appeared to be different. Many of the prominent issues between the NAE and the NAS in the 1990s had been resolved. In fact, the NAE Council passed a resolution that "enthusiastically" supported the 2013 report. Additionally, with the passage of time, a new generation of IOM leaders was able to pursue change without the pressure of historical bonds and tradition outweighing the advantages of the new proposal.[15]

Following preliminary approvals, the NAS and its leadership continued to lead the reorganization effort. In June 2013, Cicerone, NAE President Charles Vest, and IOM President Harvey Fineberg appointed a committee to examine and update the draft document describing the NAS's reorganization. The committee was chaired by joint IOM/NAS member Rick Lifton, who was both a distinguished scientist and an accomplished physician, and was further composed of representatives from across the National Academies. In creating the committee, Cicerone, Vest, and Fineberg indicated that the organization would welcome the committee's advice on whether and how the NAS should evolve "so as to continue to provide the highest service to the nation." They reported that the joint Councils of the NAS, the NAE, and the IOM had already discussed the draft proposal and expressed their enthusiasm for the concepts that were described in the document. Cicerone hoped that the committee would refine the draft document, identify potential risks and challenges that might arise during implementation, and outline the necessary steps to inform the members of the three constituent Academies and gain their support and approval.[16]

Lifton's eight-person group, known as the Joint Governance Committee (JGC), deliberated through the summer of 2013 and reported back to the NAS, the NAE, and the IOM Councils at the end of September. The committee's report represented a careful assessment of the draft report and its implications by a group with representation from all three of the affected entities (NAS, NAE, and IOM)—an invaluable step that had been overlooked in previous efforts. The members of the JGC carefully reviewed previous reorganization attempts and made a concerted effort to avoid repeating what it viewed as mistakes of the past. Based on the previous attempt under Shine's presidency, the committee concluded that the greatest hurdle would be the vote among the NAS membership. That debate had centered on whether the IOM met the definition of an Academy. The JGC tried to avoid repeating this discussion by preparing a direct response to the question as part

---

[14] "A Proposal to Better Consolidate and Align the Constituent Parts of the National Academies and to Strengthen Its Identity," Draft for Discussion by the NAS, the NAE, and the IOM Councils, February 18, 2013, IOM/NAM Records.

[15] Charles Vest to Ralph Cicerone, "NAE Council Reactions to Organizational Proposal," February 7, 2013, IOM/NAM Records.

[16] Ralph Cicerone, Charles Vest, and Harvey Fineberg to Thomas Budinger, June 17, 2003, IOM/NAM Records.

of its report. Furthermore, the committee stressed the need for substantial efforts to inform, discuss, and build consensus among NAS members before proceeding with a vote.[17]

The JGC's formal report emphasized an anomaly in the way that the branches of the NAS operated. The NAS, the NAE, and the IOM served the dual purpose of recognizing achievement through honorific membership and providing advice on matters of science, technology, and health. However, the NAS and the NAE produced studies that were issued by the NRC, whereas the IOM issued its own studies. The JGC's report highlighted the evolution of science and the interdisciplinary nature of scientific research, which necessitated a more unified organizational and reporting structure. In the future, it stated, reports on complex subjects could not be produced in isolation, instead requiring "increased breadth of expertise." Thus, it would be imperative for the NAS, the NAE, and the IOM to collaborate more closely. Over the course of the previous year, the three presidents and their respective Councils had considered these questions, which served as an impetus for change. The proposal outlined in the committee's report went much further than anything contemplated in the previous effort. The IOM would become the NAM, and its current programmatic activities would be incorporated into a new division of the NRC focused on health. Under the new structure, the NAM would be able to elect its own president and have equal representation with the NAE in NRC governance.[18]

In contrast to the high-level statements for and against the suggested IOM name change that NAS members received in 1996, the JGC's report presented a series of detailed questions and answers about the proposed changes. For example, could an organization with such a varied membership be described as an Academy? The report concluded that the membership of the IOM met the "learned individual" criterion that defined an Academy because its members were selected based on "distinguished professional achievement." Thus, the IOM was not an outlier among the NAS and the NAE in terms of the academic and professional achievements of its members. The committee also explored the question of whether a reorganization would affect the ability of the NAS to engage in activities outside the NRC framework. The committee concluded that all three Academies could continue to pursue activities outside the current NRC program and the work of its respective divisions. The report stated that "a simpler, more symmetrical and rational organizational structure, with reports issuing from the National Academies of Sciences, Engineering, and Medicine will give better clarity of our mission."[19]

Following the release of the committee's final report, a campaign to gain NAS membership support of the new organizational structure was initiated. In part, it relied on presentations at NAS regional meetings, with the goal of securing a favorable membership vote at the NAS Annual Meeting on April 29, 2014. Diane Griffin, the NAS vice president and an IOM Council member, prepared a presentation for NAS audiences that brought a sense of rigor and order to the exercise. The presentation reviewed challenges with the existing organizational structure, noting that the current structure was confusing; that it impeded the integration of science, engineering, and medicine for the next generation of research and advice; that it reduced the impact of the organization's work; and that it hindered the organization's ability to raise funds for important studies. In her presentation, Griffin outlined the proposed changes that would result in a more balanced and unified National Academy of Sciences, Engineering, and Medicine and detailed the next steps that were required.[20]

---

[17] The NAS, NAE, and IOM Joint Governance Committee to the Officers and Councilors of the National Academy of Sciences, the National Academy of Engineering, and the Institute of Medicine, September 30, 2013, IOM/NAM Records.

[18] As of 2021, the NAS was represented by more members than the NAM and the NAE on institutional governing bodies and had the final vote on institutional changes.

[19] "Report of the NAS, NAE, and IOM Joint Governance Committee, Proposals to Improve the Alignment and Impact of the NAS, NAE and IOM," September 30, 2015, IOM/NAM Records.

[20] "Future Governance of the Institute of Medicine: Communicating with IOM/NAS Members," December 3, 2014, IOM/NAM Records; Slides Prepared by Diane Griffin on "Proposed Changes in the National Academy of Sciences, National Academy of Engineering, Institute of Medicine, National Research Council," March 2015.

At the 2014 NAS Annual Meeting, 98 percent of the NAS members present voted to consider a constitutional amendment to change the name of the IOM to the NAM, establish the HMD, and grant the NAM parity with the NAS and the NAE "with respect to function, governance, and relationship to the NRC." This preliminary approval paved the way for a formal vote at the NAS Annual Meeting the following year. Discussions of the reorganization plan continued at six regional NAS meetings and at a joint meeting of the NAS, NAE, and IOM Councils.[21] All of these activities and discussions yielded positive results, and on April 28, 2015, the NAS membership voted in support of the creation of the NAM.[22] The IOM officially became an Academy on July 15, 2015.

ORGANIZATIONAL TRANSITIONS

Following this historic vote, crucial organizational details needed to be worked out. More than 1 year before the final NAS vote that approved the creation of the NAM, Fineberg had acknowledged that an organizational name change presented what he called a "significant branding challenge." What would happen to the IOM name? One idea was to retain the acronym for use by the new NRC division, but modify what it stood for, such as "Institute on Medicine and Health." In February 2015, Victor Dzau, then the IOM President, told the leaders of the NAS and NAE that the IOM name had external value and recognition among the organization's sponsors, noting that it should not be entirely discarded.[23] The NAE president, however, favored a new name, and so did some of the members of the JGC. Eventually, all parties agreed to maintain "Institute of Medicine" as the name of the new NRC division for a limited time. Ultimately, the new division would be called the Health and Medicine Division, a name that would build "on the heritage of the IOM's work in medicine while emphasizing its increased focus on a wider range of health matter." The HMD name change was implemented almost 1 year later, on March 15, 2016. (Chapter 3 Appendix Figures 3A-1 to 3A-6 illustrate the changing organizational components and names of the National Academies, the IOM/NAM, and HMD before and after the 2015 reorganization.) In the interim, describing both entities in relation to the former IOM proved a significant communications challenge.

There were also discussions about how to identify the newly expanded program of the National Academies, which had previously operated under the NRC moniker. According to Cicerone, the National Academies name would be much easier for the media to understand than the arcane workings of the NRC and its various divisions. Therefore, he suggested that the organization use the unified National Academies brand when describing the studies and convening activities carried out within NRC program divisions. Although the NRC infrastructure would continue to play a vital internal role within the National Academies, Cicerone felt that it should not be the public face of the institution. Thus, starting in 2016, reports released by NRC divisions were branded as National Academies' reports. Additionally, the seven operating divisions, including HMD, were characterized externally as National Academies' program units. The structural name of NRC was retained for internal purposes.

In considering the transition from the IOM to the NAM, decisions had to be made about which activities and components would move to the HMD and which would be retained within the NAM as part of its core program. In order to conform to a parallel structure with the NAS and the NAE, the NAM could not retain its NRC program activities. However, Dzau argued successfully that

---

[21] Slides Prepared by Diane Griffin on "Proposed Changes in the National Academy of Sciences, National Academy of Engineering, Institute of Medicine, National Research Council," March 2015.

[22] Ralph Cicerone, C. D. Mote, and Victor Dzau to All Staff, "Update on the IOM and NRC Reorganization," May 12, 2015.

[23] IOM Council Minutes, February 5, 2014, IOM/NAM Records; Ralph Cicerone, Handwritten Notes on Joint NAS, NAE, IOM Meeting, February 4, 2005, NAS-NRC Archives.

not all of the former IOM's program activities should be transferred to HMD. In discussions about the reorganization, he announced his intention for the NAM to retain the former IOM's fellowship programs, its Roundtable on Value & Science-Driven Health Care, its award programs, and select other activities that did not fit the traditional NRC mold. These types of activities were similar to those that existed uniquely within the NAS and the NAE.[24]

Questions of leadership for HMD also needed to be resolved. Dzau believed that he should serve as chair of the new division for the duration of his term, and that subsequent NAM presidents should have the right of first refusal to serve as HMD's division chair. HMD also required an Executive Director who would head the staff and report to the executive officer of the NRC. Dzau believed that this Executive Director should also report temporarily to the NAM president to reduce some of the stress and uncertainty of the transition. Preliminary plans called for Clyde Behney, a veteran IOM staffer who had served as the board director for various IOM boards and as the IOM's deputy executive officer, to fill this dual role.[25] Behney became a crucial advisor to Dzau as the NAM built its new programs, as well as a steady leader for the HMD and its staff during a time of significant upheaval.

Decisions made during the early days of the transition would establish the trajectory of the NAM as well as the HMD. Hence, all of the parties involved—leadership, members, and staff— paid close attention to the discussions on the structure of the NAM and how it would interface with the new program division. On April 24, 2015, the leaders of the NAS, the NAE, and the IOM issued what they called a management implementation plan, which summarized the decisions that had been reached in the earlier meetings. In particular, the plan specified that Dzau would chair the new NRC division for a 3-year period. Half of a newly established advisory committee for the new division would come from the NAM Council. Most of the remainder would be selected from the NAS and NAE membership. Over the course of the next 2 years, the proportion of NAM Council members on the HMD governing committee would be reduced. The plan confirmed Behney as the Executive Director of the new NRC division and indicated that he would serve simultaneously as the NAM executive officer for a transitional period of less than 1 year during the search for a permanent executive officer.[26]

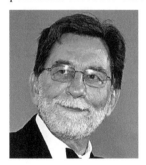

Among the most sensitive decisions were those that involved staff. People who had worked for the IOM, some for decades, would now be divided between the NAM and HMD. The shift in organizational identity was difficult for staff members who were deeply committed to the IOM's mission and proud of its heritage and body of work. Dzau determined that administrative staff (i.e., those who worked in finance and communications) should assume double duty between the NAM and the HMD until new staff could be hired for roles within the NAM. However, everyone agreed that on July 15, 2015, the programmatic staff of the former IOM (i.e., those who supported consensus studies and convening activities) would be transferred to the HMD.[27]

FIGURE 3-1 Clyde Behney. SOURCE: National Academy of Medicine.

[24] NAS Council Minutes, February 4, 2015, NAS-NRC Archives.

[25] "Reorganization Issues to Be Discussed by the Three Presidents," January 23, 2015, NAS-NRC Archives.

[26] "Reorganization of the National Academy of Medicine and the National Research Council Management Implementation Plan," April 24, 2015, NAS-NRC Archives.

[27] Ibid.

THE NATIONAL ACADEMY OF MEDICINE'S PROGRAM TAKES SHAPE

The transition did not slow the collective momentum of the organization's work. The six IOM boards that had operated under Fineberg's tenure (Food and Nutrition, Global Health, Health Care Services, Health Sciences Policy, Population Health, and Select Populations) continued their work under the HMD. Meanwhile, the NAM set about building a new programmatic approach under the leadership of Dzau. In its first 5 years, the NAM developed three novel program models—the Action Collaborative, the International Commission, and the Grand Challenge—among other approaches, and applied them to topics including global infectious disease, health equity, clinician well-being, health system reform, healthy longevity, the U.S. opioid epidemic, and more (see Chapter 7). These models were meant to supplement, rather than duplicate, the studies and convening activities carried out by the HMD. However, overlaps in subject matter and the fact that NAM and HMD leaders relied on the same pool of sponsors and volunteers, and confusion between the brands resulted in occasional tension between the two entities in the early days. Efforts were undertaken by NAM and HMD leadership to establish a collaborative and mutually supportive working relationship.

Strategic Planning

The 2015 transition effectively created two new entities—the NAM and the HMD—each of which maintained historic elements of the IOM but operated under significantly different parameters. This, along with the retirement of the strong IOM brand, required careful strategic planning to ensure the ongoing success of both entities individually, as well as the health portfolio of the entire National Academies. The first major area of strategic focus was communications—ensuring that the IOM's major stakeholders understood the practicalities of the transition as well as its rationale, and securing their confidence that they could continue to work with and rely on the restructured organization.

In addition to consumers of the former IOM's findings and recommendations—including the media, policy makers, researchers, and health practitioners—the audiences of greatest concern were financial sponsors and NAM members. Echoing a concern that had proved a formidable obstacle to the success of past attempts to create an academy, many members were concerned by what they perceived to be a new degree of separation between them and the consensus studies and convening activities that were now part of the HMD.

In response, Dzau commissioned a 2-year strategic communications plan that focused on transferring the brand attributes of the IOM to the NAM and integrating HMD's work into a holistic messaging framework. The plan called for frequent and consistent efforts to remind sponsors and members of the benefits of the transition and the continuity of the former IOM's work. These messages emphasized the benefits of the NAM's expanded leadership role within the National Academies, the possibilities for innovation conferred by its new independence, and the Academy's ongoing connection to the work that had built the IOM's reputation. The plan also called for investment in communications infrastructure to expand the NAM's networks and support health-related priorities across the organization.

Next, Dzau turned to strategic planning to support the NAM's programmatic development. Staying true to the founders' vision that the IOM should be a working organization, not a purely honorific one, he supported the development of initiatives that would advance issues important to the Academy's members. However, Dzau and the NAM Council recognized the importance of avoiding duplication or competition with the HMD. The NAM would have to chart a unique programmatic path and determine how it could add value to the work of the broader organization.

Dzau chaired an 18-month process headed by a planning committee made up of NAM members and longtime volunteers (see Box 3-1) and informed by extensive interviews with members, sponsors, policy makers, and the leaders of major health organizations. The plan, completed in the summer of 2017, resulted in new mission, vision, and value statements for the NAM, as well as three overarching strategic goals and four foundational activities to guide the growth of the organization between 2018 and 2023 (see Figure 3-2).

The first strategic goal affirmed the NAM's ongoing commitment to rigorous scientific evidence—unchanged from the principles that fueled the IOM's reputation for trustworthiness and authority over 45 years. However, the goal also acknowledged the NAM's new leadership capability as an academy coequal to the NAS and the NAE and pledged to leverage its greater autonomy and visibility in ways the former IOM could not. The second strategic goal pertained to fostering the membership of the Academy, including efforts to increase diversity and engagement as well as cultivate excellence in the next generation of health leaders who may one day become NAM members. The third and final strategic goal outlined the NAM's commitment to shaping the practice of health, medicine, and biomedical science for the rapidly evolving contexts of the future.

BOX 3-1
Members of the 2016–2017 National Academy of
Medicine Strategic Planning Committee

NAM Members and Volunteers

- Huda Akil, University of Michigan
- Robert Brook, RAND Corporation
- Sheila Burke, Harvard Kennedy School
- Victor Dzau, President, NAM
- Jack Ebeler, Health Policy Alternatives
- Eva Feldman, University of Michigan
- Elena Fuentes-Afflick, University of California, San Francisco
- Rebekah Gee, Louisiana Department of Health
- Margaret (Peggy) Hamburg, Foreign Secretary, NAM
- Jane Henney, Home Secretary, NAM
- Eve Higginbotham, University of Pennsylvania
- Steven Hyman, Broad Institute
- Carlos Jaen, The University of Texas
- Raynard Kington, Grinnell College
- Cato Laurencin, University of Connecticut
- Vivian Lee, University of Utah
- Terry Magnuson, University of North Carolina at Chapel Hill
- Michael McGinnis, Leonard D. Schaeffer Executive Officer, NAM
- Afaf Meleis, University of Pennsylvania
- Stephen Shortell, University of California, Berkeley
- Deepak Srivastava, University of California, San Francisco
- Tadataka (Tachi) Yamada, Frazier Healthcare

NAM Staff

- Kimber Bogard, Senior Officer
- Laura H. DeStefano, Director of Communications
- Morgan Kanarek, Chief of Staff
- Meg McCoy, Director of Membership and Governance

NOTE: Affiliations were accurate as of 2016.

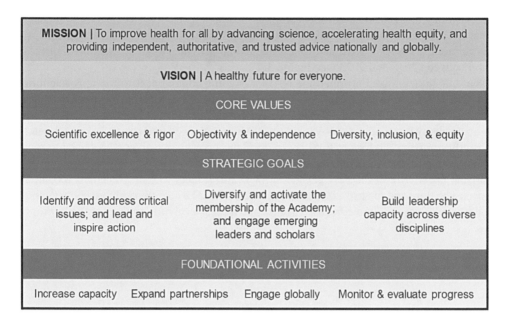

FIGURE 3-2 NAM Strategic Plan (2018–2023) at a glance.
SOURCE: National Academy of Medicine.

Following the completion of the Strategic Plan, the NAM embarked on a 5-year implementation period, reporting progress to the NAM Council annually. Meanwhile, the NAM's model was adapted by the NRC for its own strategic planning efforts, which were led by Dzau alongside National Academies' leadership. In 2022, as the implementation period for the NAM Strategic Plan neared its conclusion, Dzau called for a review and refresh of the plan. At a meeting of the NAM Council in February 2022, many Councilors expressed that the fundamentals of the 2018–2023 plan remained relevant and adaptable to current and future priorities and did not require a complete overhaul.[28]

CONCLUSION

In a succinct statement of the NAM's new programmatic approach, Dzau said that the Academy would explore "the space between knowledge and implementation" and build a nimble springboard from which to respond to urgent health crises. It would advise the nation and the world, serving to guide "the trajectory of health and health care in the United States and globally," and build momentum around "big ideas" that would inspire the health community (Dzau, 2015a). The NAM developed innovative, action-oriented program models that differed significantly from the IOM's approach and began to be adopted across the National Academies. Meanwhile, the ongoing working relationship between the NAM and the HMD sustained the legacy of the IOM and the vision of its founders.

---

[28] NAM Council Minutes, February 8–9, 2022, IOM/NAM Records.

CHAPTER 3 APPENDIX FIGURES

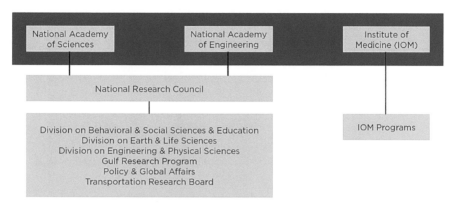

FIGURE 3A-1 National Academies' organization prior to the 2015 IOM-NAM reorganization. SOURCE: National Academy of Medicine.

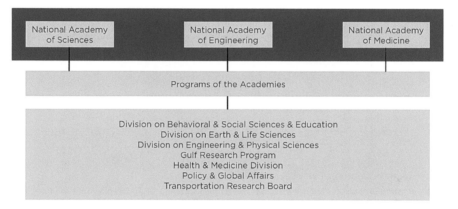

FIGURE 3A-2 National Academies organization following the 2015 IOM-NAM reorganization. SOURCE: National Academy of Medicine.

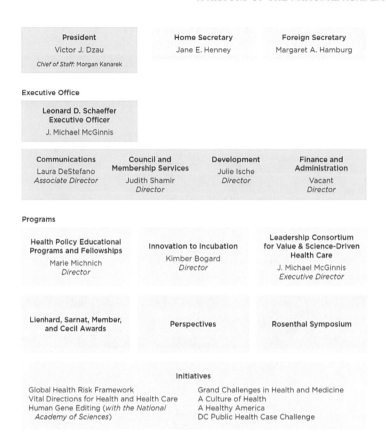

FIGURE 3A-3 NAM organizational chart, April 2016.

NOTE: This organizational chart shows the composition and staff of the NAM immediately following its reconstitution in July 2015, and is included as a snapshot of the new Academy at its inception.

SOURCE: National Academy of Medicine.

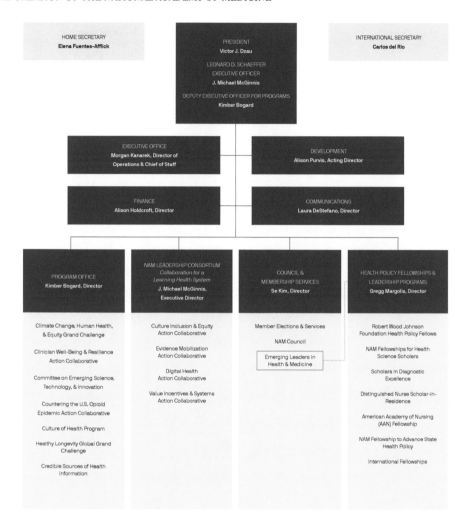

FIGURE 3A-4 NAM organizational chart, 2021.
SOURCE: National Academy of Medicine.

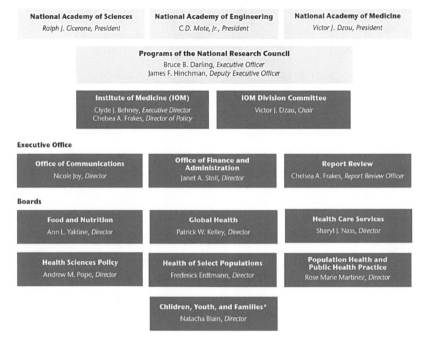

Forums, Roundtables, and Other Activities

- Food Forum
- Forum on Aging, Disability, and Independence
- Forum on Drug Discovery, Development, and Translation
- Forum on Global Violence Prevention
- Forum on Investing in Young Children Globally*
- Forum on Medical and Public Health Preparedness for Catastrophic Events
- Forum on Microbial Threats
- Forum on Neuroscience and Nervous System Disorders
- Forum on Promoting Children's Cognitive, Affective, and Behavioral Health*
- Forum on Public-Private Partnerships for Global Health and Safety
- Global Forum on Innovation in Health Professional Education
- Health Literacy Roundtable
- Medical Follow-Up Agency
- National Cancer Policy Forum
- Roundtable on Environmental Health Sciences, Research, and Medicine
- Roundtable on Obesity Solutions
- Roundtable on Population Health Improvement

- Roundtable on the Promotion of Health Equity and the Elimination of Health Disparities
- Roundtable on Translating Genomic-Based Research for Health
- Standing Committee on Aerospace Medicine and the Medicine of Extreme Environments
- Standing Committee for the Centers for Disease Control and Prevention Division of Strategic National Stockpile
- Standing Committee on Health Threats and Workforce Resilience
- Standing Committee of Medical Experts for SSA's Disability Programs
- Standing Committee on Medical and Public Health Research During Large-Scale Emergency Events
- Standing Committee on Personal Protective Equipment for Workplace Safety and Health
- Standing Committee to Support USAID's Engagement in Health Systems Strengthening in Response to the Economic Transition of Health

Joint activity with Division of Behavioral and Social Sciences and Education

FIGURE 3A-5 HMD organizational chart, 2015.

NOTES: This organizational chart shows the composition and staff of HMD immediately following its reconstitution in July 2015, and is included as a snapshot of the new division at its inception. To maintain continuity of the IOM brand following the reorganization, HMD was referred to as the "Institute of Medicine" until March 15, 2016.

SOURCE: National Academy of Medicine.

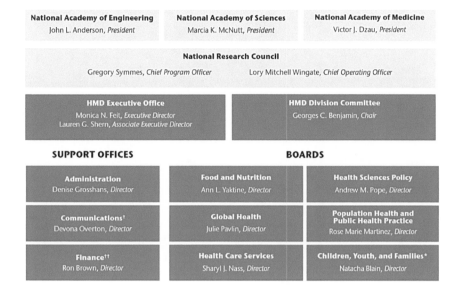

Forums, Roundtables, Standing Committees and Related Activities

- Food Forum
- Forum for Children's Well-Being: Promoting Cognitive, Affective, and Behavioral Health for Children and Youth*
- Forum on Aging, Disability, and Independence*
- Forum on Drug Discovery, Development, and Translation
- Forum on Medical and Public Health Preparedness for Disasters and Emergencies
- Forum on Mental Health and Substance Use Disorders
- Forum on Microbial Threats
- Forum on Neuroscience and Nervous System Disorders
- Forum on Regenerative Medicine
- Global Forum on Innovation in Health Professional Education
- Medical Follow-Up Agency
- National Cancer Policy Forum
- Roundtable on Environmental Health Sciences, Research, and Medicine
- Roundtable on Genomics and Precision Health
- Roundtable on Health Literacy

- Roundtable on Obesity Solutions
- Roundtable on Population Health Improvement
- Roundtable on the Promotion of Health Equity
- Roundtable on Quality Care for People with Serious Illness
- Standing Committee on Aerospace Medicine and the Medicine of Extreme Environments
- Standing Committee on Medical and Epidemiological Aspects of Air Pollution on U.S. Government Employees and their Families
- Standing Committee of Medical and Vocational Experts for the Social Security Administration's Disability Programs
- Standing Committee on Personal Protective Equipment for Workplace Safety and Health
- Standing Committee on Emerging Infectious Diseases and 21st Century Health Threats
- Standing Committee on Evidence Synthesis, and Communications in Diet and Chronic Disease Relationships
- Standing Committee for the Review of the Dietary Reference Intakes Framework

FIGURE 3A-6 HMD organizational chart, 2021.
SOURCE: National Academy of Medicine.

Part II

Impact

In its more than 50-year history, the Institute of Medicine (later the National Academy of Medicine, in collaboration with the Health and Medicine Division) produced thousands of consensus reports and other publications and hosted a vast array of public workshops and expert meetings. The following chapters describe a non-exhaustive selection of the organization's major activities and impact within three major themes: biomedical science, U.S. health care and policy, and public health in the United States and globally.

4

Biomedical Science

The Institute of Medicine's (IOM's) commitment to providing rigorous, apolitical scientific advice—as well as to the advancement of the scientific enterprise—can be traced to its roots in the National Academy of Sciences (NAS). Founded in 1863 at the height of the U.S. Civil War, at a time when the government was most interested in understanding technological advances in weaponry, the NAS was created to "investigate, examine, experiment, and report upon any subject of science" (see Chapter 1). Notably, its founding members agreed to provide advice without personal remuneration, setting a standard of volunteerism that endures to the present day among members of all three of the National Academies (Seitz, 2007). The National Academies of Sciences, Engineering, and Medicine's (the National Academies') authority and influence are built on a foundation of unparalleled access to scientific expertise, as well as their independence from the U.S. government and the private and nonprofit organizations that sponsor studies.

Although the NAS was founded under a congressional charter signed by President Abraham Lincoln, the Academy's explicit purpose was to provide advice that the government could trust to be free of partisan political influence. Thus, the organization was empowered to focus on the scientific evidence gathered and synthesized by its members. Over time, as the organization's recommendations proved to be reliable and effective, the NAS's authority and influence grew. The National Academy of Engineering and the IOM, founded as offshoots of the NAS charter in 1964 and 1970, respectively, operated with the same commitment to scientific rigor and independence and with the same reputation for trustworthy, impactful advice as previously established by the NAS.

Since its very first statement on the safety of heart transplants as the Board on Medicine in 1968 (see Chapter 1), the IOM, which became the National Academy of Medicine (NAM) in 2015 (in conjunction with the formation of the Health and Medicine Division [HMD]), has shaped national discussions related to cutting-edge medical treatments, new diagnostic tools, and scientific discoveries. Notable contributions have affected policy and practice related to organ transplantation, computed tomography (CT) scans, HIV transmission, embryonic stem cell research, and regenerative medicine, to name just a few (see Box 4-1). In addition to guiding the development and application of biomedical science and many other fields, the organization maintains a focus on the implications of scientific discoveries and technological advances for health care, health policy, and population health—including their impacts on health equity.

BOX 4-1
Highlights of Impactful Contributions to Biomedical and Health Sciences

Organ Transplantation: Following the first statement on organ transplantation in 1968, the Institute of Medicine (IOM) has revisited the science and policies guiding organ transplantation multiple times during its history. In 1997 and again in 2000, the IOM considered the science and ethics associated with non-heart beating transplantation practices and protocols. In response to the IOM's recommendations, the U.S. Secretary of Health and Human Services, Donna Shalala, appointed an advisory committee on organ transplantation in January 2001 to advise the department on policies related to procurement, allocation, and transportation of donated organs.[a] In 1999, the IOM's report *Organ Procurement and Transplantation: Assessing Current Policies and the Potential Impact of the DHHS Final Rule* studied organ procurement and transplantation policies and the implications these policies had on equity in terms of transplant wait times and geography (IOM, 1999a). In 2006, *Organ Donation: Opportunities for Action* reviewed options for increasing organ donors, including the ethics associated with living donors (IOM, 2006a). Most recently, the Health and Medicine Division (HMD) released a 2017 report called *Opportunities for Organ Donor Intervention Research,* which reviewed the "ethical, legal, regulatory, policy, and organizational issues relevant to the conduct of research in the United States involving deceased organ donors" (NASEM, 2017a).

CT Scans: During the 1970s, computed tomography (CT) scanners were being deployed as the latest imaging technology, and hospitals were competing to secure the equipment to offer this new technology to their patients. At the time, the number of CT scanners threatened to exceed the need for such expensive equipment. A 1977 IOM study urged hospitals and physicians to be cautious about the potential overuse of CT scanners, potentially contributing to rising health care costs. The report called on local health planners to assess the regional and local needs for CT scanners and ensure that the scanners would operate at maximum efficiency in an effort to cut down on waste (NRC, 1977). On May 3, 1977, President Carter saw an article describing this study in *The Washington Post,* prompting him to write a note to Secretary of Health, Education, and Welfare Joseph Califano. "Let's take similar action—stronger if possible—and include other devices as well," Carter advised (IOM, 1998a, p. 95).

HIV Transmission: In 2005, the National Institutes of Health (NIH) commissioned a review of the HIVNET 012 Perinatal HIV Prevention Study following public scrutiny and concern related to the design and conduct of the clinical trial, which was sponsored by the National Institute of Allergy and Infectious Diseases. Controversy surrounding the trial had prompted leaders of some African nations to propose ending the use of the drug nevirapine to prevent mother-to-child transmission of HIV. The IOM study, which evaluated the clinical trial, assuaged concerns around the results of the trial and the safety and efficacy of nevirapine (IOM, 2005a).

Embryonic Stem Cell Research: From 2005 to 2010 the IOM served as a national advisor in establishing guidelines for conducting research with human embryonic stem cells. Due to restrictions on federal funding in this area, privately funded research was being carried out without a set of clearly defined and unified guidelines or regulations. In 2005, the IOM released its first set of guidelines for research with human embryonic stem cells, which included ethical and scientific considerations (IOM and NRC, 2005). The IOM amended its guidelines in 2007 and 2008, and released final amendments in 2010, updating the guidelines to reflect the NIH's new role in guiding this type of research. The IOM's guidelines filled a gap and provided standards to an entire area of research that had been lacking previously (IOM and NRC, 2007a, 2008a; NRC and IOM, 2010).

Regenerative Medicine: In 2016, HMD launched a Forum on Regenerative Medicine, a convening activity that was designed "to engage in discussions that address the challenges facing regenerative medicine to improve health through the development of effective new therapies." Since its inception, the forum has held workshops related to challenges and opportunities for cellular therapies, manufacturing processes for regenerative medicine, and variability in the clinical translation of regenerative engineering products. The forum's activities are contributing to important discussions in this new and rapidly expanding field (NASEM, n.d.a; NRC and IOM,).

---

[a] Evaluation of Impact from IOM Reports (Database), IOM/NAM Records.

The following sections describe the IOM's, the NAM's, and the HMD's major contributions to four key areas: the human genome, vaccine safety and efficacy, childhood and adolescent development, and cancer. A final section details the organization's role as a scientific advisor to several departments and agencies within the U.S. federal government, as well as international partners in Africa. The activities described in this chapter were led by IOM, NAM, or HMD staff in collaboration with NAM member and non-member expert volunteers.

THE HUMAN GENOME: FROM SEQUENCING TO EDITING

Alongside the NAS, the IOM played a leading role in the human genome sequencing project from its very beginnings in the late 1980s. Today, the NAM continues to be a driving force in current discussions about the rapidly developing field of human genome editing. In 1988, the seminal report *Mapping and Sequencing the Human Genome,* which was released by the National Research Council (NRC), served as a blueprint for what would become the Human Genome Project, an historic international effort to map more than 20,000 genes that make up the human genome and determine the sequence of 3 billion chemical base pairs (Oak Ridge National Laboratory, n.d.). The committee—which was chaired by Bruce Alberts, who would later be selected as the NAS president in 1993—set goals for the complex endeavor, described organizational strategies, and even suggested funding levels. In April 2003, just 13 years after it was launched, the Human Genome Project reached completion, setting the stage for a new era of biomedical research; the potential to unlock new diagnostic and treatment options for an array of diseases and disorders; and an opportunity to create a more personalized, gene-based approach to medicine (NHGR, n.d.; see Figure 4-1). It should be noted that not all were in favor of the Human Genome Project—scientists worried before the project began that "it [may have] generated enormous reams of uninterpretable and ... useless data ... with few clues about how any of that genetic material works or can trigger disease" (Angier, 1990). Other scientists fundamentally disagreed with the entire project, noting that a better understanding of genetics would provide no insight into better understanding the human race (Langer, 2021).

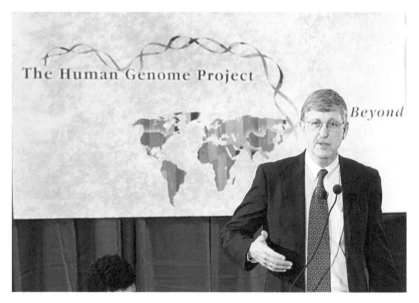

FIGURE 4-1 Francis Collins, an NAM member who was then Director of the National Institutes of Health, announces the successful completion of the Human Genome Project on April 14, 2003.
SOURCE: Ernie Branson, National Institutes of Health (CC BY 2.0).

In the field of genomics, as in many other fields, translating scientific advances into practice and ultimately into improvements in human health required building bridges between scientific research and medical practice—a role the National Academies and the IOM had played for decades. To facilitate this journey and realize the potential of this new area of scientific research, the IOM launched the Roundtable on Translating Genomic-Based Research for Health in 2007. The round-table brought together interested sponsors and stakeholders who represented academia, the pharmaceutical industry, patient and health care provider organizations, and the government for open discussions in a neutral environment (IOM, 2008e; NASEM, n.d.a). The roundtable organized its work into focus areas, which have covered a wide range of evolving topics including precision therapeutics; education, engagement, and cultural change; digital health; implementation of public health systems; and evidence for policy and practice (NASEM, n.d.a, n.d.p). From 2007 through 2015, the roundtable held 27 meetings and 22 public workshops, and it released 21 workshop summaries, commissioned several papers, and published a number of discussion papers and commentaries, all of which contributed a wealth of information to the field (NASEM, 2015). In 2014, under the auspices of the roundtable, an Action Collaborative called the Global Genomic Medicine Collaborative was launched and incorporated as a 501(c)(3) nonprofit organization with administrative support from the Global Alliance for Genomics and Health. The Action Collaborative hosted a series of international meetings in Washington, DC; Singapore; and Athens that assembled participants from more than 25 countries to develop and implement a "global toolbox" for advancing and deploying genomic medicine.[1]

In 2015, Geoffrey Ginsburg and Sharon Terry—external volunteers who served as co-chairs of the Roundtable on Translating Genomic-Based Research for Health—announced that the roundtable would be renamed the Roundtable on Genomics and Precision Health (NASEM, 2015). This change coincided with the launch of the Obama administration's Precision Medicine Initiative, which aimed "to enable a new era of medicine through research, technology, and policies that empower patients, researchers, and providers to work together toward development of individualized care" (The White House, President Barak Obama, n.d.). At this time, the roundtable updated its mission "to explore strategies for improving health through the implementation of genomics research findings, as well as other related technologies that inform individual health choices, into medicine, public health, education, and policy" (NASEM, 2016m, p. 2; NLM, n.d.). Today, the revitalized roundtable serves as an important convening activity for a diverse set of stakeholders and sponsors, contributing to the advancement of genomics and precision medicine.

During this same time period, advances in human genome editing technology became a topic of interest and concern for scientists, regulatory bodies, and the public. Genome editing, which involves laboratory methods to create changes in DNA, had recently been aided by new molecular biology research that improved both the accuracy and flexibility of the editing capabilities. These new advances held great potential for treating and possibly eradicating genetic diseases. In the laboratory, using human cells, scientists could locate a gene in which a mutation resulted in a specific disease and edit the gene to eliminate that mutation. Germline gene editing might, for example, change the genes that were responsible for diseases inherited from one or both parents, such as cystic fibrosis and sickle cell anemia. Gene editing had reached a stage at which its promise was recognized. However, these new methods had to be refined and perfected, and the ethical and societal implications had to be examined and seriously considered across the scientific community in collaboration with many other stakeholders.

In December 2015, just a few months after the creation of the NAM, an International Summit on Human Gene Editing convened in Washington, DC, at the NAS Building (see Figure 4-2). The NAM, along with the NAS, The Royal Society of the United Kingdom, and the Chinese Academy

---

[1] Evaluation of Impact from IOM Reports (Database), IOM/NAM Records.

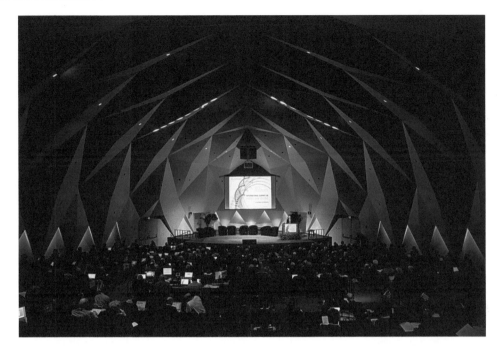

FIGURE 4-2 International Summit on Human Gene Editing in Washington, DC, in 2015.
SOURCE: National Academy of Medicine.

of Sciences, hosted the 3-day event. David Baltimore, an NAM/NAS member and Nobel laureate who had played a major role in the IOM's response to the HIV/AIDS epidemic, told an audience of more than 500 people that, "we could be on the cusp of a new era in human history." There was a sense that "we are close to being able to alter human heredity" and the question was "how, if at all, do we as a society want to use this capability."

During the final session of the conference, the 12-member organizing committee, which was chaired by Baltimore,[2] articulated some of the conclusions that had been reached at the summit. The committee noted that additional research was needed and should continue with appropriate ethical and legal oversight, warning that edited embryos or germline cells should not be used to induce pregnancy. The committee encouraged the study of gene therapies that would involve editing somatic cells within existing regulatory frameworks, calling for rigorous evaluation to facilitate a better understanding of the potential risks and benefits of this type of editing. As for editing germline cells, which would be carried by all the cells of the child and then passed on to future generations, the organizing committee said it would be "irresponsible" to proceed with the clinical use of germline editing until the safety and efficacy issues were resolved and there was a "broad societal consensus about the appropriateness of the proposed application." The committee called on the host organizations, including the NAM, to establish an ongoing international forum to continue discussions and work toward harmonized global regulations. For the NAM, this recommendation represented an opportunity to lend its voice to a major scientific global initiative from the beginning. NAM President Victor Dzau signed a statement in which he and his fellow Academy presidents welcomed the call "to continue to lead a global discussion on issues related to human gene editing" (Cicerone et al., 2015).

---

[2] David Baltimore was the President Emeritus and the Robert Andrews Millikan Professor of Biology at the California Institute of Technology during this time.

Building an international framework for human genome editing became an important part of the NAM's programmatic portfolio. The subject of human genome editing fit within with the NAM's strategic goal to "actively identify and address critical issues ... and lead and inspire action on bold ideas to impact science, medicine, policy, and health equity domestically and globally." Within the National Academies, the Human Genome Editing Initiative became a joint activity of the NAM and the NAS that was co-chaired by NAM members R. Alta Charo[3] and Richard O. Hynes.[4] The activity represented the type of collaboration that the creation of the NAM was meant to foster. In 2017, the NAS and the NAM jointly issued a consensus report called *Human Genome Editing: Science, Ethics, and Governance,* which continued the discussion from the 2015 summit. The report offered a set of principles for the governance of human genome editing, including the promotion of "well-being, transparency, due care, responsible science, respect for persons, fairness, and transnational cooperation." These principles informed the recommendation that research and clinical trials that involved somatic gene editing be limited to the prevention and treatment of disease and disability. Research involving germline genome editing should be undertaken only for the treatment or prevention of serious disease or disabilities and only when strict oversight is in place. The report concluded that all research efforts should be limited to the treatment or prevention of disease, not for human enhancements such as making a person physically stronger or altering physical appearances. The report helped lay the groundwork for the Second International Summit on Human Gene Editing, which was held in Hong Kong in 2018 (NASEM, 2017b).

Following the summit in Hong Kong—at which a Chinese scientist announced that embryonic germline editing had been used to establish a pregnancy that resulted in the birth of twins—an International Commission on the Clinical Use of Human Germline Genome Editing was launched in the spring of 2019 (NASEM, 2019a). In a statement announcing the new commission, Dzau and Sir John Skehel, the Vice-President of The Royal Society of the United Kingdom, highlighted the urgent need for a global framework to guide researchers and regulators. The NAM, the NAS, and The Royal Society of the United Kingdom, with engagement from other international academies of medicine, would work together "to develop a framework for scientists, clinicians, and regulatory authorities to consider when assessing potential clinical applications of human germline genome editing" (NASEM, 2019b).

In 2020, the NAM, the NAS, and The Royal Society issued the commission's consensus report, titled Heritable Human Genome Editing. The report concluded that human embryos whose genomes have been edited should not be used to create a pregnancy until it was established that precise genomic changes could be made reliably and without introducing undesired changes—criteria that had not yet been met. The report specified stringent preclinical and clinical requirements for establishing safety and efficacy and for undertaking long-term monitoring of outcomes. Furthermore, it called for extensive national and international dialogue before any nation decided whether to permit clinical use of heritable human genome editing and identified essential elements of national and international scientific governance and oversight for the field. A third international summit was scheduled to take place in London in 2023.

VACCINE SAFETY AND EFFICACY

One of the most widely recognized public health achievements of the 20th century is the development and widespread use of vaccines. Establishing and maintaining public trust in the efficacy and safety of vaccines, however, has required ongoing research and public communication strate-

---

[3] R. Alta Charo was the Sheldon B. Lubar Distinguished Chair and the Warren P. Knowles Professor of Law and Bioethics at the University of Wisconsin–Madison when this report was released.

[4] Richard O. Hynes was an Investigator at the Howard Hughes Medical Institute and the Daniel K. Ludwig Professor for Cancer Research at the Massachusetts Institute of Technology when this report was released.

gies. Throughout its history, the IOM has actively participated in many national vaccine conversations and reviewed research associated with the safety and efficacy of various vaccinations. Polio was one of the first diseases targeted for vaccine development, and the IOM was there to advise the nation on the implementation of a new version of the vaccine in the 1970s. The IOM took part in discussions about the widespread implementation of anthrax vaccines after terrorist attacks in 2001 and also contributed a strong, evidence-based voice in disputing a 1998 *Lancet* article that falsely connected the measles, mumps, and rubella (MMR) vaccine with autism (Wakefield et al., 1998). Over the years, the IOM became one of the nation's most trusted advisors on a topic that was often contentious and emotional for concerned parents throughout the United States. Vaccine-related work is one of the IOM's core activities, and the IOM has now released more than two dozen reports on various topics related to vaccines.

The first polio vaccine was developed by Jonas Salk and approved for use in 1955. Like the influenza vaccination, also developed by Salk, the polio vaccine used an inactive (sometimes referred to as "killed") form of the virus that was administered via injection (Science History Institute, n.d.; see Figure 4-3). Also in the 1950s, Albert Sabin developed another polio vaccine that used live-attenuated forms of the virus and was administered orally. Sabin's vaccine was approved in 1961. Despite successful trials of the new vaccine, there were concerns about the possibility that a vaccine containing a live form of the virus carried risks of causing polio (IOM, 1998a). In 1977, the IOM released a report called *Evaluation of Poliomyelitis Vaccines: Report of the Committee for the Study of Poliomyelitis Vaccines,* which studied the relative merits of the two widely available polio vaccines. The report confirmed the safety of Sabin's oral vaccine and recommended its continued use as the primary option for vaccinating children (IOM and NAS, 1977). A 1988 report titled *An Evaluation of Poliomyelitis Vaccine Policy Options* also reached the same conclusion, reiterating the value of the oral vaccine until a time when a combination vaccine that covered polio and other diseases (e.g., tetanus, diphtheria) became available (IOM, 1988c). These reports helped ease the public's fears associated with the live vaccine, and established the IOM as a trusted voice that could assuage public concern with evidence (IOM, 1998a, p. 113).

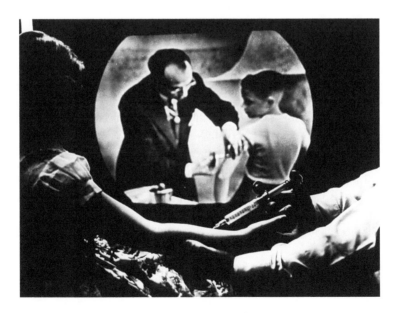

FIGURE 4-3 Children are inoculated with Jonas Salk's polio vaccine.
SOURCE: National Library of Medicine.

Over the years, the IOM encouraged the continued development of new vaccines and improvements to existing vaccines and also advised the nation on vaccine policy and disease surveillance strategies. The IOM recognized that federal and state governments needed to take the lead on combating infectious diseases and that greater efforts were needed to develop and implement surveillance strategies in collaboration with the Centers for Disease Control and Prevention (CDC). To protect against an unanticipated infectious disease outbreak, the IOM stated that the nation needed to create an "arsenal of drugs, vaccines, and pesticides." The government also needed to actively create stockpiles of selected vaccines and establish "a surge capacity for vaccine development and production that could be mobilized quickly" in the event of an infectious disease outbreak (IOM, 1992a).

In 1986, Congress passed the National Childhood Vaccine Injury Act (NCVIA) following a series of lawsuits by people who believed they had been injured by the diphtheria, pertussis, and tetanus vaccine, which had resulted in damage to the vaccine market and a deficit in public trust (CDC, n.d.a). The NCVIA called for two consensus studies to be undertaken by the IOM to determine the safety of childhood vaccines. The first, *Adverse Effects of Pertussis and Rubella Vaccines* (published in 1991), was chaired by future IOM President Harvey Fineberg, then dean of the Harvard School of Public Health (IOM, 1991e). Fineberg was a noted expert in vaccine science and policy, having co-authored an influential report titled *The Swine Flu Affair: Decision-Making on a Slippery Disease* (Neustadt and Fineberg, 1978), which sharply criticized the Ford administration's hasty response to an outbreak that did not ultimately materialize. The 1991 report was followed in 1994 by *Adverse Events Associated with Childhood Vaccines: Evidence Bearing on Causality* (chaired by NAM member Richard B. Johnston, Jr.) (IOM, 1994a).[5] The IOM reports resulted in changes to the Vaccine Injury Table, a list of conditions associated with vaccines mandated to be reported by the NCVIA (Evans, 2006).

Public concerns about vaccine safety grew exponentially with the publication of the 1998 *Lancet* article that inaccurately associated the MMR vaccine with autism. Once again, the IOM found itself as a mediator of scientific and public debate. The IOM released *Immunization Safety Review: Vaccines and Autism* in 2004, marking the culmination of an immunization safety project that had been funded by the CDC and the National Institutes of Health (NIH). The project, which was launched in 2001, convened a carefully selected committee that was composed of experts in pediatrics, neurology, genetics, public health nursing, and ethics who were not engaged in vaccine research and who had no other apparent conflicts of interest.[6] IOM President Ken Shine noted that he was "heavily criticized by the vaccine community" because the committee did not include vaccine experts, but the success of the study proved the effectiveness of using a group of "wise but disinterested people."[7] Chaired by NAM member Marie McCormick,[8] the Immunization Safety Review Committee investigated nine areas of vaccine safety over the course of 3 years. The topics included vaccines and sudden unexpected death in infancy, cancer, immune dysfunction, autism, and other neurologic concerns (NASEM, n.d.b).

When the IOM accepted the immunization safety review assignment, its first task consisted of examining a possible relationship between the MMR vaccine and autism. The public held strong opinions on the possible connections, and some parents who had children with autism were convinced that the vaccine had caused autism in their children. In a report to the IOM Council, Susanne Stoiber, IOM Executive Officer at the time, noted that these beliefs represented an "erosion of public trust in those responsible for vaccine development, licensure, scheduling and policymaking."

---

[5] Johnston was the Senior Vice President for Programs and the Medical Director of the March of Dimes Birth Defects Foundation and an Adjunct Professor of Pediatrics at the Yale University School of Medicine when this report was published.

[6] Susanne A. Stoiber to IOM Council, "Overview of IOM Program Activity," July 9, 2001, IOM/NAM Records.

[7] Private correspondence, Kenneth Shine to Laura H. DeStefano, April 18, 2020.

[8] Marie McCormick was the Sumner and Esther Feldburg Professor of Maternal & Child Health in the Department of Society, Human Development, and Health at the Harvard T.H. Chan School of Public Health during this time.

Immunization safety had become "a contentious area of public health policy, with discourse around it having become increasingly polarized and exceedingly difficult."[9]

The Immunization Safety Review Committee worked quickly and produced its first report on vaccines and autism in a 3-month period. In that timeframe, the committee conducted a careful, but expedited, review of the published and unpublished literature on the statistical linkages between the MMR vaccine and autism and also the biologic mechanisms by which the vaccine might cause autism. In its report, the committee stated that it had found "no credible evidence" linking autism to the MMR vaccine. However, it did not completely dismiss the possibility that such a link might exist. Thus, the committee urged the CDC and the NIH to study the biological mechanisms that could possibly cause the MMR vaccine and other childhood vaccines to trigger autism (IOM, 2001a).

Unfortunately, the nuances of the report and calls for additional research were overlooked by the media, and the headline became "no link found between MMR and autism." This conclusion was not readily accepted by the public and some lawmakers. As a strong believer in the MMR-autism theory, Representative Dan Burton (D-CA), who chaired the House Committee on Government Operations, was particularly dissatisfied with the committee's work and the report's findings. Burton issued subpoenas requesting recordings of the committee's deliberations, but he could find nothing concerning.[10] Meanwhile, McCormick and the IOM staff members who supported the committee received what Stoiber described as "a number of very harsh and emotional letters from parents and advocacy groups."[11] Shine stepped in and leveraged his relationship with Representative Henry Waxman (D-CA), whom Shine knew from his time at UCLA. Shine called on Waxman to help defuse the situation with Burton.[12]

Each of the Immunization Safety Review Committee's eight reports (see Box 4-2) covered a controversial and emotionally charged topic, such as possible linkages between the additive thimerisol—a preservative used in some vaccines—and neurodevelopmental disorders, including autism. In its October 2001 report, the committee reached the same conclusion on thimerosal as it did in the report evaluating the MMR vaccine: no clear evidence to establish a connection to autism or other neurodevelopment disorders (IOM, 2001b). However, the committee did support previous policy decisions to remove thimerisol from vaccines and recommended the use of thimerisol-free vaccines whenever possible.

BOX 4-2
Immunization Safety Review Reports

- *Immunization Safety Review: Vaccines and Autism* (2004)
- *Immunization Safety Review: Influenza Vaccines and Neurological Complications* (2004)
- *Immunization Safety Review: SV40 Contamination of Polio Vaccine and Cancer* (2003)
- *Immunization Safety Review: Vaccinations and Sudden Unexpected Death in Infancy* (2003)
- *Immunization Safety Review: Multiple Immunizations and Immune Dysfunction* (2002)
- *Immunization Safety Review: Hepatitis B Vaccine and Demyelinating Neurological Disorders* (2002)
- *Immunization Safety Review: Thimerosal-Containing Vaccines and Neurodevelopmental Disorders* (2001)
- *Immunization Safety Review: Measles-Mumps-Rubella Vaccine and Autism* (2001)

---

[9] Susanne A. Stoiber to IOM Council, "Overview of IOM Program Activity," July 9, 2001, IOM/NAM Records.

[10] Private correspondence, Kenneth Shine to Laura H. DeStefano, April 18, 2020.

[11] Susanne A. Stoiber to IOM Council, "Overview of IOM Program Activity," July 9, 2001, IOM/NAM Records.

[12] Interview between Kenneth Shine and Edward Berkowitz, November 2018.

In 2004, the IOM issued its capstone report in the series, *Immunization Safety Review: Vaccines and Autism*, which offered an opportunity to revisit its earlier findings concerning possible connections between the MMR vaccine and the additive thimerosal and autism. The committee reviewed the new literature that had been released during the 3-year span of its work, but the committee's conclusions did not change based on any of the newly available literature. The committee's final report upheld the conclusions in its earlier reports, and recommended that "available funding for autism research be channeled to the most promising areas" (IOM, 2004c).

The stakes were high for the IOM in its role as mediator and scientific advisor to the nation on such a controversial topic. An overwhelming majority of the public health community believed that vaccinations, although not completely without risk, were critical to preventing the spread of infectious disease and improving the nation's health, particularly among children in the first years of life. The IOM's reports strongly supported the consensus within the public health community. For IOM members the primary concern was not the safety of vaccines, but rather the barriers that prevented people from being immunized (Durch and Klerman, 1994; IOM, 2013a), which included public misinformation, fear, and lack of trust. In its 2001 report on thimerosal, the committee stated that "it is important to do everything possible to restore, maintain, and build trust in vaccines" (IOM, 2001b, p. 8). The statement served as the foundation for much of the IOM's work in vaccines. The immunization safety review series played an important part in public discourse and immunization policy decisions in the United States at a critical time. The series provided state and federal government agencies with a balanced, scientific assessment of the risks associated with vaccines, and it provided public health and medical authorities a scientific foundation to rebut controversial theories about the safety of vaccines, specifically those related to autism.[13]

Studying vaccine safety became an ongoing activity, not only because of recurring vaccine scares but also because of changes in the disease and political environments. Following the terrorist attacks of September 11, 2001, anthrax was identified as a possible biologic weapon that could be deployed against the public, as was demonstrated by several instances of contaminated mail targeting media outlets and political offices (see Figure 4-4). A vaccine against anthrax had been developed in the 1970s but had primarily only been used for people who were routinely exposed to anthrax through contact with animals. In the 1990s, during the Gulf War, the Department of Defense (DOD) had confirmed the existence of an Iraqi bioweapons program and was concerned that anthrax might be used against military personnel. At that time, the DOD began widely vaccinating members of the military and announced in 1997 that all military personnel would eventually be vaccinated against anthrax. However, questions about the vaccine's safety and efficacy persisted among the public and prompted the initiation of an IOM study in 2000. The attacks on September 11 and the anthrax mailings increased the urgency of the committee's work, in case the widespread use of the vaccine was deemed necessary as a public safety measure. The IOM's 2002 report *The Anthrax Vaccine: Is It Safe? Does It Work?*, which was chaired by NAM member Brian L. Strom,[14] concluded that the existing vaccine was safe and effective. However, it also called for the development of a better vaccine that would not require six doses and annual boosters to maintain efficacy, as was necessary with the existing vaccine (IOM, 2002e). Following the release of the report and its confirmation of vaccine safety, the DOD decided to continue its plan to vaccinate military personnel against anthrax, especially those serving in high-risk areas, and the Department of Health and Human Services (HHS) continued to purchase and maintain its supply of the vaccine.[15]

In 2011, HHS commissioned the IOM to conduct a study focused on the potential adverse effects associated with vaccines against measles, mumps, and rubella (MMR); varicella (chicken

---

[13] Impact of IOM Reports (Database), IOM/NAM Records.

[14] Brian L. Strom was a Professor and the Chair of Biostatistics and Epidemiology at the University of Pennsylvania Perelman School of Medicine when this report was published.

[15] Impact of IOM Reports (Database), IOM/NAM Records.

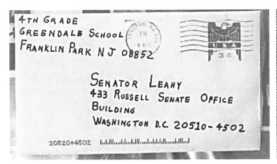
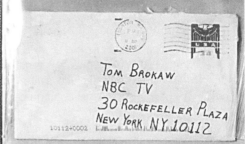

FIGURE 4-4 Anthrax-laced letters delivered to Senator Patrick Leahy and newscaster Tom Brokaw following the September 11, 2001, terrorist attacks.
SOURCE: Federal Bureau of Investigation.

pox); influenza; hepatitis A and B; human papillomavirus (HPV); meningitis; and diphtheria, pertussis, and tetanus (DPT). This report was designed to follow up and build on the IOM's previous vaccine safety work. The resulting report, *Adverse Effects of Vaccines: Evidence and Causality,* was released in August 2011. The committee, which was chaired by NAM member Ellen Wright Clayton,[16] concluded that "vaccines remain one of the greatest tools in the public health arsenal" (IOM, 2011a). The HHS applied the data and analysis presented in the report to update the National Vaccine Injury Compensation Program's (VICP's) Vaccine Injury Table, which defined specific injuries, disabilities, and illnesses that would qualify a claimant for compensation through the VICP (CDC, n.d.b; HRSA, n.d.). Following the release of the report, HHS indicated that it would use the report to provide "a scientific basis for future review and decisions on VICP claims" (CDC, n.d.b).

In late 2020, as the first-ever mRNA vaccines against COVID-19 were given emergency authorization by the Food and Drug Administration (FDA), the NAM and HMD became heavily involved in advising government, health leaders, and the public about the safety and efficacy of the vaccines, as well as their equitable allocation and distribution (see Chapter 7).

THE SCIENCE OF CHILDHOOD AND ADOLESCENT DEVELOPMENT

From early in its history, the IOM and its leadership promoted the idea that social factors were prominent influences associated with health outcomes. As research on brain development and gene–environment interactions evolved, the organization quickly identified the potential lifelong impact of these interactions, especially exposures and life circumstances from before birth through adolescence. Over time the organization cultivated a body of work dedicated to advancing the science of childhood and adolescent development with a concentration on the complex interactions across a constellation of biological, social, behavioral, and environmental factors. The IOM strongly encouraged the application of science and evidence as a basis for the funding and implementation of programs geared toward children and youth. The organization also consistently highlighted the importance of continued research in areas of childhood and adolescent development to ensure children had the opportunity to fulfill their potential and lead healthy lives.

---

[16] Ellen Wright Clayton was the Craig-Weaver Professor of Pediatrics, the Director of the Center for Biomedical Ethics and Society, and a Professor of Law at Vanderbilt University at the time.

From Neurons to Neighborhoods

In 2000, the NRC, in collaboration with the IOM,[17] issued a major report on early childhood development called *From Neurons to Neighborhoods: The Science of Early Childhood Development*. This report, which was produced by a committee chaired by NAM member Jack P. Shonkoff,[18] became one of the IOM's most recognizable reports in the field, delving into questions related to the ongoing nature versus nurture debate. Through the report's 14 chapters, the committee examined evidence surrounding "the nature and tasks of early development" and the "context of early development," with chapters dedicated to communication and learning; building friendships and interacting with peers; brain development; nurturing relationships and families; child care; and neighborhoods and communities. In presenting the report's 11 recommendations, the committee concluded that "the nation has not capitalized sufficiently on the knowledge that has been gained from nearly half a century of considerable public investment in research on children from birth to age 5" (IOM and NRC, 2000, p. 384).

What distinguished this report from previous work in this area was that it brought together the latest scientific research on brain development with recent findings in social science on environmental influences on childhood development. The report marked a step forward in assessing the relative effects of gene–environment interactions on development, and it informed policy decisions, programs, and interventions across the nation for many years to come. For example, the report was cited in several pieces of legislation after it was released (e.g., Keeping Children and Families Safe Act of 2003, the 2004 reauthorization of the Individuals with Disabilities Education Act). The report was also cited as the basis for the growing emphasis on early childhood learning programs in a 2012 *Wall Street Journal* article. Betty Holcomb of the Center for Children's Initiatives indicated that "the turn toward very early education began with a 2000 study from the National Research Council that brought together years of research arguing that the first three years of life are crucial in a child's development" (Ensign, 2012).

A decade after the release of *From Neurons to Neighborhoods*, the IOM and the NRC partnered again to hold a 2-day workshop that was designed to explore advances that had been made since the release of the report. The workshop summary that resulted from the meeting—*From Neurons to Neighborhoods: An Update* (2012)—captured presentations and discussions from breakout sessions. During the workshop, participants focused on the original report's four major themes:

1. All children are born wired for feelings and ready to learn.
2. Early environments matter and nurturing relationships are essential.
3. Society is changing and the needs of young children are not being addressed.
4. Interactions among early childhood science, policy, and practice are problematic and demand dramatic rethinking. (IOM and NRC, 2012, p. 43)

In addition to assessing progress that had been made, the workshop participants also considered outstanding challenges and opportunities to promote additional progress in early childhood development research. In his closing remarks, committee chair Shonkoff stated that he believed that the first two themes had "stood the test of time" with new research contributing to the field in those areas (IOM and NRC, 2012, p. 43). He identified the third and fourth themes as urgent needs

---

[17] *From Neurons to Neighborhoods: The Science of Early Childhood Development* was a product of the Board on Children, Youth, and Families, which was administratively positioned within the National Research Council's Division of Behavioral and Social Sciences and Education (DBASSE) when the report was released. Throughout its history, the BCYF rotated every 5 years between the IOM and the NRC's DBASSE until 2015 when it found a permanent home within DBASSE.

[18] Jack P. Shonkoff was at the Heller Graduate School of Brandeis University when this report was released.

that required additional attention in order to "dramatically improve the lives of children and their prospects for the future" (IOM and NRC, 2012, p. 44).

The National Children's Study

In October 2000, Congress passed the Children's Health Act, which authorized the "National Institute of Child Health and Human Development [NICHD] to conduct a national longitudinal study of environmental influences (including physical, chemical, biological, and psychosocial) on children's health and development" (IOM and NRC, 2008b, p. 1). The National Children's Study (NCS), which would be a collaborative effort across the U.S. government, was designed to follow approximately 100,000 children from before birth through the age of 21, representing "the largest long-term study of environmental and genetic effects on children's health ever conducted in the United States" (IOM and NRC, 2008b, p. 1). Upon request of the NICHD, the National Academies convened a joint NRC and IOM committee chaired by NAM member Samuel H. Preston[19] that was charged with evaluating the "scientific rigor of the NCS and the extent to which it is being carried out with methods, measures, and collection of data and specimens to maximize the scientific yield of the study" (IOM and NRC, 2008b, p. 2). In its report, *The National Children's Study Research Plan: A Review,* which was released in 2008, the committee provided an assessment of the strengths and weaknesses of the study design and offered specific recommendations to further improve the plan for the NCS. The committee concluded that the NCS provides "an excellent opportunity" to advance research related to gene–environment interactions and the influence of those interactions on health outcomes and childhood development (IOM and NRC, 2008b, p. 2). Following the release of the report, the NIH released a statement indicating that it would delay a planned expansion of recruitment for individuals to join the NCS that was set to begin in 2009 as a result of the IOM's report and recommendations (IOM and NRC, 2014b).

In 2013, Congress requested the National Academies to evaluate the NICHD's revised study plans, resulting in a report called *The National Children's Study 2014: An Assessment* (IOM and NRC, 2014b). Following its evaluation, the committee offered a set of recommendations focused on the "overall study framework, sample design, timing, content and need for scientific expertise and oversight" (NAP, 2014). The committee, which was chaired by NAS member Greg J. Duncan,[20] reiterated the potential value of the NCS (IOM and NRC, 2014b). However, in December 2014, following the release of the report, Francis Collins, the NIH Director, released a statement that ended the NCS. Citing budget constraints, concerns that were highlighted by the joint NRC and IOM committee, and findings from an internal NIH advisory committee, Collins stated that the NCS was not feasible, indicating optimism "that other approaches will provide answers to these important research questions" (NIH, 2014).

Health Equity and Development

Continuing its commitment to advancing the science of childhood development with an emphasis on complex biological, social, and environmental interactions, the National Academies released a report in 2019 called *Vibrant and Healthy Kids: Aligning Science, Practice, and Policy to Advance Health Equity* (NASEM, 2019d). The report was part of the NAM's Culture of Health Program (COHP; see Chapter 7), and it built on the NRC/IOM's *From Neurons to Neighborhoods* work, the 2017 HMD report *Communities in Action: Pathways to Health Equity* (also part of the COHP;

---

[19] Samuel H. Preston was in the Department of Sociology at the University of Pennsylvania when this report was published.

[20] Greg J. Duncan was in the School of Education at the University of California, Irvine, during this time.

NASEM, 2017o), and new research in neurobiological and socio-behavioral sciences. Emphasizing the importance of "early experience and life circumstances," the interactions across biological, psychosocial, and environmental factors, and the influence these interactions and experiences have on health and well-being throughout the course of life, the new report evaluated the evidence behind the causes and consequences of health inequalities for children living in the United States (NASEM, 2019d). The committee, which was chaired by NAM member Jennifer E. DeVoe,[21] concluded that "reducing health disparities by addressing their systemic root causes, including poverty and racism, is foundational to advance health equity" (NASEM, 2019c, p. 3). In an effort to reduce known disparities and improve outcomes for young children and their families, the committee developed a set of recommendations and a roadmap that government officials, policy makers, and leaders in health care, public health, social services, early care and education, and the justice system could use to apply science to early development. The committee also identified priorities for future research that included studies related to "discrimination and structural racism, trauma-informed care, and development of culturally tailored interventions" (NASEM, 2019c, p. 3).

While *Vibrant and Healthy Kids* concentrated on development that occurs during the prenatal and early childhood phases of life, the Board on Children, Youth, and Families—now a collaborative activity between HMD and the Division of Behavioral and Social Sciences and Education (DBASSE) (NASEM, n.d.c)—released a report in 2019 as part of the COHP that explored adolescent development. The report was called *The Promise of Adolescence: Realizing Opportunity for All Youth* (NASEM, 2019f). Like the *Vibrant and Healthy Kids* report, *The Promise of Adolescence* examined brain development, the complex interactions between biology and the environment, and health disparities. Following its review of the available evidence, the committee found that "changes in brain structure and connectivity that happen in adolescence present young people with unique opportunities for positive, life-shaping development, and for recovery from past adversity" (NASEM, 2019e, p. 1). To promote health equity and to ensure that adolescents have the opportunity to realize their full potential, the committee—chaired by NAM member Richard J. Bonnie[22]—made specific recommendations directed toward the education system, the health system, the child welfare system, and the justice system. In terms of future research, the committee called for further investments in research to expand data and knowledge linked to developmental processes, supportive socio-environmental factors, and understanding and overcoming inequalities for adolescents. Underscoring the need for action, the committee indicated that "our society has a collective responsibility to build systems that support and promote positive adolescent development" (NASEM, 2019f, p. 13).

Advancing Health and Well-Being Throughout Childhood and Adolescence

As with other organizational priorities of ongoing interest and importance, the IOM created two forums in 2014 that were dedicated to advancing children's health and well-being by applying science and evidence to policy making. The stated goal of the Forum on Investing in Young Children Globally was to ensure that "decision-makers around the world use the best science and evidence for investing to optimize the well-being of children and their lifelong potential" (Huebner et al., 2016). The purpose of the Forum for Children's Well-Being: Promoting Children's Cognitive, Affective, and Behavioral Health was to convene discussions that would "strive[s] to advance effective, affordable, and equitable systems that promote well-being and foster evidence-informed prevention, treatment, and implementation research and practice" (NASEM, n.d.d). Both forums

---

[21] Jennifer E. DeVoe was a Professor and the Chair of the Department of Family Medicine at Oregon Health & Science University when this report was published.

[22] Richard J. Bonnie was at the University of Virginia during this time.

brought together diverse groups of sponsors, experts, and interested stakeholders for workshops with the common goal of ensuring the best health possible for children and youth across the globe. In addition to the forums and reports described above, the Board on Children, Youth, and Families, in collaboration with other parts of the IOM and the National Academies (e.g., the NRC's DBASSE), produced numerous consensus reports focused on childhood development and well-being over the years, such as those listed in Box 4-3.

FACILITATING PROGRESS IN CANCER RESEARCH

Cancer is a collection of complex diseases that manifest themselves in different ways in different individuals at any point throughout one's lifespan. Cancer has, arguably, garnered more attention and consideration from a scientific, social, cultural, and political standpoint than any other disease in human history. The IOM started prioritizing cancer as an organizational area of interest in the 1990s when it released its first report entirely dedicated to a cancer-related topic; the report, *Oral Contraceptives and Breast Cancer,* provided a summary of the potential benefits and risks associated with oral contraceptives based on the latest available evidence and offered recommendations for future research (IOM, 1991a). In 1997, the IOM established the National Cancer Policy Board. During its existence, the board was dedicated to the study of the "prevention, control, diagnosis, treatment, and palliation of cancer." In 2005, a structural reorganization transformed the National Cancer Policy Board into the National Cancer Policy Forum. The forum continued a

---

BOX 4-3
Additional Examples of Reports on Childhood Development and Well-Being[a]

- *Feeding Infants and Children from Birth to 24 Months: Summarizing Existing Guidance* (2020)
- *Birth Settings in America: Outcomes, Quality, Access, and Choice* (2020)
- *Promoting Positive Adolescent Health Behaviors and Outcomes: Thriving in the 21st Century* (2020)
- *Transforming the Financing of Early Care and Education* (2018)
- *Parenting Matters: Supporting Parents of Children Ages 0–8* (2016)
- *Preventing Bullying Through Science, Policy, and Practice* (2016)
- *Transforming the Workforce for Children Birth Through Age 8: A Unifying Foundation* (2015)
- *Investing in the Health and Well-Being of Young Adults* (2015)
- *Confronting Commercial Sexual Exploitation and Sex Trafficking of Minors in the United States* (2013)
- *New Directions in Child Abuse and Neglect Research* (2014)
- *Child and Adolescent Health and Health Care Quality: Measuring What Matters* (2011)
- *Preventing Mental, Emotional, and Behavioral Disorders Among Young People: Progress and Possibilities* (2009)
- *Adolescent Health Services: Missing Opportunities* (2008)
- *Early Childhood Assessment: Why, What, and How* (2008)
- *Children's Health, the Nation's Wealth: Assessing and Improving Child Health* (2004)
- *Community Programs to Promote Youth Development* (2002)
- *Adolescent Risk and Vulnerability: Concepts and Measurement* (2001)
- *From Generation to Generation: The Health and Well-Being of Children in Immigrant Families* (1998)

---

[a] See https://www.nap.edu/topic/303/behavioral-and-social-sciences/children-youth-and-families.

range of activities related to cancer research, diagnosis and treatment, and public health and health policy concerns (see also Chapter 5). Since 2005, the forum has released more than 40 publications resulting from public workshops (NASEM, 2021c).

Although the IOM studied a wide range of topics related to cancer, including quality of care, palliative care (see Chapter 5), and cancer control efforts in low- and middle-income countries (see Chapter 6), a large portion of the IOM's, and subsequently the HMD's, cancer work focused on research questions that revolved around what caused cancer, how it might be prevented, and how it could be diagnosed, treated, and possibly cured using cutting-edge technologies. Over the years, the National Cancer Policy Board/Forum served as the organization's driving force for discourse on advancing cancer research—from improving clinical trials to leveraging informatics and nanotechnology in research. Box 4-4 provides examples of the research-oriented publications released by the National Cancer Policy Board/Forum.

BOX 4-4
Examples of National Cancer Policy Forum Publications
Focused on Advancing Cancer Research

- *Advancing Progress in the Development and Implementation of Effective, High-Quality Cancer Screening* (2021)
- *Drug Research and Development for Adults Across the Older Age Span* (2021)
- *Reflections on Sharing Clinical Trial Data: Challenges and a Way Forward* (2020)
- *Applying Big Data to Address the Social Determinants of Health in Oncology* (2020)
- *Enhancing Scientific Reproducibility in Biomedical Research Through Transparent Reporting* (2020)
- *Advancing Progress in the Development of Combination Cancer Therapies with Immune Checkpoint Inhibitors* (2019)
- *Improving Cancer Diagnosis and Care: Clinical Application of Computational Methods in Precision Oncology* (2019)
- *The Drug Development Paradigm in Oncology* (2017)
- *Policy Issues in the Clinical Development and Use of Immunotherapy for Cancer Treatment* (2016)
- *Appropriate Use of Advanced Technologies for Radiation Therapy and Surgery in Oncology* (2016)
- *The Role of Clinical Studies for Pets with Naturally Occurring Tumors in Translational Cancer Research* (2015)
- *Assessing and Improving the Interpretation of Breast Images* (2015)
- *Policy Issues in the Development and Adoption of Biomarkers for Molecularly Targeted Cancer Therapies* (2015)
- *Contemporary Issues for Protecting Patients in Cancer Research* (2014)
- *Implementing a National Cancer Clinical Trials System for the 21st Century* (2013, 2011)
- *Informatics Needs and Challenges in Cancer Research* (2012)
- *Facilitating Collaborations to Develop Combination Investigational Cancer Therapies* (2012)
- *Nanotechnology and Oncology* (2011)
- *Extending the Spectrum of Precompetitive Collaboration in Oncology Research* (2010)
- *Policy Issues in the Development of Personalized Medicine in Oncology* (2010)
- *Multi-Center Phase III Clinical Trials and NCI Cooperative Groups* (2009)
- *Improving the Quality of Cancer Clinical Trials* (2008)
- *Developing Biomarker-Based Tools for Cancer Screening, Diagnosis, and Treatment: The State of the Science, Evaluation, Implementation, and Economics* (2006)

NOTE: All of the publications in this list are workshop summaries or proceedings of a workshop.

In addition to the work of the National Cancer Policy Board/Forum, the organization also released numerous consensus reports and other workshop summaries that were developed to accelerate and improve cancer research. Some of the publications were generally focused on screening, drug development, and new research tools and techniques (examples described below), while others were tailored to more specific areas of cancer research, such as environmental risk factors associated with cancer. For example, in 2002, the IOM published a summary of a workshop hosted by the Roundtable on Environment Health called *Cancer and the Environment: Gene–Environment Interaction* (IOM, 2002a). The workshop, which was chaired by NAM member Paul G. Rogers,[23] initiated broad discussions about potential interactions between genes and environmental factors based on recent progress in genomic research, and it provided a venue to explore next steps for research in this area. A decade later, the IOM released *Breast Cancer and the Environment: A Life Course Approach* (2012b), which considered environmental risk factors specific to breast cancer, how those risk factors could be mitigated throughout the lifespan, and additional research needs. The environmental health section in Chapter 6 provides more information on these two reports. Another area that the IOM and HMD revisited often was cancer research and care for women. Box 4-5 provides samples of reports that were dedicated to meeting the unique needs of women in terms of cancer prevention, detection, and treatment through advances in research.

Cancer Research and Drug Development

As described below and in previous chapters, the IOM and later the HMD have had a long history with the NIH in which the IOM provided advice to the NIH on its research agenda and strategies to ensure progress and equity in scientific research. For example, in 1999 the IOM released a report called *The Unequal Burden of Cancer: An Assessment of NIH Research and Programs for Ethnic Minorities and the Medically Underserved*. The committee, chaired by NAM member M. Alfred Haynes,[24] offered the NIH a set of recommendations devised to ensure that ethnic minority and medically underserved populations were included in and benefited from NIH-funded cancer research programs (IOM, 1999b) (described in more detail in Chapter 5).

A little more than a decade after the release of *The Unequal Burden of Cancer,* the IOM continued its investigation of the NIH's cancer research infrastructure with its report, *A National Cancer*

BOX 4-5
Cancer and Women's Health

- *Ovarian Cancers: Evolving Paradigms in Research and Care* (2016)
- *Breast Cancer and the Environment: A Life Course Approach* (2012)
- *Women's Health Research: Progress, Pitfalls, and Promise* (2010)
- *Saving Women's Lives: Strategies for Improving Breast Cancer Detection and Diagnosis* (2005)
- *Improving Breast Imaging Quality Standards* (2005)
- *Meeting Psychosocial Needs of Women with Breast Cancer* (2004)
- *Mammography and Beyond: Developing Technologies for the Early Detection of Breast Cancer* (2001)
- *Information for Women About the Safety of Silicone Breast Implants* (2000)
- *Oral Contraceptives and Breast Cancer* (1991)

---

[23] Paul G. Rogers was a partner at Hogan & Hartson in Washington, DC, at the time.
[24] M. Alfred Haynes was a Former President and the Dean of the Drew Postgraduate Medical School and the Former Director of the Drew-Meharry-Morehouse Consortium Cancer Center in Rancho Palos Verdes, California, during this time.

Clinical Trials System for the 21st Century: Reinvigorating the NCI Cooperative Group Program (IOM, 2010a). As described in the report, clinical trials provided the crucial link between biomedical research findings and advances in cancer prevention, detection, and treatments in clinical practice. For more than a half century the NIH supported the nation's largest clinical trials network—the Clinical Trials Cooperative Group Program, which was established in 1955 (IOM, 2010a)—and by the early 2000s engaged "more than 3,100 institutions and 14,000 investigators who enroll more than 25,000 patients in clinical trials each year" (IOM, 2010a, pp. 2–3). Following its review, the committee, which was chaired by NAM member John Mendelsohn,[25] concluded that "one of the Program's strengths is the extensive involvement of physicians and patients from the community setting." However, the program faced significant hurdles in its "ability to conduct the timely, large-scale, innovative clinical trials needed to improve patient care" (IOM, 2010a, p. 2). In response to these findings, the committee offered four goals and a series of recommendations to enhance cancer clinical trials supported by the NIH and its National Cancer Institute (NCI). The committee's goals involved increasing efficiency, innovation, and physician and patient participation in clinical trials.

Following the release of the 2010 report, the National Cancer Policy Forum continued the conversation with two implementation-oriented workshops that resulted in publications called *Implementing a National Cancer Clinical Trials System for the 21st Century* (IOM, 2011b, 2013b). In 2014, based, in part, on the IOM's recommendations and the ongoing discussion through the National Cancer Policy Forum, the NIH restructured its role in and support of clinical trials by establishing the National Clinical Trials Network, which replaced the Clinical Trials Cooperative Group Program (NIH, n.d.b). The NCI also committed to improving the program's efficiency by shortening timelines for initiating new trials, streamlining the program's information technology system, and consolidating the nine groups that conduct adult oncology trials into four.[26]

In response to continuing advances in biomedical research, the IOM released its 2007 report, *Cancer Biomarkers: The Promises and Challenges of Improving Detection and Treatment.* The committee explored the use of biomarkers[27] as an opportunity to improve cancer outcomes through early detection, precision diagnosis, and the development and use of more personalized treatment options. The committee, chaired by NAM member Harold L. Moses,[28] concluded that "progress overall has been slow, despite considerable effort and investment" (IOM, 2007a, p. 3). In its report, the committee provided 12 recommendations that were organized into three categories related to research and tools, guidelines and standards, and methods and processes that could be employed to promote the development, validation, and adoption of biomarkers in research and, eventually, clinical practice. The committee noted that if its recommendations were implemented, they held the potential to streamline biomarker research, making "effective use of the available resources [and creating] a pathway for success that balances the need to encourage innovation while also ensuring that adequate standards for validation and qualification are met" (IOM, 2007a, p. 4). In March 2009, Senator Edward Kennedy (D-MA) sponsored a bill called the 21st Century Cancer ALERT (Access to Life-Saving Early detection, Research and Treatment) Act, which included provisions based on the IOM's report. The bill also cited the IOM's 2008 report, *Cancer Care for the Whole Patient: Meeting Psychosocial Health Needs* (U.S. Congress, Senate,, 2009) (see Chapter 5).

---

[25] John Mendelsohn was President of the University of Texas M.D. Anderson Cancer Center when this report was published.

[26] Impact of IOM Reports (Database), IOM/NAM Records.

[27] The committee defined biomarkers as "any characteristic that can be objectively measured and evaluated as an indicator of normal biological or pathogenic processes, or of pharmacological response to a therapeutic intervention" (IOM, 2007a, p. 4).

[28] Harold L. Moses was the Ingram Professor of Cancer Research, the Chair of the Department of Cancer Biology, and the Director Emeritus of Vanderbilt-Ingram Cancer Center at this time.

The IOM released two more reports that also contributed to scientific discussions about how to promote advances in biomedical research and drug development in light of new findings, recent technology innovations, and novel opportunities identified by the research community: *Large-Scale Biomedical Science: Exploring Strategies for Future Research* (IOM and NRC, 2003a) and *Evolution of Translational Omics: Lessons Learned and the Path Forward* (IOM, 2012a). Although these reports were not focused solely on cancer research, the scientific and biomedical principles described in them and the reports' recommendations were very much applicable to cancer research, its scientific underpinnings, and its applicability to cancer drug development. For example, *Large-Scale Biomedical Science* described how new tools and technologies were expanding the scope and scale of biomedical research designed to study complex biological systems. In its report, the committee, which was chaired by external volunteer Joseph V. Simone,[29] presented seven recommendations that were intended to "facilitate a move toward a more open, inclusive, and accountable approach to large-scale biomedical research, and help strike the appropriate balance between large- and small-scale research to maximize progress in understanding and controlling human disease" (IOM and NRC, 2003a, p. 11). *Evolution of Translational Omics*[30] reviewed opportunities to "strengthen omics-based test development and evaluation," with the "ultimate goal of guiding therapeutic decisions to improve patient outcomes" (IOM, 2012a, p. 4). The committee—chaired by NAM member Gilbert S. Omenn[31]—made recommendations to "enhance development, evaluation, and translation of omics-based tests while simultaneously reinforcing steps to ensure that these tests are appropriately assessed for scientific validity (NASEM, n.d.c1)." After evaluating the report's findings and recommendations, the National Cancer Institute of the NIH developed a checklist that included 30 criteria that were based on the principles set forth in the IOM report. The purpose of the checklist was to determine the readiness of an omics test for use in guiding patient care in clinical trials.[32]

Advancing Cancer Prevention and Screening

In addition to its work to support progress in cancer clinical trials and biomedical research broadly, the IOM also contributed to research related to the prevention, screening, and diagnosis of cancer (see related reports in Box 4-6). In 2003, the National Cancer Policy Board released *Fulfilling the Potential of Cancer Prevention and Early Detection,* which argued that more could be done to reduce rates of cancer. Citing the immense burden of cancer on individuals, families, and the nation, the report presented a national strategy "to realize the promise of cancer prevention and early detection" (IOM and NRC, 2003b). The committee, also chaired by Simone, explored opportunities to prevent cancer through lifestyle changes (e.g., smoking cessation, improvements in diet and exercise), improve outcomes though screening and early detection, leverage primary care settings to implement cancer prevention and control strategies, expand education and training programs, and accelerate research. The committee set forth a dozen recommendations intended to guide a national strategy that could reduce the burden of cancer in the United States. Highlighting available evidence to support screening and prevention efforts, the committee urged policy mak-

---

[29] Joseph V. Simone was with Simone Consulting in Dunwoody, Georgia, at the time.

[30] The term "omics" encompasses "multiple molecular disciplines that involve the characterization of global sets of biological molecules such as DNAs, RNAs, proteins, and metabolites. For example, genomics investigates thousands of DNA sequences, transcriptomics investigates all or many gene transcripts, proteomics investigates large numbers of proteins, and metabolomics investigates large sets of metabolites" (IOM, 2012a, p. 1).

[31] Gilbert S. Omenn was a Professor of Internal Medicine, Human Genetics, and Public Health, and the Director of the University of Michigan Center for Computational Medicine and Bioinformatics at the University of Michigan Medical School in Ann Arbor when this report was published.

[32] Impact of IOM Reports (Database), IOM/NAM Records.

BOX 4-6
Selected Key National Academies Reports on Cancer

Quality Cancer Care

- *Diagnosing and Treating Adult Cancers and Associated Impairments* (2021)
- *Childhood Cancer and Functional Impacts Across the Care Continuum* (2021)
- *Making Medicines Affordable: A National Imperative* (2017)
- *Improving Diagnosis in Health Care* (2015)
- *Delivering High-Quality Cancer Care: Charting a New Course for a System in Crisis* (2013)
- *From Cancer Patient to Cancer Survivor: Lost in Transition* (2006)
- *Improving Breast Imaging Quality Standards* (2005)
- *Childhood Cancer Survivorship: Improving Care and Quality of Life* (2003)
- *Ensuring Quality Cancer Care* (1999)

Cancer Prevention and Control

- *Guiding Cancer Control: A Path to Transformation* (2019)
- *Hepatitis and Liver Cancer: A National Strategy for Prevention and Control of Hepatitis B and C* (2010)
- *Fulfilling the Potential of Cancer Prevention and Early Detection* (2003)
- *State Programs Can Reduce Tobacco Use* (2000)
- *Taking Action to Reduce Tobacco Use* (1998)
- *Growing Up Tobacco Free: Preventing Nicotine Addiction in Children and Youths* (1994)
- *Diet, Nutrition, and Cancer: Directions for Research* (1983)

Research Policy and Infrastructure

- *Biomarkers for Molecularly Targeted Therapies: Key to Unlocking Precision Medicine* (2016)
- *Ovarian Cancers: Evolving Paradigms in Research and Care* (2016)
- *Evolution of Translational Omics: Lessons Learned and the Path Forward* (2012)
- *A National Cancer Clinical Trials System for the 21st Century: Reinvigorating the NCI Cooperative Group Program* (2010)
- *Evaluation of Biomarkers and Surrogate Endpoints in Chronic Disease* (2010)
- *Beyond the HIPAA Privacy Rule: Enhancing Privacy, Improving Health Through Research* (2009)
- *Cancer Biomarkers: The Promises and Challenges of Improving Diagnosis and Treatment* (2007)
- *Making Better Drugs for Children with Cancer* (2005)
- *Large-Scale Biomedical Science: Exploring Strategies for Future Research* (2003)
- *Mammography and Beyond: Developing Technologies for the Early Detection of Breast Cancer* (2001)
- *Extending Medicare Reimbursement in Clinical Trials* (2000)

---

ers, government agencies, health insurance companies, and others to implement evidence-based guidelines, programs, and policies.

In 2010, the IOM released a report called *Hepatitis and Liver Cancer: A National Strategy for Prevention and Control of Hepatitis B and C,* which reviewed opportunities to prevent chronic liver disease and liver cancer. The committee, chaired by external volunteer R. Palmer Beasley,[33]

---

[33] R. Palmer Beasley was the Ashbel Smith Professor and the Dean Emeritus of the University of Texas School of Public Health in Houston when this report was released.

estimated that in the United States approximately 150,000 people would die in the next decade as a result of liver disease or cancer caused by hepatitis B and C (IOM, 2010b). Although there is a vaccine against hepatitis B, preventing hepatitis C relies on strategies to eliminate exposure to the blood-borne pathogen. Like the IOM's 2003 report *Fulfilling the Potential of Cancer Prevention and Early Detection*, this new report outlined a national strategy focused on screening and prevention. Following a review of available evidence, the committee offered recommendations to improve surveillance, increase knowledge and awareness, expand rates of hepatitis B vaccination for at-risk populations, and strengthen programs for screening for, preventing, and controlling hepatitis B and C infections (IOM, 2010b). The committee also called for additional research to develop a vaccine for hepatitis C and research on the "effectiveness and safety of peripartum antiviral therapy to reduce and possibly eliminate perinatal hepatitis B virus transmission" (IOM, 2010b, p. 6).

SCIENTIFIC ADVISOR TO THE U.S. GOVERNMENT

The IOM's mission to provide evidence-based advice, often in response to developments in scientific research, requires establishing effective ongoing relationships with many federal, state, and local agencies, such as the NIH, the FDA, the Department of Veterans Affairs (VA), and many others, as well as non-profit and international organizations, such as the African Academy of Sciences. Because of the IOM's reputation and its charter under the National Academies, agencies and organizations from around the world have relied on the IOM, and now the NAM and HMD, to provide evidence-based recommendations that are unbiased and removed from partisan politics. For the past half-century, the IOM, the NAM, and the HMD have brought together the most well-respected experts to evaluate available research and to inform advances in scientific research and policy.

Advising the National Institutes of Health

As the federal government's leader in medical sciences and research, the NIH has a long history with the IOM that dates back to its origins as the Board on Medicine. At that time, NIH Director James Shannon served as an advisor in the creation of what would become the IOM (see Chapter 1). The IOM's second president, Donald Fredrickson, was also a long-time NIH employee who left his position as IOM President to serve as the NIH's Director, and David Hamburg, the IOM's third President, spent a significant portion of his career at the NIH (see Chapter 2). Numerous other NIH leaders have been elected as IOM and NAM members, including NIH Director Francis Collins and the Director of the National Institute of Neurological Disorders and Stroke, Story Landis. Additionally, many IOM/NAM members have received research funding at their home institutions through NIH research programs and grants. These close connections have fostered a productive relationship in which the NIH has sponsored numerous IOM/NAM studies and roundtables throughout the years. Leaders and researchers from the NIH were often called on by IOM committees to present and inform their deliberations. In return, the IOM served as an advisor to the NIH, often providing guidance on its research agenda, its organization, and its policies and programs. The NIH's ongoing relationship with the IOM continues today through new collaborations with the NAM such as the Action Collaborative on Countering the U.S. Opioid Epidemic (see Chapter 7). The NIH also continues to sponsor new HMD studies and participates in the division's roundtables and forums (e.g., Roundtable on Genomics and Precision Health, the Forum on Neuroscience and Nervous System Disorders, and the National Cancer Policy Forum).

The subject of the NIH's organization and how it should conduct its major research activities has arisen many times during the IOM's history. This topic has always been crucial to the academic research community, as the NIH's organizational structure in many ways shapes the funding structure and grant opportunities available to academic researchers across the United States. Looking back, during the Reagan era, the IOM studied the organization of the NIH for the first time. Released in 1984, the IOM's brief report—*Responding to Health Needs and Scientific Opportunity: The Organizational Structure of the National Institutes of Health*—advised against the creation of institutes to address such subjects as nursing and arthritis, as Congress was considering at the time. The report suggested that the NIH needed to have organizational coherence and stability, stating that there should be a "presumption—to be overridden only in exceptional circumstances—against additions at the institute level" (IOM, 1984a, p. 20).

In 1990 and 1998 the IOM returned to questions related to the NIH's structure and priority setting process. The 1990 report—*Consensus Development at the NIH: Improving the Program,* which was chaired by J. Sanford Schwartz, an NAM member and Councilor (2019–2021)[34]—reviewed the structure and function of the NIH's Consensus Development Program (IOM, 1990a). The NIH program was charged with releasing consensus statements that reviewed available evidence related to current topics in medicine and medical research, not unlike the mission of the IOM (NIH, n.d.c). The 1998 report, *Scientific Opportunities and Public Needs: Improving Priority Setting and Public Input at the National Institutes of Health,* proved to be particularly influential in the NIH's operations. In the report, the IOM committee, which was chaired by NAM member Leon E. Rosenberg,[35] called on the NIH to "strengthen its analysis and the use of health data, such as burdens and costs of disease" when setting its research priorities (IOM, 1998d, p. 5). The report also recommended ways the NIH could assess the potential for scientific progress in a particular area and means by which to balance the goals of treating illnesses and investing in research focused on prevention. The report highlighted the need for better tracking and data related to the amount of funding the NIH dedicated to research related to specific diseases. The IOM also urged the NIH's institutes and centers to develop multi-year strategic plans and encouraged the development of an office focused on gathering public input. The report noted that the organizational structure of the NIH required periodic review in "light of changes in science and health needs of the public" (IOM, 1998d, p. 11). Following the release of the report, the NIH implemented the Research, Condition, and Disease Categorization process, which was used to track and report spending on different diseases and research areas.[36]

In addition to reviewing the NIH's structure and priority setting processes, the IOM also contributed to national discussions about the environment in which all medical research on humans was conducted and the ethical questions associated with the use of chimpanzees in medical research. In 2003, the IOM released *Responsible Research: A Systems Approach to Protecting Research Participants.* The report was commissioned by HHS in response to public concern that originated from isolated but widely reported incidents involving research participants, such as the death of a volunteer in an asthma study. Injuries and deaths associated with research participation led to questions about the safety of human research funded by the NIH and other government and industry sponsors. In its report, the committee, which was chaired by NAM member Daniel D. Federman,[37] emphasized the necessity of pursuing "every promising mechanism to maximize the protection of individuals participating in research" (IOM, 2003a, p. viii). The report presented a three-part strategy that included refocusing Institutional Review Boards on "thorough ethical review and oversight of research protocols," integrating research participants into the system, and maintaining "high

---

[34] J. Sanford Schwartz was the Executive Director of the Leonard Davis Institute of Health Economics, an Associate Professor of Medicine and Health Care Systems, and the Robert D. Eilers Associate Professor of Health Care Management and Economics at the University of Pennsylvania when this report was published. J. Sanford Schwartz passed away in 2021.

[35] Leon E. Rosenberg was a Professor in the Department of Molecular Biology and the Woodrow Wilson School of Public and International Affairs at Princeton University during this time.

[36] Impact of IOM Reports (Database), IOM/NAM Records.

[37] Daniel D. Federman was the Carl W. Walter Distinguished Professor of Medicine and Medical Education at Harvard University in Boston, Massachusetts, during this time.

standards for and continuing review of Human Research Participants Protection Programs" (IOM, 2003a, p. 5). The report stated that throughout the process, the needs of the research participants—not of the institution conducting the research—should be paramount. The report stressed the importance of recognizing research participants' contributions to science and stated that injuries acquired as a result of study participation should be adequately compensated without regard to fault (IOM, 2003a).

Because chimpanzees often served as a proxy for humans in medical research, the NIH turned to the IOM and the NRC's Board on Life Sciences in December of 2011 to help determine whether the use of chimpanzees in medical research was still necessary given the availability of new research technologies, techniques, and cell lines. In its report—*Chimpanzees in Biomedical and Behavioral Research: Assessing the Necessity*—the committee indicated that the chimpanzee's genetic proximity to humans "not only make[s] it a uniquely valuable species for certain types of research" but also demands "a greater justification for conducting research using this animal model" (IOM and NRC, 2011a, p. 2). The committee, which was chaired by NAM member and Councilor (2020–2022) Jeffrey P. Kahn,[38] came to an unexpected conclusion that had a wide impact on medical research across the county, stating that "while the chimpanzee has been a valuable animal model in past research, most current use of chimpanzees is unnecessary" except for a few very specific cases (IOM and NRC, 2011a, p. 4). In January 2013, the NIH released a response on how it would implement the committee's recommendations, accepting 28 out of 29 of the recommendations.[39] By August 2016, the NIH had developed a plan to retire all of the chimpanzees used in research to a federally owned sanctuary (NIH, n.d.d; see Figure 4-5). The NIH's response and actions demonstrated the very tangible impact of the IOM's work on the conduct of medical research in the United States.

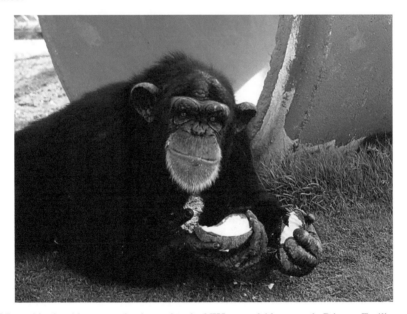

FIGURE 4-5 Pumpkin the chimpanzee is pictured at the NIH-owned Alamogordo Primate Facility, which houses chimpanzees that were previously used in biomedical research.
SOURCE: National Institutes of Health.

---

[38] Jeffrey P. Kahn was with the Johns Hopkins University Berman Institute of Bioethics at this time. Jeffrey P. Kahn concluded his term as Councilor in 2021 but assumed the seat of J. Sanford Schwartz after his passing, also in 2021.

[39] "Impact of IOM Reports and Activities, Documented April–June 2014," in IOM Council Minutes, July 1, 2014; "Inspiring Action," IOM Council Minutes, April 15, 2015,

Continuing its service as an advisor to the NIH, the IOM released *The CTSA Program at NIH: Opportunities for Advancing Clinical and Translational Research* in 2013. The NIH had commissioned the IOM to review its Clinical and Translational Science Awards Program (CTSA). The CTSA Program had been established in 2006 "to provide integrated intellectual and physical resources for the conduct of original clinical and translational research" and to expedite the translation of basic and clinical research "into clinical and community practice" (IOM, 2013c, p. 1). In the program's first 7 years, it grew from 12 to 61 research sites. The program aimed to link these sites and their research, creating a national consortium that promoted the application of best practices in clinical and translational research. A CTSA Consortium Coordinating Center at Vanderbilt University served as a central hub for disseminating research and other resources to the participating sites. The committee was chaired by Alan I. Leshner, an active NAM member who served on its Council from 2007 to 2012 and sat on HMD's Division Committee from 2018 to 2021.[40] During its review, the committee identified widespread support of the CTSA program, and noted that it had succeeded in establishing the CTSA sites as "academic focal points for clinical and translational research" (IOM, 2013c, p. 4). The task ahead involved transforming the CTSA program and its sites into a "tightly integrated network" (IOM, 2013c, p. 4) in which researchers actively engaged in "substantive and productive collaborations" (IOM, 2013c, p. 4). The committee concluded that the CTSA program was fulfilling its mission and "should be the national leader for advancing innovative and transformative clinical and translational research to improve human health" (IOM, 2013c, p. 13). In response to the IOM's report, the NIH's National Center for Advancing Translational Sciences (NCATS) Advisory Council released a report in May 2014 called the "NCATS Advisory Council Working Group on the IOM Report: The CTSA Program at NIH" (NCATS, 2014, p. 1). The advisory committee's report was drafted to respond to the IOM's recommendations and "to provide guidance on programmatic changes needed to implement the report's recommendations" (NCATS, 2014, p. 1).

Food and Drug Administration: Promoting the Development and Regulation of Safe Medical Products

For more than a century, the FDA has had the difficult task of approving new drugs and therapies to protect the public without unduly delaying access to potentially life-saving treatments. Over the years, many of the FDA's leaders were also IOM members and served in IOM leadership roles, including Jane Henney and Margaret Hamburg, who served as IOM's Home and Foreign Secretaries, respectively. IOM members Rob Califf, Lester Crawford, Charles E. Edwards, Scott Gottlieb, Jere Goyan, Don Kennedy, David Kessler, Mark McClellan, and Frank E. Young also served as FDA commissioners over the years. Although the FDA had sponsored IOM reports previously, the IOM's relationship with the FDA solidified in the beginning of the 21st century when the IOM was called on to provide an unbiased assessment of the FDA's regulation of drugs following a turbulent period in the history of pharmaceutical policy and drug safety.

In the last two decades of the 20th century, the FDA faced sharp political and public criticism over the slow speed of its drug approval process. During the peak of the HIV/AIDS epidemic in the 1980s, delays in the drug approval process were widely publicized and protestors accused the FDA of blocking access to experimental drugs that held promise to treat HIV/AIDS (Aizenman, 2019). During the next decade, House Speaker Newt Gingrich called the FDA the "leading job killer in America," and pharmaceutical companies threatened to move their operations overseas. In an effort to reduce the length of time required for the drug review process, Congress passed the Prescription

---

[40] Alan I. Leshner was with the American Association for the Advancement of Science in Washington, DC, when this report was published.

Drug User Fee Act in 1992, which allowed the pharmaceutical industry to pay the FDA user fees. While the 1992 act did shorten the drug approval process, there were concerns of unintended safety consequences associated with approving drugs that had not been fully evaluated in larger numbers of people in the general population (Applebaum, 2005; Wadman, 2005).

During the first few years of the 21st century, a number of serious drug safety issues came to light that amplified criticism of the FDA. On September 30, 2004, Merck withdrew the anti-inflammatory Vioxx—a drug used by at least two million people with arthritis and other painful conditions—due to reports of increased risks of heart attacks and strokes. The Senate Finance Committee investigated the withdrawal and found evidence that Vioxx had caused at least 88,000 heart attacks, of which 30 to 40 percent were fatal. David Graham of the FDA's Office of Drug Safety told the senators that "Vioxx is a terrible tragedy and a profound regulatory failure." In April 2005, the FDA asked Pfizer to withdraw Bextra, another popular drug used to treat rheumatoid arthritis and osteoarthritis, because of risks it posed to the heart, stomach, and skin (Wadman, 2005).[41] Safety concerns with other classes of drugs also arose at this time. Anti-depressants such as Paxil were linked to suicides among adolescents. Crestor, a cholesterol medication used by 2.8 million people, was associated with a muscle-destroying condition called rhabdomyolosis. Hormone replacement therapies used by hundreds of thousands of women over several decades were linked to increased risk of breast cancer, heart disease, stroke, and blood clots.

In 2005, the FDA commissioned an IOM report to evaluate the existing systems for drug approval and post-market surveillance and to "make recommendations to improve risk assessment, surveillance, and the safe use of drugs" (IOM, 2006g, p. 3). Throughout the study, the committee and its deliberations were closely monitored by interested stakeholders including the media, the FDA, and Congress. The committee's first public meeting included testimony from Janet Woodcock, Deputy Commissioner of Operations at the FDA, who told the committee that the system had "obviously broken down to some extent." Woodcock cautioned, however, that risk-free drugs were not possible. "One of the questions on the table, really," she said, "is how much uncertainty are we willing to tolerate."[42] On September 22, 2006, the IOM released the committee's much anticipated report, *The Future of Drug Safety: Promoting and Protecting the Health of the Public*. In its findings, the committee—chaired by NAM member and Councilor (2012–2018) Sheila P. Burke[43]—highlighted the overall consensus among stakeholders that improvements were needed in the drug approval process, signaling an openness to change. In an effort to guide that change, the committee offered 25 detailed recommendations to strengthen the pre- and post-approval phases in the areas of organizational culture, science and expertise, regulation, communication, and resources. The committee encouraged a lifecycle approach to the drug safety system in which newly available data would continuously inform a more complete risk and benefit profile of approved drugs that could then be used to update regulatory decisions in a more transparent way (IOM, 2006g).

To promote continuous open dialog about drug development among stakeholders, including the FDA, NIH, pharmaceutical companies, academic researchers, and patient organizations, the IOM launched the Forum on Drug Discovery, Development, and Translation in 2005 (IOM, 2010g). In its 15-year history, the forum has held almost 50 meetings and released 30 publications. In its early days, the forum's work continued and expanded on many of the discussions initiated after the release of the 2006 *Drug Safety* report, including a 2007 workshop that focused on the implication of the report's recommendations and the next steps for the FDA in fulfilling those recommendations (IOM, 2007c). The forum also tackled overarching topics related to the development of medical

---

[41] "Timeline and Key Stakeholders," IOM Committee on the Assessment of the U.S. Drug Safety System, Background Information, May 9, 2005.

[42] "Transcript," *The Nightly Business Report*, June 8, 2005, IOM/NAM Records.

[43] Sheila P. Burke was the Deputy Secretary and the Chief Operating Officer of the Smithsonian Institution in Washington, DC, during this time.

products such as understanding and communicating uncertainty on product risks and benefits (IOM, 2007d), advancing regulatory sciences, and examining real-world evidence (NASEM, 2016a). Over the years, the forum's work stretched beyond the borders of the United States and served as a venue to discuss global topics related to drug development including drug-resistant tuberculosis and the harmonization of global drug regulation (IOM, 2013f). Following the transition from the IOM to HMD, the forum established four thematic priorities to guide its activities: innovation and reform of the drug discovery and development enterprise, science across the drug development and discovery lifecycle, clinical trials and clinical product development, and infrastructure and workforce (NASEM, 2019i). In a 2015 congressional report, Senators Lamar Alexander (R-TN) and Richard Burr (R-NC) cited the forum "as a foundational resource in identifying and addressing the challenges facing the U.S. clinical trials enterprise."[44]

In an effort to improve post-market evaluation and regulation of drugs, following the enactment of the Food and Drug Administration Act of 2007, the FDA called on the IOM to "convene a committee to evaluate the scientific and ethical issues involved in conducting studies of the safety of approved drugs" (IOM, 2012c, p. 4). The committee released a letter report in July 2010 that offered a framework for evaluating data from post-market studies. The committee's final report, *Ethical and Scientific Issues in Studying the Safety of Approved Drugs,* which was released in 2012, concluded that the "FDA's current approach to drug oversight in the post-marketing setting is not sufficiently systematic and does not ensure continued assessment of benefits and risks of drugs associated with a drug over its lifecycle" (IOM, 2012c, p. 14). The committee, which was co-chaired by NAM members Ruth R. Faden[45] and Steven N. Goodman,[46] offered 22 recommendations and called on the FDA to establish a standardized, yet flexible, regulatory framework to make the agency's "decision-making process more predictable, transparent, and active" (IOM, 2012c, p. 14). Echoing sentiments from the 2006 report, the committee encouraged the FDA to "embrace more fully a lifecycle approach to drug safety oversight" (p. 1), emphasizing the importance of post-market review as a critical part of ensuring the safety of medical products used by millions of Americans every day.

Veterans Health Administration: Occupational and Environmental Exposures During Military Service

The VA operates the largest direct service health care system in the United States, the Veterans Health Administration (VA, n.d.a). Some of the more than 9 million American veterans who seek care through the VA each year are living with the aftereffects of exposure to dangerous environments and hazardous substances that were encountered during military service. These types of exposures to chemicals, radiation, and other pollutants and health hazards, including risk factors for posttraumatic stress disorder (see Chapter 6) and traumatic brain injury that might occur during the course of military service, are considered a unique type of occupational health concern. As with other types of occupational and environmental exposures to hazardous substances, the long latency period between exposure during military service and the manifestation of disease makes establishing causality difficult. As demonstrated in the following sections, the recognition and study of hazardous exposures unique to military service has expanded over time with each war and military conflict and have sometimes been associated with increasing pressure from veterans, their families,

---

[44] Impact of IOM Reports (Database), IOM/NAM Records.

[45] Ruth R. Faden was the Philip Franklin Wagley Professor of Biomedical Ethics and the Executive Director of the Berman Institute of Bioethics at the Johns Hopkins University in Baltimore, Maryland, at this time.

[46] Steven N. Goodman was a Professor of Medicine and Health Research and Policy and the Associate Dean for Clinical and Translational Research at the Stanford University School of Medicine in Stanford, California, when this report was published.

and advocates. The studies evolved from WWII exposures associated with nuclear and chemical weapons testing to Agent Orange exposure during the Vietnam War to air pollutants from burn pits that were used to dispose of waste during conflicts in Iraq and Afghanistan. Working with the VA to study veterans' health and the possible linkages with exposure to hazards as part of military service was a core activity of the IOM's Medical Follow-Up Agency (MFUA) for more than 70 years.

Founded by Michael DeBakey in 1946 within the NRC, the Medical Follow-Up Agency conducted ongoing clinical studies designed to evaluate injuries and disease associated with veterans' service in World War II. In 1955 the MFUA initiated a long-term effort to create a twins registry that would include verified sets of twins, both of whom had served in World War II. During its more than half-century existence, the registry grew to include nearly 16,000 twin pairs and served as the basis for numerous epidemiologic and heritability studies, including psychological studies and studies of a range of diseases such as cancer, Alzheimer's disease, and Parkinson's disease (Gatz and Butler, 2020). Access to the registry was strictly managed through a committee, and proposed research studies had to meet Institutional Review Board requirements. The comprehensive nature of the registry and the records associated with it made the registry "one of the most valuable longitudinal cohorts of aging men available" (IOM, 2003k, p. 115).

In 1988, the MFUA moved from the NRC to the IOM where it evolved to focus more broadly on epidemiologic studies of veteran populations and their health concerns. The MFUA's work was not entirely free of controversy, which stemmed, in part, from veterans' disability compensation programs in which payments varied according to the severity of the injury. The VA looked to the IOM to review the evidence associated with exposures during military service, and the VA would then use the IOM's findings to inform decisions regarding the compensation programs and which diseases would be covered (Panangala et al., 2014). Determining compensation for occupational diseases was particularly challenging because it was sometimes hard to separate health problems caused by military service from those that were associated with a person's lifestyle (e.g., lung diseases and cancer) or with other occupational exposures (e.g., agriculture, mining, manufacturing).

Although the MFUA conducted numerous epidemiologic studies of veterans over the years, there were times when the agency concluded that epidemiologic studies were not feasible. Following World War II, a number of soldiers were present at the sites where atmospheric tests of nuclear weapons were conducted between 1945 and 1962. In subsequent years, these veterans, who were referred to as "atomic veterans" were concerned about possible adverse reproductive outcomes for their spouses and possible genetic defects and disease for their children and grandchildren. In 1994, the VA asked the IOM to assess the feasibility of conducting epidemiological studies to evaluate possible effects in the spouses, children, and grandchildren of the atomic veterans. The challenge with diseases caused by radiation was that they were "generally indistinguishable from those that occur naturally in the population from other causes." In 1995, the IOM released *Adverse Reproductive Outcomes in Families of Atomic Veterans: The Feasibility of Epidemiologic Studies,* which was authored by a committee chaired by external volunteer William J. Schull.[47] The committee concluded that epidemiological studies among the families of atomic veterans would be infeasible (Miller, 1995). For example, finding and engaging a large enough sample size of children and grandchildren of atomic veterans to study was difficult. Additionally, establishing the levels of radiation that the veterans had been exposed to would have been challenging, and the estimates that were available suggested that the exposures during the weapons testing were generally below common forms of additional background radiation exposures (e.g., living at a high altitude, receiving CT scans) (IOM, 1995).

Some of the IOM's epidemiologic studies evaluated direct hazard exposures that resulted from

---

[47] Willliam J. Schull was the Director of the Center of Demographic and Population Genetics at the School of Public Health at the University of Texas at Houston when this report was released.

classified experiments involving military personnel. During World War II, War Department officials were concerned by the threat of chemical weapons. In an effort to protect soldiers in war zones from mustard gas and an arsenic-containing agent called lewisite, the War Department initiated a chemical defense research program that tested protective clothing against these gases. In the studies, military personnel wearing the test clothing were exposed to mustard gas or lewisite in a gas chamber until the soldier developed erythema, indicating a failure of the clothing. At the conclusion of the research program, more than 60,000 military personnel had been involved in the testing. Over time, some of the veterans who had participated in the tests began experiencing health problems they thought could be related to their exposures to the poisonous gases. Some sought benefits from the VA, only to have their claims denied because of the secrecy of the test programs. Eventually the VA identified seven conditions, including asthma and chronic bronchitis, that might be related to participation in the tests. In 1991, the VA asked the IOM "to assess the strength of association between exposure to these agents and the development of specific diseases" (IOM, 1993a, p. 2).

The IOM released *Veterans at Risk: The Health Effects of Mustard Gas and Lewisite* on January 6, 1993. The study committee found it difficult to draw conclusions from the thousands of scientific reports it reviewed and testimony from the affected veterans it heard during its open information-gathering sessions. However, the evidence did support a causal relationship between exposures to the poisonous gases and a variety of diseases that included respiratory diseases and cancers, skin diseases and cancer, various eye conditions and diseases, leukemia, psychological disorders, and reproductive dysfunction. The committee also uncovered evidence that the participants' exposure may have been higher than originally reported. The committee was dismayed by the lack of follow-up health assessments and epidemiologic studies, which diminished the availability of data. In its report, the committee noted that the secrecy surrounding the program and testing "impeded well-informed health care for thousands of people" (IOM, 1993a, p. 8). The committee, chaired by NAM member and Foreign Secretary (1994–1998) David P. Rall,[48] recommended that the VA establish a program to identify, notify, evaluate, and follow veterans who had participated in this chemical defense research program and had been exposed to mustard gas and lewisite (IOM, 1993a; Pechura, 1993).

Subsequent wars and conflicts led to different types of occupational exposures and health concerns for veterans who had served their country. For Vietnam veterans, exposure to Agent Orange and other herbicides used on the battlefield created the potential for long-term health problems (see Figure 4-6). In 1991, Congress passed a law that called on the IOM to complete a biennial review of available medical and scientific literature related to exposure to the herbicides that were used in the Vietnam War (see Box 4-7). To conduct the work, the IOM appointed a new committee to review the available literature for each update, and the committees were sometimes asked to focus on specific health outcomes that might be related to exposure. For example, the 1996 update identified "limited or suggestive" evidence of the presence of spina bifida in children of fathers who were Vietnam veterans with exposure to herbicides. This finding supplemented findings from previous updates that highlighted "sufficient evidence of an association" between exposure to herbicides and soft-tissue sarcoma and Hodgkin's disease.

Unlike other IOM activities, the ongoing mechanism by which the Agent Orange series revisited the literature identified new connections as the veterans aged and as new diseases were manifested. It also allowed for amending previous findings based on new evidence. For example, the 2012 update indicated "limited or suggestive" evidence of linkages between exposure and strokes (IOM, 2014a), and the 2014 update concluded that Parkinson's-like symptoms and Parkinson's disease were associated with exposure, while also downgrading the spina bifida evidence

---

[48] David P. Rall was a retired Director of the National Institute of Environmental Health Sciences at the National Institutes of Health in Washington, DC, at the time.

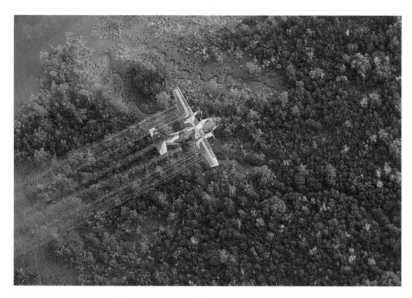

FIGURE 4-6 U.S. Air Force UC 123K plane spraying delta area with dioxin-tainted herbicide/defoliant Agent Orange, in Vietnam War defensive measure 20 miles southeast of Saigon.
SOURCE: Photo by Dick Swanson/The LIFE Images Collection/Getty Images (CC BY 2.0).

from the 1996 update to "inadequate/insufficient" (NASEM, 2016b). The findings from this series of reports improved the medical care that Vietnam veterans received by increasing the awareness of VA clinicians who cared for these patients. The findings also improved the veterans' disability compensation system by improving the accuracy and completeness of the list of diseases and con-

---

BOX 4-7
Examples of the Institute of Medicine's Veterans and Agent Orange Reports

- *Veterans and Agent Orange: Update 11 (2018)*
- *Veterans and Agent Orange: Update 2014 (2016)*
- *Veterans and Agent Orange: Update 2012 (2014)*
- *Veterans and Agent Orange: Update 2010 (2012)*
- *Veterans and Agent Orange: Update 2008 (2009)*
- *Veterans and Agent Orange: Update 2006 (2007)*
- *Veterans and Agent Orange: Update 2004 (2005)*
- *Veterans and Agent Orange: Length of Presumptive Period for Association Between Exposure and Respiratory Cancer (2004)*
- *Veterans and Agent Orange: Update 2002 (2003)*
- *Characterizing Exposure of Veterans to Agent Orange and Other Herbicides Used in Vietnam: Final Report (2003)*
- *Veterans and Agent Orange: Herbicide/Dioxin Exposure and Acute Myelogenous Leukemia in the Children of Vietnam Veterans (2002)*
- *Veterans and Agent Orange: Update 2000 (2001)*
- *Veterans and Agent Orange: Herbicide/Dioxin Exposure and Type 2 Diabetes (2000)*
- *Veterans and Agent Orange: Update 1998 (1999)*
- *Veterans and Agent Orange: Update 1996 (1996)*
- *Veterans and Agent Orange: Health Effects of Herbicides Used in Vietnam (1994)*

ditions associated with exposures to herbicides, and therefore, eligible for compensation (IOM, 1996a). The last report in the series was released in November 2018 and served as the 11th biennial update (NASEM, 2018a).

During the Vietnam War era, between 1962 and 1973, the military conducted testing that was referred to as Project SHAD (Shipboard Hazard and Defense). The goal of the tests was to assess the susceptibility of naval ships to chemical and biological agents that could be deployed in war time. It is estimated that approximately 6,000 Navy and Marine Corps personnel were exposed to various agents during these tests, and not all of them were made aware of the testing at the time (IOM, 2007b). In 2002, the VA commissioned the IOM to conduct an epidemiologic study after numerous veterans who had been exposed to hazardous agents during Project SHAD raised health concerns that could be connected to their exposures. The IOM and the National Academies went on to release two reports: *Long-Term Health Effects of Participation in Project SHAD (Shipboard Hazard and Defense)*[49] (IOM, 2007b) and *Assessing Health Outcomes Among Veterans of Project SHAD (Shipboard Hazard and Defense)* (NASEM, 2016c).

The first study, which was released in 2007, "found no difference in all-cause mortality between SHAD veterans and the comparison group, but there was an increased risk of death from heart disease among some SHAD veterans" (IOM, 2007b, p. 2). Subsequent survey results also determined that SHAD participants reported "poorer overall physical and mental health" (NASEM, 2016c, p. 1). The second study, which was released in 2016, analyzed 7 years of additional data and some newly available diagnostic data. The findings from the follow-up report generally aligned with findings from the first report, but "it did not find an elevation in heart disease mortality" (NASEM, 2016c, p. 1). Following the two studies, the committee, which was chaired by external volunteer David J. Tollerud,[50] concluded that "the results of the analyses provide no evidence that the health of SHAD veterans overall or those in the exposure groups is significantly different from that of similar veterans who did not participate in these tests" (NASEM, 2016c, p. 9).

Beyond the epidemiologic studies conducted by the MFUA that focused primarily on WWII and Vietnam era veterans, MFUA and the IOM's other boards also conducted studies relevant to the health of U.S. veterans following exposures to hazardous materials and physical and psychological stressors during more recent military conflicts. For example, in the early 1990s, the United States deployed nearly 700,000 military personnel to the Persian Gulf region to fight in and support Operation Desert Shield and Operation Desert Storm. Upon returning home, some of the veterans reported health concerns that they attributed to their military service and exposures during that time. As public scrutiny increased and symptoms were documented in 25 to 35 percent of veterans who served (IOM, 2013d), Congress and the VA commissioned the IOM to conduct a range of studies to understand the long-term health outcomes of service in the Gulf War. The studies were designed to evaluate best practices for collecting and analyzing data, provide comprehensive literature reviews on the health effects of specific exposures, conduct ongoing and long-term review of the health effects of serving in the Gulf War, and recommend treatment strategies. In the quarter century following the end of the Gulf War, the IOM, and subsequently the HMD, released more than two dozen reports dedicated to the health of Gulf War veterans (see Box 4-8). The series of reports covered a variety of potential exposures that military personnel encountered from different types of radiation (e.g., depleted uranium) and chemicals (e.g., insecticides, combustible products) to infectious diseases to physical and psychological consequences of serving in the Gulf War. Many of these exposures were unique to military service when compared to occupational and environmental

---

[49] This report was authored by three IOM staff members—William F. Page, Heather A. Young, and Harriet M. Crawford—with oversight from an advisory panel that was chaired by Daniel H. Freeman, Jr.

[50] David J. Tollerud was a Professor and the Chair of the Department of Environmental and Occupational Health Sciences at the University of Louisville School of Public Health and Information Sciences when this report was released.

BOX 4-8
Gulf War and Health Reports

- *Gulf War and Health: Volume 11: Generational Health Effects of Serving in the Gulf War* (2018)
- *Gulf War and Health: Volume 10: Update of Health Effects of Serving in the Gulf War, 2016* (2016)
- *Considerations for Designing an Epidemiologic Study for Multiple Sclerosis and Other Neurologic Disorders in Pre and Post 9/11 Gulf War Veterans* (2015)
- *Gulf War and Health: Volume 9: Long-Term Effects of Blast Exposures* (2014)
- *Gulf War and Health: Volume 9: Long-Term Effects of Blast Exposures* (2014)
- *Chronic Multisymptom Illness in Gulf War Veterans: Case Definitions Reexamined* (2014)
- *Gulf War and Health: Treatment for Chronic Multisymptom Illness* (2013)
- *Gulf War and Health: Volume 8: Update of Health Effects of Serving in the Gulf War* (2010)
- *Gulf War and Health: Volume 7: Long-Term Consequences of Traumatic Brain Injury* (2009)
- *Gulf War and Health: Updated Literature Review of Depleted Uranium* (2008)
- *Epidemiologic Studies of Veterans Exposed to Depleted Uranium: Feasibility and Design Issues* (2008)
- *Gulf War and Health: Volume 6: Physiologic, Psychologic, and Psychosocial Effects of Deployment-Related Stress* (2008)
- *Gulf War and Health: Volume 5: Infectious Diseases* (2007)
- *Amyotrophic Lateral Sclerosis in Veterans: Review of the Scientific Literature* (2006)
- *Gulf War and Health: Volume 3: Fuels, Combustion Products, and Propellants* (2005)
- *Gulf War and Health: Volume 4: Health Effects of Serving in the Gulf War* (2006)
- *Gulf War and Health: Updated Literature Review of Sarin* (2004)
- *Gulf War and Health: Volume 2: Insecticides and Solvents* (2003)
- *Gulf War Veterans: Treating Symptoms and Syndromes* (2001)
- *Gulf War and Health: Volume 1: Depleted Uranium, Pyridostigmine Bromide, Sarin, and Vaccines* (2000)
- *Gulf War Veterans: Measuring Health* (1999)
- *Adequacy of the Comprehensive Clinical Evaluation Program: Nerve Agents* (1997)
- *Adequacy of the VA Persian Gulf Registry and Uniform Case Assessment Protocol* (1998)
- *Adequacy of the Comprehensive Clinical Evaluation Program: A Focused Assessment* (1997)
- *Health Consequences of Service During the Persian Gulf War: Recommendations for Research and Information Systems* (1996)
- *Health Consequences of Service During the Persian Gulf War: Initial Findings and Recommendations for Immediate Action* (1995)

---

exposures in other types of more traditional occupational settings, requiring long-term assessment to fully understand the health effects of these exposures.

The Gulf War and Health series of reports shaped the VA's policies related to the benefits and services that are provided to Gulf War veterans, and in some cases the VA expanded benefits available to veterans as a direct result of the reports' findings. For example, the VA classified certain symptoms and illnesses identified in the IOM's reports (e.g., ALS, functional gastrointestinal illnesses, certain medically unexplained illnesses) as "Gulf War Presumptive Illnesses," which resulted in an expedited benefits application process for veterans with these illnesses and symptoms (VA, 2016, n.d.b). In 2013, citing Volume 7 of the IOM's Gulf War and Health series, the VA expanded available benefits for veterans who had experienced traumatic brain injuries and added five conditions associated with service-related traumatic brain injuries to its list of presumptive illnesses: Parkinson's disease, certain types of dementia, depression, unprovoked seizures, and certain diseases of the hypothalamus and pituitary glands.[51] The VA also used the series of reports and the findings included in the reports to increase the available funding for research. For example, following the release of the 2013 and 2014 reports on chronic multi-symptom illnesses, the VA allocated $2.8 million to assess possible treatments for the conditions experienced by Gulf War veterans.[52] In 2016, following the release of the tenth volume of the Gulf War and Health series, the VA extended the deadline for veterans seeking benefits for illnesses associated with service in the Gulf War by 5 years to 2021. In making its decision, which was based on the report's finding, the VA noted that "symptoms could manifest in Gulf War veterans at any point, and there was no basis for stopping veterans from seeking benefits at the end of 2016."[53]

Following the terrorist attacks of September 11, 2001, the United States deployed military forces to Afghanistan and Iraq to lead and support armed conflicts that lasted nearly two decades. During these conflicts the military used open air burn pits to dispose of waste (e.g., plastic, metal, wood, solvents, medical waste, human waste, petroleum) (NASEM, 2017c; see Figure 4-7); one of these pits, located outside of Baghdad, was used to burn "up to 200 tons of waste per day in 2007" (IOM, 2011c). The emissions from these burn pits raised questions about possible adverse health effects for military personnel exposed to these pits during their military service. On two separate occasions, the VA asked the IOM and then the HMD to conduct studies related to the burn pits.

In 2011, the IOM released *Long-Term Health Consequences of Exposure to Burn Pits in Iraq and Afghanistan,* which concluded that there was insufficient evidence available to provide concrete conclusions regarding the long-term health effects of burn pit exposure. The committee, also chaired by Tollerud,[54] recommended "more efficient data-gathering methods" along with another study that would "evaluate the health status of service members from their time of deployment over many years to determine their incidence of chronic diseases" (IOM, 2011c). In 2010, prior

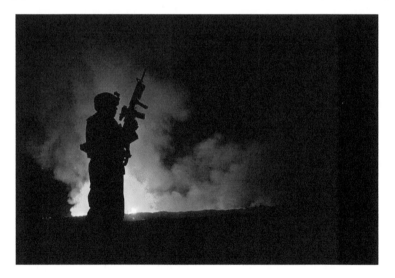

FIGURE 4-7 U.S. Marine Corps Sgt. Robert B. Brown, with Combat Camera Unit, Regimental Combat Team 6, watches over the civilian firefighters at the burn pit as smoke and flames rise into the night sky behind him in Camp Fallujah, Iraq.
SOURCE: U.S. Marine Corps photo by Cpl. Samuel D. Corum (CC BY-NC-ND 2.0).

---

[51] Impact of IOM Reports (Database), IOM/NAM Records.

[52] Ibid.

[53] Ibid.

[54] David J. Tollerud was a Professor and the Chair of the Department of Environmental and Occupational Health Sciences at the University of Louisville School of Public Health and Information Sciences when this report was released.

to the release of the IOM's report, Congress banned the use of open air burn pits, and in 2013, the VA established a registry at the direction of Congress to better document personnel who had been exposed (NASEM, 2017c). In 2017, the HMD released a second report called *Assessment of the Department of Veterans Affairs Airborne Hazards and Open Burn Pit Registry,* which reviewed the design of the registry and the use of its data. In its report, the committee, which was chaired by NAM member David A. Savitz,[55] provided a set of recommendations directed at improving the registry in terms of "addressing the future medical needs of the affected groups ... and collecting, maintaining, and monitoring information collected" (NASEM, 2017c, p. 13).

The MFUA remained part of the IOM until 2015, when it was transferred to the HMD following the creation of the NAM. However, today MFUA's activities are limited and only represent a small fraction of the work it once did. In many ways, the MFUA's work was unique among the IOM's portfolio. For example, some of the work was ongoing in nature (e.g., Agent Orange series) and some of it involved original research that was conducted by statisticians and epidemiologists on the MFUA staff who collaborated with clinical investigators from academic medical centers (Berkowitz and Santangelo, 1999). The MFUA maintained its twins registry and also established a cohort catalog, a "collection of study populations of former military personnel assembled as part of proposed or completed research dating back to the 1940s" (Butler, n.d.). Under HMD, the MFUA became part of the Board on Military and Veterans Health.

Advising Other Government Agencies

In addition to its work with the NIH, the FDA, the VA, the IOM, the NAM, and the HMD built and maintained strong relationships with numerous other government agencies throughout its history. For example, the IOM provided advice to the CDC through its *Leading Health Indicator* reports, which the agency used to guide its Health People reports—the national agenda for improving the public's health (see Chapter 6). The IOM and the HMD also offered guidance to the National Highway Traffic Safety Administration in its Crisis Standards of Care reports as well as through the work of the organization's Forum on Medical and Public Health Preparedness for Disasters and Emergencies (see Chapter 6). In terms of providing advice intended to advance research and the implementation of research findings in government policy, the IOM and now the HMD have also provided advice to the National Institute for Occupational Safety and Health (NIOSH), the National Aeronautics and Space Administration (NASA), and the Social Security Administration (SSA), as described below.

Advising NIOSH

NIOSH, a branch of the CDC, has the mission "to develop new knowledge in the field of occupational safety and health and to transfer that knowledge into practice" (CDC, n.d.c), which supports its vision for "safer, healthier workers." In 2005, NIOSH provided support for the IOM to establish the Standing Committee on Personal Protective Equipment (PPE) for Workplace Safety and Health, which was designed "to provide strategic guidance in addressing PPE issues for a wide range of workers" (NASEM, 2019g, p. 20). PPE is deployed to protect workers exposed to a variety of environmental and occupational hazards, including chemicals, radiation, particulate matter in the air, heights, infectious pathogens, and anything else that may pose a risk to worker health and safety. PPE, such as protective clothing, respirators, face masks, safety harnesses, and lift-assistance devices, is used in any occupational setting where hazards exist— from hospitals and nursing homes to construction sites, mines, and farms. Over the years, the standing committee has held more than two dozen meetings to

---

[55] David A. Savitz was the Vice President for Research, a Professor of Epidemiology, and a Professor of Obstetrics and Gynecology at Brown University in Providence, Rhode Island, when this report was published.

support NIOSH in fulfilling its research-oriented mission as it relates to PPE. The standing committee has hosted a number of public workshops and meetings, and several ad hoc consensus studies have spun off of the work of the standing committee (NASEM, n.d.e) (see Box 4-9).

In addition to the standing committee, NIOSH also commissioned the IOM, in partnership with other divisions within the National Academies, to conduct a series of evaluative studies to review a selected group of research programs at NIOSH. Over the course of 3 years (2006–2009), the IOM, with the NRC, released eight reports that provided in-depth reviews of specific NIOSH research programs (e.g., traumatic injury, health hazards, PPE, mining safety and health, and construction) (see Box 4-9). The committees conducting the program reviews also examined the "relevance and impact of NIOSH's work" in fulfilling its vision and mission (IOM and NRC, 2009a). To complete this work and develop recommendations to improve the NIOSH research programs, the assigned committees used a common evaluation framework and scoring criteria for assessing the relevance

---

BOX 4-9
A Sample of Reports Commissioned to Advise the National
Institute for Occupational Safety and Health

- *Reusable Elastomeric Respirators in Health Care: Considerations for Routine and Surge Use* (2019)
- *Integration of FDA and NIOSH Processes Used to Evaluate Respiratory Protective Devices for Health Care Workers: Proceedings of a Workshop* (2017)
- *Developing a Performance Standard for Combination Unit Respirators: Workshop in Brief* (2015)
- *The Use and Effectiveness of Powered Air Purifying Respirators in Health Care: Workshop Summary* (2015)
- *Occupational Health Nurses and Respiratory Protection: Improving Education and Training: Letter Report* (2011)
- *Preventing Transmission of Pandemic Influenza and Other Viral Respiratory Diseases: Personal Protective Equipment for Healthcare Personnel, Update 2010* (2011)
- *Certifying Personal Protective Technologies: Improving Worker Safety* (2011)
- *Evaluating Occupational Health and Safety Research Programs: Framework and Next Steps* (2009)
- *Traumatic Injury Research at NIOSH: Reviews of Research Programs of the National Institute for Occupational Safety and Health* (2009)
- *The Health Hazard Evaluation Program at NIOSH: Reviews of Research Programs of the National Institute for Occupational Safety and Health* (2009)
- *Evaluating Occupational Health and Safety Research Programs: Framework and Next Steps* (2009)
- *Construction Research at NIOSH: Reviews of Research Programs of the National Institute for Occupational Safety and Health* (2009)
- *The Personal Protective Technology Program at NIOSH: Reviews of Research Programs of the National Institute for Occupational Safety and Health* (2008)
- *Agriculture, Forestry, and Fishing Research at NIOSH: Reviews of Research Programs of the National Institute for Occupational Safety and Health* (2008)
- *Mining Safety and Health Research at NIOSH: Reviews of Research Programs of the National Institute for Occupational Safety and Health* (2007)
- *Preparing for an Influenza Pandemic: Personal Protective Equipment for Healthcare Workers* (2007)
- *Measuring Respirator Use in the Workplace* (2007)
- *Assessment of the NIOSH Head-and-Face Anthropometric Survey of U.S. Respirator Users* (2007)
- *Hearing Loss Research at NIOSH: Reviews of Research Programs of the National Institute for Occupational Safety and Health* (2006)

and impact of the institute's work. The final report in the series—*Evaluating Occupational Health and Safety Research Programs: Framework and Next Steps*—was released in 2009. It provided detailed information on the framework and scoring criteria the committees used, as well as a handful of recommendations that could be applied to continuously evaluate and improve research, surveillance, and efforts to translate research into policy and practice.

Advising NASA

The IOM's mission to improve health for all (later adopted by the NAM and HMD) has not been limited to U.S. borders, nor even to the boundaries of Earth's atmosphere or orbit. In 2000, NASA commissioned an IOM study "to develop a vision for space medicine for long-duration space travel" (IOM, 2001c). The resulting 2001 report, *Safe Passage: Astronaut Care for Exploration Missions,* called on NASA to establish "a comprehensive health care system for astronauts to capture all relevant epidemiological data" and institute "a long-term, focused health care research strategy to capture all necessary data on health risks and their amelioration" (IOM, 2001c, p. 1). This committee, which was chaired by NAM member John R. Ball,[56] and its resulting report marked the start of a long-term relationship between the IOM and NASA that included NASA's sponsorship of the Standing Committee on Aerospace Medicine and the Medicine of Extreme Environments (NASEM, n.d.f). The standing committee was designed to support NASA in considering scientific, technical, and policy factors related to areas such as "the development of optimal aerospace medicine healthcare as an evolving multidisciplinary and international enterprise; health maintenance and care policies related to aerospace medicine; [and] clinical research requirements and clinical strategies" (NASEM, n.d.f).

Building on the standing committee's work, NASA also sponsored a range of IOM studies that focused on risk reduction, the health of humans in space, and long-term health outcomes for those who had traveled to space previously (see Box 4-10). For example, in 2008, the IOM released a letter

---

BOX 4-10
A Sample of Reports Commissioned to Advise the
National Aeronautics and Space Administration

- *Review of NASA's Evidence Reports on Human Health Risks: 2017 Letter Report* (2018)
- *Review of NASA's Evidence Reports on Human Health Risks: 2016 Letter Report* (2017)
- *Review of NASA's Evidence Reports on Human Health Risks: 2015 Letter Report* (2016)
- *Review of NASA's Evidence Reports on Human Health Risks: 2014 Letter Report* (2015)
- *Review of NASA's Evidence Reports on Human Health Risks: 2013 Letter Report* (2014)
- *Health Standards for Long Duration and Exploration Spaceflight: Ethics Principles, Responsibilities, and Decision Framework* (2014)
- *A Review of NASA Human Research Program's Scientific Merit Assessment Processes: Letter Report* (2012)
- *Review of NASA's Human Research Program Evidence Books: A Letter Report* (2008)
- *Review of NASA's Space Flight Health Standards: Letter Report* (2007)
- *A Risk Reduction Strategy for Human Exploration of Space: A Review of NASA's Bioastronautics Roadmap* (2006)
- *Integrating Employee Health: A Model Program for NASA* (2005)
- *Review of NASA's Longitudinal Study of Astronaut Health* (2004)
- *Safe Passage: Astronaut Care for Exploration Missions* (2001)

---

[56] John R. Ball was an Executive Vice President Emeritus of the American College of Physicians in Havre de Grace, Maryland, during this time.

report called *Review of NASA's Human Research Program Evidence Books: A Letter Report*, which was developed to advise NASA on its plan "to assemble the available evidence on human health risks of spaceflight and moves forward in identifying and addressing gaps in research" (IOM, 2008a, p. 1). Ultimately, NASA developed a set of 30 "evidence reports" that compiled evidence linked to space travel-related risks such as cardiovascular disease, cancer, radiation syndrome, cognitive and behavioral conditions, psychiatric disorders, and bone fractures and osteoporosis. In 2013, NASA asked the IOM, and subsequently the HMD, to review the evidence reports in terms of "quality of the evidence, analysis, and overall construction of each report" (IOM, 2008a; NASEM, 2017d). Each year between 2014 and 2018, the IOM, and then the HMD, released a letter report that reviewed a subset of NASA's 30 evidence reports, identifying gaps in the content of the reports and suggesting opportunities and sources for strengthening the reports (NASEM, 2017d). In its final letter report, the committee commended NASA's evidence reports, stating that the collection "will contribute to improving the health and performance of future astronauts and enhancing future human spaceflight endeavors" (NASEM, 2017d, p. 47).

Advising SSA

The Social Security Act of 1935 established what became the SSA, which was developed to administer retirement and disability benefits in the United States. Under the umbrella of SSA disability benefits, SSA manages the Social Security Disability Insurance (SSDI) program, which was established under the Eisenhower administration in 1956, and the Supplemental Security Income (SSI) program, which was signed into law by Nixon in 1972. As the programs evolved, the SSA built a relationship with the National Academies, including the IOM and now the HMD, to provide advice related to the improvement of the SSA disability determination process. For example, in 1987 the IOM released its first report commissioned by SSA: *Pain and Disability: Clinical, Behavioral, and Public Policy Perspectives*. In its report, the committee—chaired by NAM member Arthur Kleinman[57]— reviewed available evidence on pain and described how the SSA could evaluate claims related to chronic pain (IOM, 1987). In 2004, the SSA commissioned the IOM "to study its medical procedures and criteria for determining disability and to make recommendations for improving the timeliness and accuracy of its disability decisions" (IOM, 2007e, p. 1). The committee, which was chaired by NAM member and Councilor (2003–2005) John D. Stobo,[58] produced a report that was released in 2007 called *Improving the Social Security Disability Decision Process*. The 2007 report followed an interim report released in 2006 and provided 11 recommendations to improve the processes used to make decisions regarding eligibility for disability benefits. Box 4-11 includes a list of additional reports that were commissioned to advise the SSA and the administration of its disability programs.

At the request of SSA, the HMD also formed the Standing Committee of Medical and Vocational Experts for the Social Security Administration's Disability Programs, which was tasked with surveying, collecting, and analyzing "literature, clinical practices, and published studies related to disability" (NASEM, n.d.g). The standing committee was also established to provide a neutral venue for "discussions of disability issues and the SSA's sequential evaluation process" (NASEM, n.d.g). To fulfill this objective, the committee was specifically asked to organize conferences in the Baltimore, Maryland, or Washington, DC, areas to engage the public. The standing committee serves as another mechanism by which the HMD can serve the SSA in its efforts to ensure that its disability programs are built on a strong foundation of the most up-to-date evidence and meet the needs of the programs' beneficiaries.

---

[57] Arthur Kleinman was a Professor of Medical Anthropology and Psychiatry at the Harvard Medical School and on the Faculty of Arts and Sciences at Harvard University at the time.

[58] John D. Stobo was the President of the University of Texas Medical Branch at Galveston when this report was released.

BOX 4-11
A Sample of Reports Commissioned to Advise
the Social Security Administration

- *Functional Assessment for Adults with Disabilities* (2019)
- *Opportunities for Improving Programs and Services for Children with Disabilities* (2018)
- *Health-Care Utilization as a Proxy in Disability Determination* (2018)
- *Speech and Language Disorders in Children: Implications for the Social Security Administration's Supplemental Security Income Program* (2016)
- *Informing Social Security's Process for Financial Capability Determination* (2016)
- *Psychological Testing in the Service of Disability Determination* (2015)
- *Mental Disorders and Disabilities Among Low-Income Children* (2015)
- *Cardiovascular Disability: Updating the Social Security Listings* (2010)
- *HIV and Disability: Updating the Social Security Listings* (2010)
- *Improving the Social Security Disability Decision Process* (2007)
- *The Dynamics of Disability: Measuring and Monitoring Disability for Social Security Programs* (2002)

BUILDING CAPACITY OF INTERNATIONAL SCIENCE ACADEMIES

The IOM also serves as an advisor to peer organizations around the globe, with the African Science Academy Development Initiative (ASADI) illustrating this aspect of the IOM's work with particular clarity. In 2004 the Bill & Melinda Gates Foundation awarded the National Academies a 10-year, $20 million grant "to strengthen the capability of African science academies to provide independent, evidence-supported advice to inform African government policy making and public discourse related to improving human health" (NASEM, n.d.h). Oversight of the initiative was shared between the NRC's Policy and Global Affairs division and the IOM, which created a new board called the Board on African Science Academy Development. Unlike other IOM boards, the new board would not conduct consensus studies or initiate roundtables or forums; instead it would offer advice and support to 14 African science academies with an emphasis on developing "infrastructure, personnel, relationships between the academy and its government, and rigorous procedures for providing policy advice" (NASEM, n.d.h).

The stated goal of the ASADI was "to develop African science academies so that they are regarded as trusted sources of credible scientific advice in each nation" (NASEM, n.d.h). The project originally concentrated on science academies in seven countries, with Nigeria, South Africa, and Uganda competitively selected to participate in the program "at the most intensive level," with an emphasis on capacity building. As the academies matured and achieved greater degrees of independence and proven capacity, they "graduated" from the program. The Academy of Science of South Africa, for example, achieved financial self-sustainability and graduated from the program in 2011. The Ugandan Academy remained in the program until 2014, when the ASADI grant ended. The ASADI sent staff and members from the National Academies to each of the countries to work directly with local personnel, sharing knowledge, insights, and best practices. Throughout the lifespan of ASADI, the National Academies needed to maintain a careful balance in offering advice and encouraging growth and independence among the African science academies without heavily influencing the direction of the academies or dictating to the host countries, unconsciously echoing past imperialist and colonialist administrations.

As part of the ASADI, an annual conference was hosted by one of the African academies. The primary goals of the conferences were to "enhance cooperation among African science academies, strengthen relationships among representatives of the academies and the policymaking community, and foster a greater understanding and appreciation of the value of evidence-based policy advice" (NASEM, n.d.h). The conferences also provided an opportunity for National Academies' staff to further engage with staff from the African academies. Not all of the ASADI activities took place in Africa. Officials from the African science academies also visited the United States to observe the IOM and the National Academies in action. In September 2009, the Board on African Science Academy Development, working in collaboration with the Network of African Science Academies, hosted a week-long training program in Washington, DC, for 23 African program and research staff. The participants engaged in sessions on how the IOM conducts its work and develops evidence-based recommendations in the United States, as well as discussions of the various models of convening activities the IOM uses, such as forums, roundtables, and consensus studies, to fulfill its mission as advisor to the nation.[59]

CONCLUSION

Improvements in human health—from disease prevention to cure—depend on advances in biomedical research and the translation of research findings into clinical and public health policy and practice. Throughout its history, the IOM was fully committed to advancing scientific research in order to realize better health outcomes and well-being across the life course for all populations. Over the years, the IOM was called on to provide recommendations in a wide range of scientific areas, such as those described in this chapter—including human genome research, vaccine safety and efficacy, childhood and adolescent development, and cancer. Thanks to the dedication and expertise of the IOM's leadership, members, and committee members, the IOM was able to provide unbiased evidence-based recommendations on how best to facilitate progress in research to a range of government agencies, nonprofit organizations, and international partners. Through its forums, roundtables, and standing committees, the IOM was also able to bring together representatives from academia, government, the pharmaceutical and health care industries, and other interested stakeholders and experts to have conversations that might not otherwise be possible. Today, the NAM and the HMD continue the IOM's legacy to facilitate and promote the acceleration of biomedical research and its translation, whenever possible, while also maintaining responsible and equitable research practices that comply with agreed-upon ethical standards and regulations.

---

[59] "IOM Council Board Report: Board on African Science Academy Development," September 2011, IOM/NAM Records.

5

U.S. Health Care and Policy

"Human beings, in all lines of work, make errors. Errors can be prevented by designing systems that make it hard for people to do the wrong thing and easy for people to do the right thing." —To Err Is Human (IOM, 2000a)

This quote, from the preface of *To Err Is Human: Building a Safer Health System,* focuses on a single piece of health care quality: preventing medical errors. However, it signals a broader theme that has underpinned nearly all of the Institute of Medicine's (IOM's), and subsequently the National Academy of Medicine's (NAM's) and the Health and Medicine Division's (HMD's), work—a recognition that the system as a whole needs to be improved in order to realize the quadruple aim of satisfactory patient experience, improved population health, sustainable costs, and improved clinician well-being. The IOM, and later the NAM and the HMD, have produced a robust body of work aimed at understanding and influencing the complex and evolving contexts and components that make up the U.S. health care system. Throughout its history, the organization has taken a leading role in guiding improvements related to quality, access, value, and measurement with the goal of establishing a continuously improving health system.

This chapter contains examples of areas in which the IOM made distinctive contributions that helped shape and refine the policies, processes, and outcomes of U.S. health care related to quality and safety, health care professional education and patient empowerment, health care reform and the availability of health insurance, and health care for complex illnesses and conditions. Underlying all of the work highlighted in this chapter is a foundational theme of quality—from providing high-quality cancer and end-of-life care to enhancing the health care workforce and the health information technology (IT) infrastructure employed across the health care system. The activities described in this chapter were facilitated by IOM, NAM, or HMD staff alongside expert volunteers from among the NAM membership as well as externally.

BUILDING A CULTURE OF HEALTH CARE QUALITY

To Err Is Human, published in 2000, became one of the IOM's most recognizable studies and put the organization on the map as the ultimate authority on health care quality. But the origins of the IOM's focus on quality began many years earlier, with a study in response to the Omnibus Budget Reconciliation Act of 1986. As Medicare spending continued to grow through the 1970s and 1980s, the program came under increasing political scrutiny, and questions about how Medicare costs could be contained while also maintaining quality began to emerge (Davis and Burner, 1995; IOM, 1990b). The 1986 legislation included a provision that called for a study to define quality and develop a strategy for setting priorities to ensure that care delivered through Medicare met that definition. To complete the task, the IOM assembled a committee that worked from 1987 to 1990 to draft a three-part series of reports with a set of recommendations that offered an "ambitious and far-reaching strategic plan for assessing and assuring the quality of medical care for the elderly during the next decade" (IOM, 1990b, p. xi).

The first volume in the series—*Medicare: A Strategy for Quality Assurance*—was released in 1990. It highlighted "a broad concern among the health professions about the quality of health care" coupled with a "rising dissatisfaction about the health care system on the part of the public and policymakers" (IOM, 1990b, p. 1). The report, although centered on the Medicare program, considered quality of care across the health care system more broadly. The committee, which was chaired by NAM member and Councilor (2002–2004) Steven A. Schroeder,[1] defined health care quality as "the degree to which health services for individuals and populations increase the likelihood of desired health outcomes and are consistent with current professional knowledge" (p. 4). In conjunction with the definition, the committee identified three main categories of quality deficiencies: overuse of unnecessary and inappropriate services, underuse of needed services, and "poor technical or interpersonal performance by practitioners and institutions" (p. xvi). According to the committee, neither Medicare nor the health care system had a "direct mandate to measure, assure or improve the quality of care" (Lohr and Harris-Wehling, 1991, p. 6). The report influenced medical practice and policy in the United States and expressed the IOM's general vision of what the health care system should be.

When Kenneth Shine arrived as president of the IOM in 1992, he queried members about what priority topics the IOM should explore in the coming years. A significant number indicated that they would like to see the IOM become more active in the area of health care quality. At the time, Shine noted, Ford Motor Company was leveraging "quality" as a value to outsell Japanese car makers, and "everyone thought their doctor and hospital was quality."[2] Under Shine's leadership, therefore, the IOM launched a 3-year initiative on health care quality. This initiative was unique in that the request came from the IOM members rather than the government. Expansive in its thinking, the IOM Council envisioned the initiative cutting across all of the IOM's boards. To define the scope and structure of the initiative, the IOM established a steering committee—chaired by external volunteer Walter J. McNerney[3]—that prompted the IOM Council to issue a white paper. The IOM printed 5,000 copies and widely disseminated the white paper to IOM members; congressional staff; key government stakeholders at the federal, state, and local levels; and health professional and consumer groups.[4] The paper noted that the U.S. health care system was in a state of transition, moving from a "traditional" model—in which physicians had considerable

---

[1] Steven A. Schroeder was the Chair of the Division of General Internal Medicine at the University of California, San Francisco, when this report was released.

[2] Private correspondence, Ken Shine to Laura H. DeStefano, April 18, 2020.

[3] Walter J. McNerney was a Professor of Health Policy and a Consultant at the J.L. Kellogg Graduate School of Management at Northwestern University.

[4] IOM Council Minutes, April 11–12, 1994, IOM/NAM Records.

autonomy—to a managed care model. As this transition proceeded, the paper emphasized that the nation could not lose sight of the "urgent need to monitor and improve the quality of health and the effectiveness of health care" (IOM, 1994c, p. viii).[5]

The steering committee continued to meet through 1995, while the IOM explored options to expand its health care quality portfolio.[6] The key development from these efforts was the creation of the National Roundtable on Health Care Quality in 1995. The roundtable offered a "nonadversarial environment to explore ongoing rapid changes in the medical marketplace and the implications of those changes for the quality of health and health care in this nation" (IOM, 1998b, p. 5). The members of the roundtable, who came from government, academia, private industry, and the health media, initiated a variety of quality-related activities that included workshops, commissioned papers, and "periodic statements for the nation on quality of care matters" (IOM, 1998b, p. 5).

In the fall of 1996, the roundtable held a workshop on measuring quality. Although technical in nature, the workshop promulgated a new "process improvement" approach to quality that reversed previous assumptions. For example, this new approach suggested that quality controls could save money rather than cost money in the long run. Furthermore, quality needed to be incorporated into ongoing processes, rather than measured retrospectively. "Integrating Strategies for Health Care Improvements" became the subject of a second workshop the following year. In 1998, the roundtable released a statement outlining major conclusions from its work. The "Statement on Quality of Care" built on the IOM's previous work related to Medicare and on the 1994 white paper from the IOM Council (IOM, 1998b). The statement highlighted the pressing need for improvements and indicated that health care quality in the United States would not improve until the nation "undertook a major, systematic effort to overhaul how we deliver health care services, educate and train clinicians, and assess and improve quality" (IOM, 1998b, p. 10).

The work of the National Roundtable on Health Care Quality and the IOM Council affirmed that health care quality was an appropriate focus for future IOM activities. At the beginning of 1997, Board on Health Care Services Chair and NAM member Don Detmer[7] suggested the IOM's efforts represented an "incomplete conceptual framework" with strategies that were too "imprecise to shape the future meaning of health care quality in our nation." Shine emphasized the need for consistency in the IOM's role in quality discussions and believed that the intersection between quality and value might be a good place for additional IOM work.[8] The IOM proceeded by launching a Special Initiative on Health Care Quality that included a Quality Initiative Coordinating Committee, which was designed to oversee the IOM's health care quality activities and ensure the consistency Shine envisioned.[9]

By March 1998, the Board on Health Care Services had prepared a proposal for a Committee on Quality of Health Care in America, which stemmed from a perceived lack of information on the prevalence of health care quality problems and how changes to care delivery might improve quality. The Board felt that the existing roundtable efforts were important, but that it was necessary to undertake a consensus study, with its ability to draw conclusions and make formal recommendations. The Executive Committee of the IOM Council approved the ambitious study in February 1998, and on August 11, 1998, Shine wrote to William C. Richardson, head of the Kellogg Foun-

---

[5] "America's Health in Transition: Protecting and Improving the Quality of Health and Health Care," in materials to accompany IOM Council Meeting, July 19, 1994, IOM/NAM Records.

[6] "America's Health Care in Transition: Protecting and Improving Health and the Quality of Health Care," memo describing the key points of the Institute of Medicine Special Initiative, December 1999, IOM/NAM Records.

[7] Don Detmer was the Vice President of Health Sciences at the University of Virginia during this time.

[8] IOM Council Minutes, January 6–7, 1997, IOM/NAM Records.

[9] "Draft Charge to the Quality Initiative Coordinating Committee," in materials for IOM Council Meeting, January 6–7, 1997, IOM/NAM Records.

dation, confirming his appointment as chair of the committee.[10,11] Janet Corrigan, Senior Board Director of the Board on Health Care Services and a well-respected quality expert in her own right, would serve as the Director of the IOM's Quality of Health Care in America project. Under Richardson and Corrigan's leadership, the committee was organized into two subcommittees that worked semi-autonomously, holding independent meetings and information-gathering sessions: the Subcommittee on Quality Improvement Strategies for Health Care in the United States—chaired by NAM member Donald Berwick[12]—and the Subcommittee on Creating an External Environment for Quality—co-chaired by external volunteer J. Cris Bisgard[13] and NAM member Molly Joel Coye.[14] The committee with its subcommittees would eventually produce two reports: *To Err Is Human: Building a Safer Health System* (IOM, 2000a) and *Crossing the Quality Chasm: A New Health System for the 21st Century* (IOM, 2001d).

To Err Is Human: Building a Safer Health System

Released on November 29, 1999, the committee's first report, *To Err Is Human,* illuminated the scale of medical errors and patient safety gaps in the United States. In the report's preface, Committee Chair Richardson set the tone of the report, stating that humans in all lines of work made errors, but many could be prevented "by designing systems that make it hard for people to do the wrong thing and easy for people to do the right thing" (IOM, 2000a, p. ix). The report highlighted specific examples of startling medical errors that resulted in death (e.g., a chemotherapy overdose, use of incorrect drugs) or significant injury (e.g., amputation of the wrong limb). By extrapolating data from studies on adverse events in hospitals, the committee indicated that between 44,000 and 98,000 deaths could be attributed to medical errors, representing the eighth leading cause of death in the United States, noting that more people died from medical errors than died from motor vehicle accidents, breast cancer, AIDS, or workplace injuries.

Despite the magnitude of the problem, the committee stated that a cycle of inaction had developed, and emphasized that the status quo was unacceptable. Patients were being harmed by "the same health care system that is supposed to offer healing and comfort" (IOM, 2000a, p. 3). The report indicated that safety needed to be built into the care process using a systems approach to patient safety. The committee's stated goal was to disrupt the cycle of inaction and offer a roadmap that would lead to improvements over the next 10 years. The committee made recommendations in four major areas: national efforts to "enhance the knowledge base about safety," mandatory and voluntary reporting efforts to identify and learn from errors, efforts to "raise standards and expectations for improvements in safety," and efforts to create safety systems and implement safe practices at the delivery level (p. 6). The committee acknowledged that significant changes would be required across the health care system to create a culture of safety. However, the estimated costs associated with preventable medical errors in terms of lives lost (as many as 98,000) and dollars spent ($17–$29 billion) indicated a resounding need for change.

---

[10] Board on Health Services, For Action, New Project, "Quality of Health Care in America," March 10, 1998, IOM/NAM Records.

[11] Kenneth I. Shine to William Richardson, August 11, 1998, IOM/NAM Records.

[12] Donald Berwick was the President and the Chief Executive Officer of the Institute for Healthcare Improvement during this time. Berwick served as a member of the NAM Council from 2002 to 2007 and on the HMD's Division Committee from 2016 to 2019.

[13] J. Cris Bisgard was the Director of Health Services at Delta Airlines at the time.

[14] Molly Joel Coye was the Senior Vice President and the Director of the Lewin Group's West Coast office during this time.

To Err Is Human's Impact

Upon its release, *To Err Is Human* received more media coverage than any report up to that point in the IOM's history. The IOM for the first time had hired a public relations firm to boost the exposure of the report.[15] Television networks ran stories on the release of the report, as did nearly all of the nation's major newspapers. Coverage also extended beyond the United States, reaching Germany and England. The coverage came in waves, with many media outlets and newspapers running follow-up stories. As the report attracted media, it was also evaluated by the health care community. The Blue Cross Blue Shield Association applauded the report, and the American Medical Association issued a favorable statement. However, not all responses were positive. Troyen Brennan, who was affiliated with Brigham and Women's Hospital, wrote a critical article in the *New England Journal of Medicine* in April 2000, highlighting potential flaws in the report's methodology and questioning the practicality of its recommendations (Brennan, 2000).[16] Lucian Leape, a committee member and professor at Harvard's School of Public Health at the time, defended the IOM's report in a July 2000 *JAMA* article, concluding that the report had "galvanized a national movement to improve patient safety" (Leape, 2000).

The report garnered immediate attention from the White House and President Clinton (Pear, 2000). Clinton made it clear that health care quality would become a policy priority for his administration. Following the meeting with Richardson and IOM staff, Clinton ordered a series of executive actions. He required that the private health insurance plans that participated in the Federal Employee Health Benefits Program implement quality improvement and patient safety initiatives. He also instructed federal agencies that administered health plans, such as the Department of Veterans Affairs (VA) and the Centers for Medicare & Medicaid Services (CMS), to evaluate and implement error reduction technologies where feasible. He announced the reauthorization of the Agency for Healthcare Research and Quality (AHRQ), and Congress then appropriated $50 million annually for patient safety research through AHRQ.[17] The IOM developed a close working relationship with John Eisenberg, then the Director of AHRQ. Clinton also directed the Office of Management and Budget to develop additional error prevention and health care quality initiatives. The White House cited the IOM report as the basis for these actions,[18] which would initiate some of the systematic changes the committee had envisioned in order to promote a safer health care system. The report also fed into the work of the National Quality Forum (NQF), which had been established less than 1 year prior, in 1999.

Congress was also quick to respond to the report. Senator James Jeffords (R-VT) asserted that the number of fatalities and injuries associated with medical errors must be reduced, stating that the Senate Committee on Health, Education, Labor, and Pensions would spearhead a "comprehensive approach to improving patient safety." His colleague Arlen Spector (R-PA) called the report "a matter of enormous importance" and vowed that the Appropriations Subcommittee on Labor, Health and Human Services and Education would hold hearings to determine how much money should be appropriated to respond to the problem (Goldstein, 1999; Pear, 1999; *Philadelphia Inquirer*, 1999). The Senate Appropriations Committee included language in the appropriations bill for fiscal year 2001 that instructed the AHRQ to initiate "the development of guidance on the collection of uniform data on patient safety." Meanwhile, states also pursued laws to reduce medical errors. For example, Florida established a Commission on Excellence in Health Care to develop a statewide strategy for improving health care delivery through "meaningful reporting standards." The state of

---

[15] Private correspondence, Kenneth Shine to Laura H. DeStefano, April 18, 2020.

[16] IOM Council Minutes, October 17–18, 2000. IOM/NAM Records.

[17] Impact of IOM Reports (Database), IOM/NAM Records.

[18] "Clinton-Gore Administration Takes New Steps to Improve Health Care Quality and Ensure Patient Safety," December 7, 1999, White House news release, IOM/NAM Records.

Washington passed a law that required its Department of Health to publicly disclose information it received regarding medical errors, and by 2007, at least 23 states had implemented similar requirements for reporting medical errors.[19]

In July 2005, President George W. Bush enacted the Patient Safety and Quality Improvement Act of 2005, which cited the IOM's report *To Err Is Human* as its impetus (see Figure 4-8). The overarching purpose of the legislation was to "improve patient safety by encouraging voluntary and confidential reporting of events that adversely affect patients" (AHRQ, n.d.). One of the provisions of the law established Patient Safety Organizations (PSOs), which would be designed "to collect, aggregate, and analyze confidential information reported by health care providers." Three years after the law was enacted, the Department of Health and Human Services (HHS) released regulations for the PSOs, which had been recommended by the IOM report. In 2008, a *New York Times* article credited *To Err Is Human* as the catalyst for the growing patient safety movement in the United States (Sack, 2008).

Crossing the Quality Chasm, 2001

The IOM released the Committee on Quality of Health Care in America's second report—*Crossing the Quality Chasm: A New Health System for the 21st Century*—on March 1, 2001. While *To Err Is Human* concentrated specifically on medical errors and patient safety, the new report "focused more broadly on how the health care delivery system can be designed to innovate and improve care." According to the report, the health care system required fundamental change; incremental improvements would not be sufficient. Despite many technological advances, "a highly fragmented delivery system that largely lacks even rudimentary clinical information capabilities" resulted in "poorly designed care processes characterized by unnecessary duplication of services and long waiting time and delays" (IOM, 2001d, p. 3).

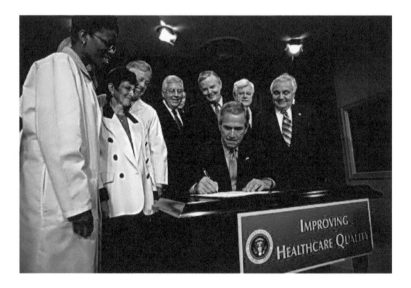

FIGURE 5-1 President George W. Bush signs the Patient Safety and Quality Improvement Act of 2005, at a signing ceremony on Friday, July 29, 2005, at the Eisenhower Executive Office Building in Washington, DC. SOURCE: White House photo by Eric Draper, White House Archives.

[19] Impact of IOM Reports (Database), IOM/NAM Records.

In its report, the committee envisioned a redesigned health care system that would be safe, effective, patient-centered, timely, efficient, and equitable—a mantra that would be repeated often in health policy circles and would become recognized as the six dimensions of quality. The redesigned health care system would need to ensure that health care delivery was evidence-based, leveraged available health information technologies, realigned payment structures with quality goals, and engaged and prepared health care professionals. To achieve this vision, the committee offered 10 guiding principles:

1. "Care is based on continuous healing relationships.
2. Care is customized according to patient needs and values.
3. The patient is the source of control.
4. Knowledge is shared and information flows freely.
5. Decision making is evidence-based.
6. Safety is a system property.
7. Transparency is necessary.
8. Needs are anticipated.
9. Waste is continuously decreased.
10. Cooperation among clinicians is a priority" (IOM, 2001d, pp. 8–9).

The committee's recommendations added specificity to its general framework. For example, the committee called on Congress to establish a "Health Care Quality Innovation Fund" to invest in projects that would lead to improved quality. The committee also called on the AHRQ to identify 15 or more of the most common, top-priority conditions and then work with stakeholders to create care processes and action plans to ensure the delivery of consistent, quality-based care for the identified conditions.

Crossing the Quality Chasm's *Impact*

Following the release of the report, most of the major television and newspaper outlets featured stories on it, all of which included reference to the previous report, *To Err Is Human*. Committee members were interviewed and widely quoted in the articles, and Molly Joel Coyle participated in a series of radio interviews that reached listeners in the major metropolitan areas across the United States.[20] Together the committee's two reports "laid out a vision for how the health care system and related policy environment must be radically transformed in order to close the chasm between what we know to be good quality care and what actually exists in practice" (NASEM, n.d.i). *To Err Is Human* had captured the nation's attention in a way the IOM had never done before, and put the IOM at the center of a media storm of unprecedented size. The IOM declaration that preventable medical errors killed more people than many of the leading causes of death caught the nation's attention. *Crossing the Quality Chasm* followed up on the success of the first report and defined strategies that should be used to reinvent the U.S. health care system to ensure that high-quality care was readily available in communities across the country (NASEM, n.d.i).

In response to the IOM's work and its two new quality reports, the Robert Wood Johnson Foundation (RWJF) partnered with the Institute of Healthcare Improvement to create a $26 million, five-part demonstration project called "Pursuing Perfection: Raising the Bar for Health Care Performance," which operated from 2001 to 2008. The demonstration project sought to "improve the performance of the seven participating health care institutions" and "demonstrate to the broader

---

[20] Saira Moini to Janet Corrigan, Linda Kohn, Shari McGuire, Susan Turner-Lowe, and Barbara Rice, March 20, 2001, transmitting "Dissemination Plans and Reports," March 19, 2001, CQHCA Files, IOM/NAM Records; "Fax Alert, U.S Health Care System Is Experiencing a Quality Gap, Says IOM," Radio Interviews Friday, March 2, 2001, CQHCA files, IOM/NAM Records; Draft Script, News/Broadcast Network, Inc., February 28, 2001.

provider community that ideal care is attainable" (RWJF, 2010, p. 1). Upon completion of the project, RWJF concluded that "the organizations transitioned from 'devoted but average performers' to national leaders in health care improvement" (p. 1). One of the grantees, the Henry Ford Health System's Behavioral Health Services, set a goal of eliminating deaths by suicide among its patient population by completely redesigning care delivery around the IOM's six dimensions of health care quality. Approximately 11 years after the implementation of the redesign, the average annual rate of suicide in the health care system's patient population dropped 80 percent—from approximately 110 per 100,000 in 1999 to approximately 36 per 100,000 in 2010—which included one year in which the health care system met its goal of zero suicides (2009) (Coffey and Coffey, 2016).

To Err Is Human and *Crossing the Quality Chasm* continue to have an impact on health care quality and safety nearly two decades after the first report was released. This continued impact is due, in part, to the ongoing commitment and subsequent studies released by the IOM, the NAM, and the HMD (described below), which over the years have led to important policy changes and an increased commitment to quality across the U.S. health care system overall. Citing widespread public and private patient safety efforts and initiatives that were sparked by *To Err Is Human* and *Crossing the Quality Chasm,* AHRQ released a report in 2014 that indicated that hospitals and health care providers nationwide made fewer mistakes in treating patients between 2010 and 2013, sparing at least 50,000 lives and saving $12 billion in health care spending (AHRQ, 2015). The report indicated that there was a cumulative decrease of 1.3 million hospital-acquired infections, representing a 17 percent decline during the same timeframe.

The Quality Chasm Series

Having established itself as a leader in the promotion of health care quality in the United States, the IOM launched a new initiative that focused on "operationalizing the vision described in the Quality Chasm report." The initiative included a new series of reports and activities that would be geared toward implementing the IOM's vision for health care quality and a culture of safety. The timing of this initiative coincided with an increased national focus on health care quality and safety, as well as patient-centered care and evidence-based medicine in an effort to reduce unnecessary costs while increasing value throughout the U.S. health care system. During this timeframe, numerous programs and initiatives were launched throughout the health care system. For example, CMS initiated a series of pay-for-performance initiatives in the early 2000s based on guidance from organizations such as the NQF and the National Committee for Quality Assurance (NCQA) (CMS, 2005). At this time, organizations and agencies such as the NQF, the NCQA, the Institute for Healthcare Improvement, The Joint Commission, the AHRQ, the CMS, and many others were also looking for opportunities to establish and apply measures that could be used to improve the health care system. As health information technologies and electronic medical records were being implemented more broadly, these new technologies allowed for the possibility of more robust data collection and analysis to serve as the foundation to guide future improvements (Burstin et al., 2016; Chassin and Loeb, 2011; IHI, 2018; The Joint Commission, n.d.).

The first three reports in the series were released in 2003. Picking up on a recommendation from *Crossing the Quality Chasm,* the first report—*Priority Areas for National Action: Transforming Health Care Quality*—identified 20 priority areas for the AHRQ, which could be used to guide public and private health care sectors toward improving the quality of health care being delivered in the United States (IOM, 2003h). The authoring committee of this report was chaired by NAM member George J. Isham.[21] The next three reports released in the series looked at improving leader-

---

[21] George J. Isham was the Medical Director and the Chief Health Officer at HealthPartners, Inc., in Minneapolis during this time.

ship in health care quality, implementing successful health care demonstration projects on a larger scale, and improving health professional education (see Box 5-1).

In January 2004, the IOM hosted a "Quality Chasm Summit," which was designed to demonstrate that the redesign of the health care system described in the Quality Chasm report was both possible and already under way in some communities. The summit examined "a discrete subset of the priority areas"[22] from the IOM's 2003 report that included "asthma, chronic heart failure, major depression, diabetes, and pain control in advanced cancer" (IOM, 2004a, p. ix). In planning the summit, the committee, which was chaired by NAM member Reed V. Tuckson,[23] identified six cross-cutting themes that served as the basis of working sessions during the summit: "measurement, information and communications technology, care coordination, patient self-management support, finance, and community coalition building" (p. 2). The overarching goal of the summit was to foster change and establish momentum, moving beyond the blueprints and guidance laid out in the reports. During the summit, leaders from 24 national-level organizations, referred to as national champions, committed to supporting continued community efforts to improve health care quality while also translating those local efforts to a larger scale.

Eventually the Quality Chasm series grew to include a dozen reports that were released between 2003 and 2015 (see Box 5-1). Following the creation of the NAM and the HMD in 2015, the focus on health care quality carried over to both organizations. The desire to apply the ideas developed in the Quality Chasm series on a global scale led to the 2018 publication of *Crossing the Global Quality Chasm: Improving Health Care Worldwide,* which was developed under the auspices of the HMD. The report followed from the World Health Organization's sustainable development goals and argued that quality needed to become as "central an agenda as universal health coverage itself." The report noted that the problems identified in the Quality Chasm series, such as fragmentation, misaligned financing, and poor training, applied not only to the U.S. health care system but to many of the health care systems around the globe. The nations of the world needed to come together "to close the enormous gaps that remain between what is achievable in human health and where human health stands today" (NASEM, 2018b) with a focus on the six dimensions of quality defined in *Crossing the Quality Chasm.* The committee, which was co-chaired by

---

BOX 5-1
The Institute of Medicine's Quality Chasm Series

- *To Err Is Human: Building a Safer Health System* (2000)
- *Crossing the Quality Chasm: A New Health System for the 21st Century* (2001)
- *Priority Areas for National Action: Transforming Health Care Quality* (2003)
- *Leadership by Example: Coordinating Government Roles in Improving Health Care Quality* (2003)
- *Fostering Rapid Advances in Health Care: Learning from System Demonstrations* (2003)
- *Health Professions Education: A Bridge to Quality* (2003)
- *Patient Safety: Achieving a New Standard for Care* (2004)
- *Keeping Patients Safe: Transforming the Work Environment of Nurses* (2004)
- *Quality Through Collaboration: The Future of Rural Health* (2005)
- *Improving the Quality of Health Care for Mental and Substance-Use Conditions* (2006)
- *Preventing Medication Errors* (2007)
- *Improving Diagnosis in Health Care* (2015)

---

[22] Ann Greiner to Bruce Alberts, March 19, 2003, Files of the Quality Chasm Summit, IOM/NAM Records.
[23] Reed V. Tuckson was the Senior Vice President of Consumer Health and Medical Care Advancement at UnitedHealth Group in Minnetonka, Minnesota, during this time.

Donald Berwick alongside external volunteer Sania Nishtar,[24] stated that quality improvements would "require investment, responsibility, and accountability on the part of health system leaders" at the global level (p. 6).

The findings and recommendations from the IOM's Quality Chasm Series resulted in a variety of impacts, from the local to the national level, with the common goal of improving patient safety and health care quality in the United States. The IOM's 2007 report, *Preventing Medication Errors* (IOM, 2007f), which was drafted by a committee co-chaired by NAM member J. Lyle Bootman[25] and external volunteer Linda R. Cronenwett,[26] resulted in a range of notable changes based on its recommendations. For example, in February 2008, the BayCare Health System and University of Southern Florida Health announced that they would "lead the deployment of free, web-based electronic prescribing to all physicians in the Tampa Bay area as the regional sponsors of National ePrescribing Patient Safety Initiative (NEPSI)." The purpose of NEPSI was to remove the barriers to electronic prescribing as a mechanism to reduce errors associated with handwritten prescriptions. On the federal level, the Medicare Electronic Medication and Safety Protection (E-MEDS) Act of 2007 was introduced in both the House and Senate in response to the IOM's recommendation to implement electronic prescribing for all prescriptions by 2010. In July 2008, HHS Secretary Michael Leavitt announced a new program in which Medicare would provide incentive payments to health care providers who used e-prescribing. Extrapolating data presented in the IOM report, HHS estimated that the new program could save Medicare as much as $156 million over a period of 5 years due to reductions in medication errors and increased efficiencies associated with e-prescribing.[27]

As the NAM established its new programs and ongoing activities in 2015, the organization continued the IOM's focus on quality, which became a cross-cutting theme that was a core part of its work. For example, the NAM's Action Collaborative on Clinician Well-Being and Resilience focused on supporting the well-being of the health care workforce, as burnout among health care workers has been shown to lead to low-quality care and an increase in medical errors (NAM, n.d.b). In 2019, the NAM published a consensus report that built on the work of the CWB Action Collaborative titled *Taking Action Against Clinician Burnout: A Systems Approach to Professional Well-Being* (NASEM, 2019h). The report cited *To Err Is Human* as a foundation for the study and a model for systemic change that was needed in the area of clinician well-being. The NAM's other programs (e.g., the NAM Leadership Consortium: Collaboration for a Value & Science-Driven Health System, Future of Nursing 2020–2030 Initiative, Vital Directions for Health and Health Care Policy Initiative) also featured high-quality health care as an underlying driver to realizing improvements in health and well-being for populations across the United States. The NAM's programs are discussed in more detail in Chapter 7.

Safety and Quality of Abortion Care

The IOM first examined the public health impact of abortion in 1975, just 2 years after the U.S. Supreme Court's decision in *Roe v. Wade* legalized abortion in the United States. *Legalized Abortion and the Public Health: Report of a Study* contained a comprehensive analysis of the scientific evidence that was available at the time (IOM, 1975). The organization did not revisit the subject until 2018, when the National Academies released a study on *The Safety and Quality of Abortion*

---

[24] Sania Nishtar was the founder of Heartfile, a health policy organization in Islamabad, Pakistan.

[25] J. Lyly Bootman was the Dean and a Professor at the University of Arizona College of Pharmacy and the Founding and the Executive Director of the University of Arizona Center for Health Outcomes and PharmacoEconomic (HOPE) Research at the time.

[26] Linda R. Cronenwett was a Professor and the Dean of the School of Nursing at the University of North Carolina at Chapel Hill when this report was published.

[27] Impact of IOM Reports (Database), IOM/NAM Records.

Care in the United States that examined the current state of the science, drawing on evidence from randomized clinical trials, systematic reviews, and epidemiological studies. The report found that the quality of abortion care varied according to where a patient lived and noted that state regulations aimed at limiting access to abortion threatened the provision of safe care (NASEM, 2018j).[28]

A VALUE AND SCIENCE-DRIVEN HEALTH SYSTEM

Recognizing the intricate connections across evidence, quality, and value and the need for a more permanent convening activity to explore these connections and catalyze change across the health care system, the IOM launched the Roundtable on Evidence-Based Medicine in April 2005. J. Michael McGinnis, then a senior scholar and visiting fellow, assumed leadership of the roundtable. The roundtable's mission was to create a neutral venue in which stakeholders, such as health care providers, employers, payers, and researchers, could discuss ways to generate and apply better data to clinical decision making, thus improving quality and assuring value. The roundtable's mission complemented the six dimensions of quality, with particular emphasis on greater efficacy in health care services. In 2010, the Roundtable on Evidence-Based Medicine evolved into the Roundtable on Value & Science-Driven Health Care. The new iteration of the roundtable developed a charter to guide its activities that included a vision, goals, and a set of core concepts and principles. The roundtable promoted science-driven health care, indicating that, "to the greatest extent possible, the decisions that shape the health and health care of Americans ... will be grounded on a reliable evidence base, will account appropriately for individual variations in patient needs, and will support the generation of new insights on clinical effectiveness" (IOM, 2011d, pp. xi–xii).[29]

The overarching goal of the roundtable was to foster a "learning health system" that cultivated and supplied "the best evidence for the collaborative health care choices of each patient and provider" (p. xi). Throughout its 10-year history the roundtable released 20 publications, most of which comprised the roundtable's Learning Health System series (NAM, 2017a). The series featured summaries of presentations and discussions from the roundtable's workshops, as well as papers from leading experts. During this time, the roundtable also released numerous discussion papers and commentaries designed to stimulate advances and the implementation of science in health care. Over the course its work, the roundtable established six "innovation collaboratives" in areas such as best practices, clinical effectiveness research, and digital learning, which were developed to encourage information sharing and accelerate change.[30]

Best Care at Lower Cost

Building on the work of the Roundtable on Value & Science-Driven Health Care, the IOM convened a committee, chaired by NAM member Mark D. Smith,[31] to offer recommendations on how to transform the U.S. health care system into a learning health care system. The study examined the challenges and opportunities related to quality and safety, health outcomes, cost and value, and access and equity. The committee highlighted the rapid growth of biomedical research, advances in innovative treatments and therapies, and the ability to manage chronic conditions that were once fatal. However, the committee concluded that the health care system continued to fall

---

[28] In June 2024, the U.S. Supreme Court overturned the *Roe v. Wade* decision, threatening access to safe abortion care for millions of women in the United States, particularly women of color, poor women, and women living in rural areas (see https://www.nationalacademies.org/news/2022/06/decision-to-overturn-roe-v-wade-could-worsen-reproductive-health-in-u-s-exacerbate-health-inequities).

[29] "IOM Program Plan & Operations Overview 2005," pp. 10–11, IOM/NAM Records.

[30] See https://nam.edu/programs/value-science-driven-health-care.

[31] Mark D. Smith was the President and the Chief Executive Officer at the California Health Care Foundation at the time.

short in fundamental ways; for example, clinical practice and education lagged behind scientific research, and care continued to be fragmented and uncoordinated, resulting in an estimated $750 billion in unnecessary health care spending in 2009 (IOM, 2013e). The committee summarized three "imperatives" for change: "the rising complexity of modern health care, unsustainable cost increases, and outcomes below the system's potential" (NAM, n.d.a).

The committee's 2013 report, *Best Care at Lower Cost: The Path to Continuously Learning Health Care in America,* emphasized that it was possible to improve health care quality and reduce costs by realizing a vision in which "science and informatics, patient-clinician partnerships, incentives, and culture are aligned to promote and enable continuous and real-time improvement in both the effectiveness and efficiency of care" (IOM, 2013e, p. 17). The committee offered 10 recommendations along with specific strategies that could be employed to fulfill its vision for a continuously learning health care system. The recommendations reinforced messages from previous IOM work. While they seemed idealistic in some ways, many of them depended on creating tools to apply and disseminate already existing knowledge.

Measuring What Matters

Achieving a learning health care system requires access to high-quality data from defined quality measures. In 2015 the IOM released *Vital Signs: Core Metrics for Health and Health Care Progress.* The committee, which was chaired by NAM member David Blumenthal,[32] was tasked with reviewing existing quality measures, identifying gaps in those measures and systems, and establishing priorities for measures that would contribute to a "continuously learning and improving health system" (NASEM, n.d.j). The study was conducted at a time when the number of measures was expanding rapidly and policy makers were focused on "measuring the value of health services and rewarding providers who improved it." The committee concluded that "although many of these measures provide useful information, their sheer number, as well as their lack of focus, consistency, and organization, limits their overall effectiveness in improving performance of the health system" (IOM, 2015a). To remedy the situation, the committee identified "a set of standardized measures required at national, state, local, and institutional levels" and recommended steps "to implement and refine" the measures. The 15 core measures—which included life expectancy, overweight and obesity, and addictive behavior—were meant to be "parsimonious, outcomes-oriented, reflective of system performance, meaningful and had utility at multiple levels." Through its recommendations, the committee's overarching goal was to ensure "better health at lower cost for all Americans" (Blumenthal and McGinnis, 2015; IOM, 2015a,b).

Health Information Technology and Digital Infrastructure

Measuring quality and health outcomes with the goal of improving clinical decision making and overall health care required a robust health IT infrastructure. From early discussions of health IT, the IOM supported the introduction, use, and integration of electronic medical records, data collection systems, and telemedicine as a mechanism to improve health care. For example, in 1991 the IOM released a report called *The Computer-Based Patient Record: An Essential Technology for Health Care.* The committee that produced the report, which was chaired by Don Detmer,[33] concluded that electronic records should be "the standard for medical and all other records related to health care" (IOM, 1997a, p. 50). The IOM also examined the potential benefits of telemedicine and how new technologies could be implemented to expand access to care in the 1996 report

---

[32] David Blumenthal was the President of The Commonwealth Fund during this time.

[33] Don E. Detmer was a Professor of Surgery and Business Administration and the Vice President for Health Sciences at the University of Virginia when this report was released.

Telemedicine: A Guide to Assessing Telecommunications for Health Care, which was drafted by a committee chaired by John Ball.[34] This report presented a framework for assessing the quality, accessibility, and cost of these technologies (IOM, 1996b). Despite the potential benefits of health IT solutions, the IOM recognized the importance of maintaining privacy when capturing and using electronic data in health care and research in a number of reports, including *Health Data in the Information Age: Use, Disclosure, and Privacy* (IOM, 1994b), *Protecting Data Privacy in Health Services Research* (IOM, 2000n), and *Ensuring the Integrity, Accessibility, and Stewardship of Research Data in the Digital Age* (NAS et al., 2009).

Health IT and data collection efforts in the digital age were also discussed by the Roundtable on Value & Science-Driven Health Care. For example, the roundtable held a workshop in 2010 that resulted in a workshop summary called *Digital Infrastructure for the Learning Health System: The Foundation for Continuous Improvement in Health and Health Care* (IOM, 2011j). Workshop participants discussed how advances in health information technology could reshape the delivery of health care in fundamental ways, from communication between care providers and patients to instant access to the most up-to-date evidence base. In addition to the potential benefits, the summary and workshop participants also considered potential security risks, privacy concerns, and possible interoperability issues associated with the wide-scale implementation of health IT systems.

In 2012, the IOM released *Health IT and Patient Safety: Building Safer Systems for Better Care*—a consensus report that bridged the IOM's interests in quality and safety with the appropriate use of technology in a learning health care system. The committee, chaired by NAM member Gail L. Warden,[35] recognized that health IT was not a panacea for the system's problems. As the report noted, "designed and applied inappropriately, health IT can add an additional layer of complexity to the already complex delivery of health care" (IOM, 2012d, p. 2). If, however, the technologies were "designed, implemented, and used appropriately, [they could] be a positive enabler to transform the way care is delivered (IOM, 2012d, p. 2). The report called for a coordinated effort to better understand the possible safety risks of health IT by encouraging better information flow, establishing mechanisms for reporting and investigating injuries and deaths connected with health IT failures, and taking proactive steps to "ensure that health IT is developed and implemented with safety as a primary focus" (IOM, 2012d, p. 13). In 2013, HHS released its "Health IT Patient Safety Action and Surveillance Plan," which was built on the IOM's recommendations and was designed to guide health IT activities across HHS and improve health care safety through the implementation of health IT. The plan, which also called for private-sector collaboration, included an appendix that compared the recommendations from the IOM report with HHS's proposed actions (ONC, 2013).

The NAM Leadership Consortium

When the NAM was created in 2015, the Roundtable on Value & Science-Drive Health Care evolved into the NAM Leadership Consortium: Collaboration for a Value & Science-Driven Health System, becoming one of the NAM's largest and most active programs. The Consortium provides "a trusted venue for national leaders in health and health care to work cooperatively toward their common commitment to effective, innovative care that consistently adds value to patients and society" (NAM, n.d.c). The initial membership of the consortium included several members of the former IOM roundtable, including NAM member Mark McClellan, a past commissioner of the FDA and administrator of CMS, as the chair (see Box 5-2). The consortium continued the roundtable's tradition of holding workshops, operating standing forums called "innovation collaboratives," and publishing discussion papers and commentaries through the *NAM Perspectives* platform. The consortium also expanded its portfolio to include NAM special publications (see Chapter 7).

---

[34] John R. Ball was the Chair, the President, and the Chief Executive Officer of the Pennsylvania Hospital in Philadelphia during this time.

[35] Gail L. Warden was the President Emeritus of the Henry Ford Health System in Detroit when this report was released.

BOX 5-2
Initial Membership of the National Academy of Medicine
Leadership Consortium: Collaboration for a Value &
Science-Driven Health System (October 2015)

- Mark McClellan (*Chair*), Brookings Institution
- Raymond Baxter, Kaiser Permanente
- Paul Bleicher, Optum Labs
- David Blumenthal, The Commonwealth Fund
- Paul Chew, Sanofi U.S.
- Carolyn Clancy, Office of the Under Secretary for Health
- Patrick Conway, Centers for Medicare & Medicaid Services
- Susan DeVore, Premier Healthcare Alliance
- Judith Faulkner, Epic Systems Corporation
- David Feinberg, Geisinger Health System
- Joseph Fifer, Healthcare Financial Management Association
- Thomas Frieden, Centers for Disease Control and Prevention
- Patricia Gabow, Denver Health
- Atul Gawande, Brigham and Women's Hospital; Harvard University
- James Heywood, PatientsLikeMe
- Kathy Hudson, National Institutes of Health
- Paul Hudson, AstraZeneca
- Brent C. James, Intermountain Healthcare
- Craig A. Jones, Vermont Blueprint for Health
- Gary Kaplan, Virginia Mason Health System
- Darrell Kirch, Association of American Medical Colleges
- Richard E. Kuntz, Medtronic, Inc.
- Richard Larson, Massachusetts Institute of Technology
- Peter Long, Blue Shield of California Foundation
- Peter Lurie, Food and Drug Administration
- James L. Madara, American Medical Association
- Mary D. Naylor, University of Pennsylvania
- William D. Novelli, Georgetown University
- Sam Nussbaum, WellPoint, Inc.
- Jonathan B. Perlin, HCA
- Richard Platt, Harvard Pilgrim Health Care Institute
- Richard J. Pollack, American Hospital Association
- Chesley Richards, Centers for Disease Control and Prevention
- Michael Rosenblatt, Merck & Co., Inc.
- John W. Rowe, Columbia University
- Leonard D. Schaeffer, University of Southern California
- Joe Selby, Patient-Centered Outcomes Research Institute
- Mark D. Smith, California Health Care Foundation
- Harrison C. Spencer, Association of Schools and Programs of Public Health
- Marta Tellado, Consumer Reports
- David Torchiana, Partners HealthCare System, Inc.
- Reed V. Tuckson, UnitedHealth Group
- Debra Whitman, AARP

Ex Officio

- Francis Collins, National Institutes of Health
- Karen DeSalvo, Department of Health and Human Services
- Richard Kronick, Agency for Healthcare Research and Quality
- James Macrae, Health Resources and Services Administration
- Stephen Ostroff, Food and Drug Administration
- David Shulkin, Department of Veterans Affairs
- Andrew Slavitt, Centers for Medicare & Medicaid Services
- Jonathan Woodson, Department of Defense

By 2021, the Leadership Consortium had converted its former "innovation collaboratives" to "Action Collaboratives" under the new NAM model (see Chapter 7). Those Action Collaboratives included:

- Culture, Inclusion, and Equity: Advancing a culture of health equity and engagement that places the needs of people and communities at its core.
- Evidence Mobilization: Supporting the conditions necessary for transforming real-world experiences into valuable data that are routinely used to improve population and patient-level health.
- Digital Health: Fostering improvements and innovation in digital infrastructure so that health technology is developed and applied in ways that consistently lead to better population and patient-level health.
- Value Incentives and Systems: Supporting payment systems that incentivize value and population health.

In 2021, the Consortium undertook a comprehensive sector-by-sector assessment of the health system's response to the COVID-19 pandemic, with an emphasis on determining opportunities for improvement (described further in Chapter 7).

HEALTH DISPARITIES AND HEALTH EQUITY

As the IOM developed its Quality Chasm series, it also undertook a parallel effort to study one of the six dimensions of quality identified in *Crossing the Quality Chasm*—equity. Although the IOM had considered disparities in health care previously (IOM, 1991b, 1993b, 1996c, 2000c), this new initiative would be the first time the IOM delved deeply into health disparities and potential solutions to ensure greater equity across the U.S. health care system. Health equity would emerge as one of the organization's ongoing priorities that would be examined across a wide range of reports, workshops, and other activities.

In 1999, Congress requested an IOM study focused on "understanding and reducing racial and ethnic disparities in health care." The goal of the study was to assess racial and ethnic differences in health care that could not be attributed to factors such as insurance coverage or the ability to pay. The study would also concentrate on the role of bias, discrimination, and stereotyping in health outcomes.[36] The resulting report, *Unequal Treatment: Confronting Racial and Ethnic Disparities in Health Care*, was released in 2002 and would be recognized as one of the IOM's seminal works. During its deliberations, the committee, which was chaired by NAM member and Councilor (1985–1987) Alan R. Nelson,[37] identified a large body of evidence that indicated that racial and ethnic minorities in the United States received lower quality health care, were less likely to receive routine medical care, and experienced higher rates of morbidity and mortality than non-minority populations. For example, African Americans had higher rates of mortality from heart disease, cancer, diabetes, and AIDS than any other racial or ethnic group.[38] The committee found evidence that "stereotyping, biases, and uncertainty on the part of healthcare providers can all contribute to unequal treatment" (IOM, 2003b, p. 1). The conditions in which clinical encounters took place— which included "high time pressure, cognitive complexity and pressures for cost-containment"—

---

[36] Susanne A. Stoiber to Mary Ann Mink, Supervisory Contract Specialist, Office of Minority Health, June 22, 2000, IOM/NAM Records.

[37] Alan R. Nelson was a retired physician and serving as a special advisor to the Chief Executive Officer of the American College of Physicians-American Society of Internal Medicine when this report was released.

[38] National Academy of Sciences, "Understanding and Reducing Racial and Ethnic Disparities in Health Care," Proposal No. 00-IOM-170-01, June 2000, IOM/NAM Records.

could "enhance the likelihood that these processes will result in care poorly matched to minority patients' needs" (IOM, 2003b, p. 1).

Eliminating disparities required a range of solutions that took into account the underlying complexities and causes of unequal treatment (IOM, 2003b). The committee offered 19 recommendations that included increasing awareness, better data collection and monitoring, and specific interventions at the health system level and also at the legal, regulatory, and policy levels. For example, the committee called for increasing the "proportion of underrepresented U.S. racial and ethnic minorities" (p. 2) in the health care workforce and cross-cultural education for health care professionals. The committee also believed that expanded patient education could lead to greater empowerment and more engagement in decision making.

Like many of the IOM's previous reports, *Unequal Treatment* received notable attention from the media with coverage from several of the nation's major news outlets. Following the release of the report, the W.K. Kellogg Foundation announced a $3.6 million initiative to "increase the diversity of America's health professions education programs at all levels of preparation." This initiative included funding for a follow-up IOM study to identify barriers that prevent schools and universities from recruiting and admitting minority candidates. This study ultimately resulted in the 2004 IOM report *In the Nation's Compelling Interest: Ensuring Diversity in the Health Care Workforce* (described below). The *Unequal Treatment* report was also the basis of legislation called the Health Equity and Accountability Act of 2009, which was introduced by Donna Christensen, U.S. Virgin Islands Delegate. The bill included several provisions that were directly in line with recommendations from the report, such as charging the CMS Office of Mental Health to consider reimbursement programs that reward quality care provided to minority populations and bolstering the HHS Office for Civil Rights to strengthen accountability.[39]

In addition to health disparities associated with racial and ethnic minorities, the IOM also explored disparities experienced by lesbian, gay, bisexual, and transgender (LGBT) populations in its 2011 report, *The Health of Lesbian, Gay, Bisexual, and Transgender People: Building a Foundation for Better Understanding*. The report, which was drafted by a committee chaired by NAM member Robert Graham,[40] found that as these populations became more "visible in society and more socially acknowledged," there was an overall lack of information available about the health status and health needs of these populations (IOM, 2011e). In its deliberations, the committee found evidence indicating that LGBT youth had higher rates of substance use, depression, and suicide than heterosexual populations. To fill existing knowledge gaps and ensure better access to high-quality, patient-centered care, the report developed a research agenda that laid out specific priority areas (e.g., social influences, health care inequalities, transgender health needs) across the lifespan. The committee concluded that "building the evidence base on LGBT health issues will not only benefit LGBT individuals but also provide new research on topics that affect heterosexual and non-gender-variant individuals as well" (p. 6).

The 2011 release of *The Health of Lesbian, Gay, Bisexual, and Transgender People* resulted in numerous actions at the federal level to improve research and reduce health disparities for these populations. For example, HHS announced new draft standards for the collection of health data and included LGBT populations for the first time, highlighting the "need for collection of gender identity and sexual orientation data on federally supported surveys," which had been emphasized by the IOM report. The National Institutes of Health (NIH) also took action based on the report, creating a cross-NIH coordinating group in 2011 called LGBT Research Coordinating Committee and releasing a funding opportunity announcement for research related to sexual and gender minorities.

---

[39] Impact of IOM Reports (Database), IOM/NAM Records.

[40] Robert Graham was the Professor of Family Medicine and Robert and Myfanwy Smith Chair in the Department of Family Medicine at the University of Cincinnati College of Medicine when this report was released.

In 2016, the agency also designated sexual and gender minorities as a health disparities population in research and developed a strategic plan to guide the NIH's research related to these populations over a 5-year period from 2016 to 2020. At a state level, in 2014, New York Governor Andrew Cuomo announced that New York State would launch a new multi-agency program to improve data collection for LGBT New Yorkers, citing the IOM's report as a factor in creating this new effort.[41]

Recognizing that health disparities went beyond the health care delivery system, the IOM also looked at disparities that occurred in health research. For example, the NIH commissioned an IOM study to evaluate its research programs for ethnic minorities and the medically underserved. *The Unequal Burden of Cancer: An Assessment of NIH Research and Programs for Ethnic Minorities and the Medically Underserved* was released in 1999 and indicated that "not all segments of the United States population" had received the full benefits of advances in understanding and treating cancer. The committee, which was chaired by M. Alfred Haynes,[42] made a series of recommendations on how to remedy these disparities and called on the NIH's Office of Research on Minority Health to play a more active role in "coordinating, planning" and facilitating research regarding cancer among ethnic minority and medically underserved populations (IOM, 1999b). In 2006, the IOM released a second report assessing the NIH's research programs, *Examining the Health Disparities Research Plan of the National Institutes of Health: Unfinished Business*. The report assessed the NIH's research plan to determine if it was providing the intended structure and coordination across the NIH's institutes and research programs to reduce, and ultimately eliminate, health disparities. In its report, the committee, chaired by NAM member Gerald E. Thomson,[43] provided a series of recommendations to improve the NIH's strategic planning process to close gaps related to planning, coordination, and funding allocation in connection to disparities research funded by the NIH (IOM, 2006b).

To establish a more permanent convening body to promote health equity, the IOM established the Roundtable on the Promotion of Health Equity in 2007. The roundtable sought to "promote health equity and eliminate disparities" through activities and discussion aimed at "advancing the visibility and understanding of the inequities in health and health care among racial and ethnic populations; amplifying research, policy, and community-centered programs; and catalyzing the emergence of new leaders, partners and stakeholders." Throughout its history, the roundtable held more than two dozen meetings that looked at housing, incarceration, drug control policies, and culture as factors related to health equity as well as equity concerns of specific populations such as African Americans, Native Americans, older adults, people with disabilities, and people living in rural communities. In 2010, the roundtable hosted a workshop to assess progress that had been made in eliminating health disparities during the previous decade. The workshop brought together representatives from Walgreens and the HHS's Office of Minority Health, who subsequently established an important working collaboration to improve health for the uninsured. As a result of this collaboration, Walgreens contributed more than $10 million in vouchers for free flu vaccinations during the 2011 flu season that were then distributed by HHS to approximately 350,000 eligible individuals in 15 communities across the United States (Infection Control Today, 2010).

Continuing to explore options for eliminating disparities and ensuring health equity, the HMD released a five-part series in 2016 and early 2017 that examined social risk factors that could influence health outcomes for Medicare beneficiaries (see Box 5-3). The committee was also asked to provide a set of methods that could be used to account for these risk factors in Medicare payment programs. Together, the reports defined a conceptual framework that included specific indicators

---

[41] Impact of IOM Reports (Database), IOM/NAM Records.

[42] M. Alfred Haynes was the Former President and the Dean of the Drew Postgraduate Medical School and the Former Director of the Drew-Meharry-Morehouse Consortium Cancer Center in Rancho Palos Verdes, California.

[43] Gerald E. Thomson was the Lambert and Sonneborn Professor of Medicine Emeritus and the Senior Associate Dean Emeritus at the Columbia University College of Physicians and Surgeons during this time.

BOX 5-3
The Institute of Medicine's Reports on Social
Risk Factors and Medicare Payments

- *Accounting for Social Risk Factors in Medicare Payment: Identifying Social Risk Factors* (January 2016)
- *Systems Practices for the Care of Socially At-Risk Populations* (April 2016)
- *Accounting for Social Risk Factors in Medicare Payment: Criteria, Factors, and Methods* (July 2016)
- *Accounting for Social Risk Factors in Medicare Payment: Data* (October 2016)
- *Accounting for Social Risk Factors in Medicare Payment* (January 2017)

---

for social risk factors along with health care outcomes that could be employed by Medicare's quality measures and payment programs. The committee also provided guidance on data sources and data collection methods that could be used by Medicare and reviewed strategies adopted by high-performing health care systems to improve quality of care and health outcomes for socially at-risk populations. In the final report, the committee, which was chaired by NAM member Donald M. Steinwachs,[44] concluded that "accounting for social risk factors [in Medicare payment programs] is necessary but insufficient by itself to achieve health equity" (NASEM, 2017e). The committee urged caution in modifying payment programs, noting that "quality measurement and payment policies affect the lives of real patients." However, the committee believed that accounting for social risk factors in combination with other strategies could promote greater equity for Medicare beneficiaries.

Meanwhile, following the 2015 IOM-NAM transition, the NAM established its Culture of Health Program, supported by the RWJF, to advance the evidence base for policies that support equitable good health for everyone in America (described in Chapter 7). The Program's definition of a culture of health, or a state in which everyone has "the opportunity to be healthy and reach their full potential no matter who they are or where they live" became not only the credo of the Program, but also a centering value for all of the NAM's programmatic activities (NAM, n.d.k). In 2018, "accelerating health equity" was explicitly added to the NAM's mission statement as an outcome of its strategic planning process (NAM, 2017d).

Health Literacy

In 2004, the IOM released a report called *Health Literacy: A Prescription to End Confusion.* The report initiated the IOM's ongoing examination of health literacy—one of the many factors that can contribute to health disparities and impede the realization of health equity. For example, studies indicate that individuals with lower levels of health literacy have less knowledge about managing chronic illnesses and health-promoting behaviors, decreased ability to actively participate in health decision making, lower compliance with prescribed therapies, and poorer overall health status (IOM, 2004b). Data also suggest a linkage between lower levels of health literacy and increased health care utilization (e.g., increased number of hospitalizations and emergency room visits) and health care expenditures. In its report, the IOM committee, which was chaired by NAM member

---

[44] Donald M. Steinwachs was a Professor at the Johns Hopkins Bloomberg School of Public Health at the time these reports were released.

David Kindig,[45] adopted the definition of health literacy as "the degree to which individuals have the capacity to obtain, process, and understand basic health information and services needed to make appropriate health decisions" (IOM, 2004b; Ratzan and Parker, 2000). Health literacy stemmed from a combination of social and individual factors that were mediated by education, culture, and language.

The 2004 report estimated that as many as 90 million people in the United States might not be able to fully understand or act upon complex health information, not only affecting health outcomes but also hampering the health care system's ability to provide effective, high-quality health care (IOM, 2004b). The report offered eight recommendations to improve health literacy in the United States, calling upon the government, private funders, educators, and the health care system to take action. For example, secondary schools should "incorporate health-related tasks, materials, and examples into existing lesson plans," and health care professional educators should "incorporate health literacy into their curricula and areas of competence" (p. 15). The committee concluded that "without improvements in health literacy, the promise of scientific advances for improving health outcomes will be diminished" (p. 3) The report served as the basis for multiple pieces of legislation introduced in Congress, including the National Health Literacy Act of 2007 and the Promoting Health as Youth Skills in Classrooms and Life Act of 2011.[46]

Following the release of the report, the IOM launched the Roundtable on Health Literacy in 2005 to provide a long-term platform to bring together a variety of experts and stakeholders in a neutral setting "to support the development, implementation, and sharing of evidence-based health literacy practices and policies" (NASEM, n.d.k). The roundtable envisioned "a society in which the demands of the health and health care systems are respectful of and aligned with people's skills, abilities, and values." With more than a dozen sponsors and almost 30 members, the roundtable hosted nearly 40 public meetings and released more than 30 publications. The roundtable's activities explored a wide range of topics that intersected with health literacy, including oral health; behavioral and mental health; oncology; aging; palliative care; and immigrants, refugees, and migrant workers. The roundtable also reviewed specific topics such as health literacy and informed consent, discharge instructions, and medication labels. In October 2012, as a result of the 2004 report, *Health Literacy: A Prescription to End Confusion,* and the roundtable's ongoing work, the U.S. Pharmacopeial Convention (USP) released universal standards for simplifying the content and appearance of prescription labels. The USP credited the IOM's work for inspiring the new, patient-friendly standards, which USP leadership began developing after participating in a 2007 roundtable workshop.[47]

Following the creation of the HMD, the Roundtable on Health Literacy continued its work and began partnering with other HMD roundtables and forums to cover cross-cutting topics of interest to a wider audience of stakeholders. For example, in 2016, the roundtable collaborated with the Roundtable on the Promotion of Health Equity to host a workshop that resulted in a publication called *People Living with Disabilities: Health Equity, Health Disparities, and Health Literacy: Proceedings of a Workshop,* which considered the "intersections of health equity, health disparities, health literacy, and people living with disabilities" (NASEM, 2018c, p. 1). In 2019, the Roundtable on Health Literacy co-hosted a workshop with the National Cancer Policy Forum on health literacy and communication strategies in oncology. The workshop examined "opportunities, methods, and strategies to improve the communication of information about cancer care at the level of the clinic visit, the health care organization, and the community" (NASEM, n.d.l).

---

[45] David Kindig was at the Wisconsin Public Health & Health Policy Institute of the University of Wisconsin–Madison during this time.

[46] Impact of IOM Reports (Database), IOM/NAM Records.

[47] Ibid.

THE HEALTH CARE WORKFORCE AND INFORMAL CAREGIVERS

An integral part of the IOM's vision for improving health and health care quality in the United States involved an emphasis on the health care workforce and a reconfiguration of the relationship between health care providers and patients. The IOM recognized that fulfilling the six dimensions of quality—ensuring care that is safe, effective, patient-centered, timely, efficient, and equitable—required modifications to the education and training for health care providers, as well as the composition of the health care workforce. However, health care providers and the health care system were not solely responsible for all facets of care; informal caregivers and the day-to-day care they provided could also affect health outcomes and overall well-being, especially for older adults. Actively engaging and empowering patients, their caregivers, and loved ones as partners was crucial to achieving high-quality care and better health outcomes and quality of life.

Education and Training for Health Care Providers

Over the years, the IOM examined many aspects of the health care workforce in determining how to provide the best care possible to meet specific needs of populations. For example, in the nation's efforts to fortify the workforce for the aging baby boomer population, the IOM reviewed the composition of the workforce and the skillsets needed to care for an older population. In the spring of 2008, the IOM released *Retooling for an Aging America: Building the Health Care Workforce,* a report that evaluated the current health care workforce in light of the health care needs of an aging population. The committee, which was chaired by NAM member John W. Rowe,[48] concluded that the workforce was neither large enough nor adequately trained to care for the unique needs of older Americans. The committee recommended ways in which the workforce, as well as informal caregivers such as family members and friends, could be better trained. The report also highlighted the need for programs to recruit and retain geriatric specialists, including physicians and nurses (IOM, 2008b).

The 2008 report spurred a wide range of policy discussions and actions that were geared toward better preparing the health care system and workforce for the needs of the quickly aging population. For example, a provision of the Patient Protection and Affordable Care Act (ACA), which was signed by President Obama in March 2010, expanded the Geriatric Academic Career Awards program to include advanced practice registered nurses, clinical social workers, pharmacists, and psychologists. The provision was directly in line with the IOM report's recommendation, which had called for inclusion of health professionals from disciplines other than allopathic and osteopathic in the award program. Also in line with the IOM's recommendations, other provisions in the legislation supported family caregiver training through federally funded geriatric education centers and additional training for the direct care workforce.[49] Recognizing the severity of the situation, the VA established a task force to address the health care workforce challenges presented by the aging veteran population and also released their Geriatrics and Extended Care Strategic Plan, which leveraged the IOM's recommendations but also considered the unique nature of the VA's beneficiaries, 52 percent of whom were over the age of 65.[50]

The IOM took a closer look at the mental health and substance abuse workforce for older adults in its 2012 report, *The Mental Health and Substance Use Workforce for Older Adults: In Whose Hands?* This follow-on study, which was chaired by NAM member Dan G. Blazer,[51] estimated that

---

[48] John W. Rowe was a Professor in the Department of Health Policy and Management at the Mailman School of Public Health of Columbia University at the time.

[49] Impact of IOM Reports (Database), IOM/NAM Records.

[50] Ibid.

[51] Dan G. Blazer was the J.P. Gibbons Professor of Psychiatry and Behavioral Sciences and the Vice Chair for Education and Academic Affairs at the Duke University Medical Center in Durham, North Carolina, when this report was released.

the population over the age of 65 would reach more than 72 million by 2030, and that approximately one in five older adults would have at least one mental health or substance use concern (e.g., dementia, depression, alcohol abuse). In its report, the committee called for urgent action and leadership to establish a better prepared workforce, noting that no single solution would be sufficient to ensure the availability of a well-trained cadre of health care professionals (IOM, 2012e).

Throughout its history, the IOM also focused more broadly on education and training for health care providers. For example, in 2002 the IOM hosted the Health Professions Education Summit, which was designed to explore strategies to update education and training for health care professionals to align with care delivery in the 21st century. The summit, which was organized by a committee co-chaired by external volunteer Edward M. Hundert[52] and NAM member Mary Wakefield,[53] resulted in a publication called *Health Professions Education: A Bridge to Quality* (IOM, 2003c). Following up on that theme, the IOM released a report in 2009 called *Redesigning Continuing Education in the Health Professions,* which considered continuing education across the health professions and also the possibility of establishing a national institution for continuing education (IOM, 2010c).

In 2004, the IOM assessed the diversity of the health care workforce in its report, *In the Nation's Compelling Interest: Ensuring Diversity in the Health Care Workforce.* The report noted that the diversifying population of the United States required a more diverse health care workforce. Available evidence indicated that greater diversity was "associated with improved access to care for racial and ethnic minority patients, greater patient choice and satisfaction, and better educational experiences for health professions students" (IOM, 2004d, p. 1). Therefore, the committee, which was chaired by NAM member Lonnie R. Bristow,[54] made recommendations to change admissions policies and practices, provide better financial support, and shift institutional climates to encourage greater diversity among the health care workforce in the United States.

As the health care system evolved and more emphasis was placed on collaborative, team-based care, interest in interprofessional education (IPE) models and the linkages across IPE, safety, quality, cost, and patient outcomes and satisfaction grew. In response to a request from the sponsors of the IOM's Global Forum on Innovation in Health Professional Education, the IOM convened a committee to analyze "the available data and information to determine the best methods for measuring the impact of interprofessional education on specific aspects of health care delivery and the functioning of health care systems." In 2015, the IOM released *Measuring the Impact of Interprofessional Education on Collaborative Practice and Patient Outcomes,* which called on relevant stakeholders to "commit resources to a coordinated series of well-designed studies" that assessed the association between "interprofessional education and collaborative behavior" (IOM, 2015c, p. 5). To inform the development of the necessary studies, the committee, which was chaired by external volunteer Malcolm Cox,[55] created a conceptual model that included the "education-to-practice continuum, a broad array of learning, health, and system outcomes, and major enabling and interfering factors" (IOM, 2015c, p. 28).

In 2014, the IOM released a report on a specific topic in the education and training for health care providers—the financing of graduate medical education in the United States. The report, *Graduate Medical Education That Meets the Nation's Health Needs,* indicated that approximately $15 billion of public funding had been used to support graduate medical education through Medicare, Medicaid, the VA, and the HHS's Health Resources and Services Administration (IOM, 2014b).

---

[52] Edward M. Hundert was the President of Case Western University at the time of the summit.

[53] Mary Wakefield was the Director of the Center for Rural Health at the School of Medicine and Health Sciences at the University of North Dakota at this time.

[54] Lonnie R. Bristow was a retired physician and the former President of the American Medical Association at this time.

[55] Malcolm Cox was an Adjunct Professor at the Perelman School of Medicine of the University of Pennsylvania at the time.

However, the committee, chaired by Donald M. Berwick,[56] concluded that given that level of funding over almost a half-century, there was "a striking absence of transparency and accountability for producing the types of physicians that today's health care system requires" (IOM, 2014b, p. 16). Although the committee recommended maintaining the current level of funding for graduate medical education, it stated that significant amendments were required to develop a physician workforce that is better suited to meet the dynamic health care needs of the nation. The report offered six goals and four recommendations that the CMS, Congress, and other stakeholders could use to reform the governance and financing of graduate medical education through Medicare (Sklar, 2014).

In addition to education and training for the health care workforce, the IOM also considered the environment in which health care professionals and students worked and the impact that those environments had on the delivery of high-quality care and patient safety. The IOM's report *Keeping Patients Safe: Transforming the Work Environment of Nurses* reviewed the environments in which nurses work (e.g., hospitals, nursing homes, clinics) and made recommendations for how to improve working conditions for nurses in order to promote greater patient safety (IOM, 2004h). In August 2012, Massachusetts implemented one of the report's recommendations and became the 17th state to enact a ban on mandatory overtime for nurses.[57]

In 2003, the Accreditation Council for Graduate Medical Education (ACGME) implemented national standards that "mandated an 80-hour weekly average for all residents along with implementing other minimum requirements for time off from the hospital" (IOM, 2009a, p. 28). Following the release of these common duty hour standards, there was an uptick in interest and scrutiny on resident work hours in hospitals. In 2007, Congress directed HHS to commission an IOM study "to examine the relationship between resident duty hours and patient safety" (p. 29). During its deliberations, the committee considered a range of possible consequences of resident duty hours on patient safety—for example, the potential effects of reducing time spent in hospitals on residents' educational experience, the impact of increasing the number of handovers during patient care, and the potential risks associated with long hours and sleep deprivation. In 2008, the IOM released a report called *Resident Duty Hours: Enhancing Sleep, Supervision, and Safety*. Although the report was controversial in the medical field, it led to significant changes in the way future physicians were trained. The committee, which was chaired by NAM member and Councilor (1997–2002) Michael M. E. Johns,[58] stated that the current restrictions on work hours, which allowed residents to work 30-hour shifts and up to 80 hours per week, resulted in fatigue that could jeopardize patient safety by increasing the risk for medical errors. The committee recommended that residents not be allowed to work more than 16-hour shifts and that greater emphasis be placed on handovers from one shift to the next (IOM, 2009a). In 2011, the ACGME updated its resident duty hours guidelines once more, implementing the IOM's recommendation to limit residents' shifts to 16 hours for first-year residents (Choma et al., 2013). However, by 2021, ACGME had removed the 16-hour requirement, stating that it was "incompatible with the actual practice of medicine and surgery in many specialties, excessively limiting in configuration of clinical services in many disciplines, and potentially disruptive of the inculcation of responsibility and professional commitment to altruism and placing the needs of patients above those of the physician" (ACGME, 2021, p. 52).

The Future of Nursing

With more than 3 million registered nurses in the United States in the first decade of the 21st century, nurses make up the largest contingent of the health care workforce. During the past century,

---

[56] Donald M. Berwick was the former President and the Chief Executive Officer of the Institute for Healthcare Improvement.

[57] Impact of IOM Reports (Database), IOM/NAM Records.

[58] Michael M. E. Johns was the Chancellor at Emory University when this report was released.

the role of nurses in the health care system has evolved, with shifts in scope of practice, advances in technology, health care provider shortages, greater emphasis on primary care and preventive services, and an increased strain on the health care system due to an aging population. The IOM emphasized the importance of nurses in the health care workforce and the care that they provide in its report *Nursing and Nursing Education: Public Policies and Private Actions* (IOM, 1983). More than two decades later, the organization launched an initiative designed to maximize the value and contributions of nurses to the health care workforce and system. In the 21st century, the IOM, the RWJF, and many other stakeholders recognized the vital role of nurses in providing high-quality care and also the need to expand and enhance the nursing workforce. In 2009, the IOM introduced a joint initiative with the RWJF to assess the future of nursing in the United States. The initiative—which was chaired by NAM member Donna Shalala, the former HHS Secretary and future U.S. Congresswoman[59]—was the first time the IOM had partnered with another organization to complete a consensus study. The initiative was supported by a blend of IOM and RWJF staff, who were engaged throughout the study process.[60] The staff worked jointly with the committee to develop a research strategy and communications plan to ensure that the report would have the greatest possible reach and potential for change. In conducting its work, the committee held three regional forums—in Los Angeles, Philadelphia, and Houston—that focused on acute care, care in the community, and education, respectively. Each of the forums resulted in a separate publication that informed the overall consensus study and the committee's final report.

The committee's report, *The Future of Nursing: Leading Change, Advancing Health,* was released in September 2010. It offered a blueprint for transforming the nursing profession in three key areas—education, practice, and leadership—with an emphasis on enhancing the profession to achieve greater quality, access, and value throughout the health care system. To realize this transformation, nurses needed to "practic[e] to the full extent of their education and training," "achieve higher levels of education and training," and "be full partners ... in redesigning [health] care in the United States," working as equal partners with other health care professionals (IOM, 2011f). The committee also called for better data to support "effective workforce planning and policy making" (IOM, 2011g, p. 4). In its work, the committee examined the varied educational pathways that led to a registered nurse license (e.g., community colleges, universities) and recommended that 80 percent of nurses should hold a baccalaureate degree by 2020 and that the number of nurses with doctorates should double by that time in an effort to expand the number of nurse educators.[61]

The 2010 Future of Nursing initiative and consensus report attracted wide attention across the health care industry, in political spheres, and from the media. After its release, the report became the most downloaded IOM report of all time and the second most downloaded report of all time across the entire National Academies.[62] Shortly after the release of the report, the RWJF, in partnership with the AARP, launched a "Future of Nursing: Campaign for Action" initiative. The campaign sought to organize "action coalitions" in all 50 states to help realize the report's recommendations at the state level, where decision and policy making about licensing and education frequently occur. Major themes of the campaign included advancing education, developing and leveraging nursing leadership, and promoting nursing diversity. The recommendations from the IOM report, combined with the implementation efforts of the Campaign for Action, resulted in policy change in numerous states related to scope of practice for nurses. For example, several states removed barriers to prac-

---

[59] Shalala served as the U.S. Representative for Florida's 27th congressional district from January 3, 2019, to January 3, 2021.

[60] Donna Shalala and Linda Bolton to Members of the Robert Johnson Foundation Initiative on the Future of Nursing, at the Institute of Medicine, July 1, 2009, Future of Nursing Files, IOM/NAM Records.

[61] Harvey Fineberg to Risa Lavizzo-Mourey, September 30, 2010, Future of Nursing Files, IOM/NAM Records.

[62] National Academies internal data, December 2021.

tice for advanced practice registered nurses (APRNs), ensuring that APRNs could practice without direct physician supervision.[63]

The RWJF-AARP Campaign for Action also led to a 2014 request from the RWJF for the IOM to assess changes in the field of nursing over the previous 5 years and review progress made by the RWJF-AARP campaign.[64] The resulting consensus study—*Assessing Progress on the Institute of Medicine Report* The Future of Nursing—was released in December 2015 as a report of the National Academies of Sciences, Engineering, and Medicine following the creation of the NAM and the HMD. The committee, which was chaired by NAM member Stuart H. Altman,[65] concluded that much had changed in the health care industry since the release of the previous report and that the campaign had made "significant progress toward implementing the [report's] recommendations" (NASEM, 2016e). However, more work was needed to fulfill the promise of the report's recommendations. In order to promote continued progress, the new report offered recommendations related to removing barriers to practice and care, achieving higher levels of education, promoting diversity, collaborating and leading in care delivery and redesign, and improving workforce data infrastructure (NASEM, 2016e).[66]

With 2020 approaching, the timeline set in the original Future of Nursing Initiative, the National Academies launched a new consensus study to "extend the vision for the nursing profession into 2030 and ... chart a path for the nursing profession to help our nation create a culture of health, reduce health disparities, and improve the health and wellbeing of the U.S. population in the 21st century" (NASEM, n.d.m). Supported by the RWJF, the committee, which was co-chaired by Wakefield[67] and fellow NAM member David R. Williams,[68] hosted three regional town hall events reviewing themes related to education, research, and practice; payment and care for complex health and social needs; and high tech to high touch.

The Future of Nursing 2020–2030: Charting a Path to Achieve Health Equity was released on May 11, 2021 (NASEM, 2021e). The report's key finding was that "nursing in the next 10 years will demand a larger, more diversified workforce prepared to provide care in different settings, to address the lasting effects of COVID-19, to break down structural racism and the root causes of poor health, and to respond to future public health emergencies" (NASEM, 2021b). The committee identified several key needs to help the nursing workforce reach its full potential and advance health equity in the United States: strengthening nurse education; promoting diversity, equity, and inclusion in nursing education and the workforce; investing in school and public health nurses; protecting nurses' health and well-being; preparing nurses for disaster and public health emergency response; and increasing the number of PhD-prepared nurses (NASEM, 2021b).

The Role of Informal Caregivers

In conjunction with physicians, nurses, physical and occupational therapists, social workers, and other health care professionals, informal caregivers, such as family, friends, and neighbors, are

---

[63] Impact of IOM Reports (Database), IOM/NAM Records.

[64] Robert Wood Johnson Foundation and AARP, "Future of Nursing: Campaign for Action—Campaign Overview," n.d., in Future of Nursing Files, IOM/NAM Records; Clyde Behney to Melanie Adams, Robert Wood Johnson Foundation, September 16, 2014, Institute of Medicine, Board on Health Sciences Policy, "Evaluation of the Future of Nursing Campaign for Action," September 2014, Proposal 10002323, Future of Nursing Files, IOM/NAM Records.

[65] Stuart H. Altman was the Sol C. Chaikin Professor of National Health Policy at the Heller Graduate School of Social Policy of Brandeis University in Weston, Massachusetts, when the report was released.

[66] Victor Dzau to Stuart Altman, March 25, 2015, Future of Nursing Files, IOM/NAM Records.

[67] Mary K. Wakefield was the Visiting Distinguished Professor in the Practice of Health Care at Georgetown University and also the Visiting Professor and a Distinguished Fellow at The University of Texas at Austin during this time.

[68] David R. Williams was the Florence and Laura Norman Professor of Public Health and the Chair of the Department of Social and Behavioral Sciences at the Harvard T.H. Chan School of Public Health at the time.

playing an increasingly important and varied role in the day-to-day care of older adults. In 2016, the HMD explored the role of family caregivers in its report *Families Caring for an Aging America*. During its deliberation, the committee found that more than 17.7 million people in the United States took care of an older adult due to that individual's physical, mental, or cognitive health status or limitations. The care that informal caregivers provide ranges from occasional assistance with simple household tasks to long-term care that involves coordinating medical care and medication schedules for a loved one with complex conditions such as terminal cancer or dementia. The committee noted that family caregivers were often the key to ensuring access to needed health care and community-based services. While informal caregivers can play a crucial role in the health and well-being of older adults, this potentially stressful role can take a toll on the caregivers. An extensive body of evidence indicates that caregivers for older adults face an increased risk of depression, anxiety, emotional distress, social isolation, chronic illnesses, and impaired health behaviors, as well as an increased risk for experiencing economic harms, such as loss of income.

In its report, the committee, which was chaired by external volunteer Richard Schulz,[69] offered 11 recommendations focused on ways federal and state government agencies could better meet the needs of informal caregivers and support them in their role. For example, the committee suggested expanded funding and wider implementation of "evidence-based caregiver services" and the "adoption of federal policies that provide economic support to working caregivers" (NASEM, 2016f, p. 3). The committee also called on the health care system to identify and engage caregivers and "provide them [with] evidence-based supports and referrals to services in the community" (NASEM, 2016g, p. 10). The committee concluded that "today's emphasis on person-centered care needs to evolve into a focus on person- and family-centered care" (NASEM, 2016g, p. 35), noting that "if the needs of caregivers are not addressed, we risk compromising the well-being of our elders and their families" (NASEM, 2016g, p. 258).

COMPLEX AND SERIOUS HEALTH CONDITIONS

Throughout its history, the IOM provided guidance on how the nation should approach complex and serious diseases and health conditions, such as cancer, cognitive decline and dementia, and dying (described below). In 2016, the HMD created an institutional structure for ongoing discussions related to care for complex and serious health conditions, with the creation of the Roundtable on Quality Care for People with Serious Illness. The roundtable was developed to foster an "ongoing dialogue about critical policy and research issues," with the explicit purpose of advancing the findings and recommendations from previous reports such as *Dying in America* (IOM, 2015d). With more than 30 sponsors, the roundtable released 7 publications in its first 3 years, all of which cut across themes from the IOM, the NAM, and the HMD's bodies of work in a timely way. For example, the roundtable hosted workshops related to quality measures for serious illnesses, pain management and opioids, health equity, palliative care, and better integration of patients and caregivers into care for serious illnesses.

Cancer

Coordinating and advancing cancer research (described in Chapter 4) and improving the delivery of cancer care constituted an important priority for the IOM from its very start. For example, when President Richard Nixon declared war on cancer in 1971—suggesting a national plan to cure cancer—IOM President John Hogness testified before Congress. In his testimony, Hogness

---

[69] Richard Schulz was the Director of the University Center for Social and Urban Research at the University of Pittsburgh when this report was released.

emphasized that cancer encompassed many complex diseases and was not a single disease that could easily be cured. He offered advice on how best to conduct Nixon's campaign without interrupting promising ongoing research related to the causes and treatments of the various different types of cancer.

Twenty-six years after Hogness's statement on cancer policy, the IOM established the National Cancer Policy Board in March 1997. The board was developed to initiate studies related to the "prevention, control, diagnosis, treatment, and palliation of cancer" (IOM, 1999c, p. 1). One of the board's first tasks was a study that resulted in a 1999 report called *Ensuring Quality Cancer Care*. The report, issued by the board rather than a separate study committee, exposed a wide gap between an ideal system of cancer care and current delivery mechanisms, which were deemed to be ad hoc and fragmented in nature. In the field of breast cancer, for example, the report identified quality problems related to the "underuse of mammography to detect cancer early, lack of adherence to standards for diagnosis …; inadequate patient counseling regarding treatment options; and underuse of radiation therapy and adjuvant chemotherapy after surgery" (IOM, 1999c, p. 216).

The report offered 10 recommendations to establish a cohesive national cancer care system that would ensure access to high-quality care. The committee, which was chaired by NAM member Peter Howley,[70] called for the development and implementation of evidence-based guidelines, as well as a core set of quality measures. The report also laid out the elements of quality cancer care, which included an agreed-upon care plan that outlines the goals of care, access to high-quality clinical trials, coordinated care and services, and access to psychosocial services and compassionate care. In terms of data, the committee recommended a national data system that provided quality benchmarks, studies focused on care management, the care received by recently diagnosed individuals, and the care received by specific populations (e.g., racial and ethnic minorities, older adults).[71]

Following this first report on the quality of cancer care, the IOM conducted other studies related to cancer care with an emphasis on the psychosocial needs of patients and survivors throughout their journey. A cancer diagnosis could be devastating, and the effects of a diagnosis and treatment went beyond the health care system, sometimes creating or exacerbating problems related to employment, schooling, transportation, family dynamics and relationships, caregiving roles, and mental health concerns such as depression and anxiety. The IOM's first cancer report to specifically investigate the psychosocial needs of patients was its 2004 report *Meeting Psychosocial Needs of Women with Breast Cancer* (IOM and NRC, 2004). In 2006, the IOM released *From Cancer Patient to Cancer Survivor: Lost in Transition*, which was drafted by a committee chaired by NAM member Sheldon Greenfield.[72] The report considered the psychosocial, functional, and health needs of individuals who had completed primary cancer treatment and had entered a new phase of life as a cancer survivor (IOM and NRC, 2006). The report informed the Comprehensive Cancer Care Improvement Act of 2007, which was introduced by U.S. Representatives Lois Capps (D-CA) and Tom Davis (R-VA) and 25 other co-sponsors. The bill sought to implement the recommendations of the IOM report and included provisions for providing Medicare coverage of comprehensive cancer care planning, establishing a Medicare hospice care demonstration program, and providing grants for programs related to palliative care and symptom management for patients with cancer, clinician education, and other related research areas.[73]

In its 2008 report *Cancer Care for the Whole Patient: Meeting Psychosocial Health Needs*

---

[70] Peter Howley was the George Fabyan Professor and the Chair of the Department of Pathology at the Harvard Medical School during this time.

[71] "Findings and Recommendations—Cancer Care Report," in materials for National Cancer Policy Board, 7th Meeting, July 30–31, 1998, Woods Hole, IOM/NAM Records.

[72] Sheldon Greenfield was the Director of the Center for Health Policy Research at the University of California, Irvine, when the report was released.

[73] Impact of IOM Reports (Database), IOM/NAM Records.

the IOM expanded on its 2004 report, delving into the complexities of the psychosocial needs for all patients with cancer, not just those with breast cancer. These psychosocial needs can easily be overlooked by a health care system focused on providing cutting-edge treatments to save or prolong life. The committee, which was chaired by NAM member and Councilor (2011–2017) Nancy E. Adler,[74] concluded that high-quality cancer care was not possible without providing comprehensive care that also addresses patients' and families' psychosocial needs (IOM, 2008c). During a March 2008 congressional briefing on the report, the National Cancer Institute's (NCI's) Director of the Division of Cancer Control and Population Sciences, Robert Croyle, stated that the IOM's report had served as the basis of several NCI programmatic decisions related to continuing funding for centers of excellence in patient-centered communications, supporting community cancer centers, administering patient experience surveys, pursuing measurement of patient outcomes, and encouraging research focused on the whole patient. In 2013, Congressman Steve Israel (D-NY) introduced the Improving Cancer Treatment Education Act of 2013, which was developed to provide comprehensive treatment education for patients with cancer under Medicare, citing two IOM reports: *Cancer Care for the Whole Patient* (IOM, 2008c) and *Ensuring Quality Cancer Care* (IOM, 1999c).[75]

In 2005, a structural reorganization converted the National Cancer Policy Board into the National Cancer Policy Forum (NASEM, n.d.n). As with the IOM's other roundtables and forums, the National Cancer Policy Forum was a convening activity that was designed to bring together interested experts and stakeholders in a neutral environment to host public workshops and facilitate discussion regarding high-priority concerns across the field. The forum grew to include 20 sponsors and 44 members in 2021 (NASEM, 2021c). In the years between 2005 and 2019, the forum released 44 workshop summaries that covered a broad range of topics related to cancer science and research, diagnosis and treatment, and public health and health policy concerns related to cancer. The forum's work was cross-cutting and touched on topics the IOM had reviewed more broadly in other studies, such as the health impacts of obesity, the health of children and adolescents, care quality and value, health disparities, and health IT and patient privacy (NASEM, 2021d).

In 2013, the IOM revisited the quality of cancer care in the United States, releasing a report called *Delivering High-Quality Cancer Care: Charting a New Course for a System in Crisis,* which incorporated work from the National Cancer Policy Forum (IOM, 2013g). In its report, the committee, which was chaired by NAM member Patricia A. Ganz,[76] concluded that the cancer care system was "in crisis due to a growing demand for cancer care, increasing complexity of treatment, a shrinking workforce, and rising costs" (IOM, 2013g, p. 1). To respond to this crisis and echoing themes from the 1997 quality report, the committee developed a six-part conceptual framework that involved actively engaged patients at the center of care and an adequately trained and coordinated team-based workforce that provided evidence-based care and employed a learning health IT system. The framework also called for translating available evidence into "clinical practice, quality measurement, and performance improvement," while ensuring cancer care that was both accessible and affordable (IOM, 2013h, p. 11). The report emphasized the importance of a continuum of cancer care, from prevention and risk reduction to screening, diagnosis, and treatment to survivorship and end-of-life care.

As with many of the IOM's health care quality-focused reports, *Delivering High-Quality Cancer Care* was the source of initiatives to improve the quality of care delivered to patients with cancer in the United States. Citing the IOM's report and its recommendations. In 2015, CMS released a request for applications through its Center for Medicare & Medicaid Innovation that called for new

---

[74] Nancy E. Adler was a Professor of Medical Psychology and the Vice-Chair of the Department of Psychiatry at the University of California, San Francisco, during this time.

[75] Impact of IOM Reports (Database), IOM/NAM Records.

[76] Patricia A. Ganz was a Distinguished University Professor at the University of California, Los Angeles, Schools of Medicine and Public Health, and the Director of Cancer Prevention and Control Research at the Jonsson Comprehensive Cancer Center.

models of oncology care aimed at "testing the effects of better care coordination, improved access to practitioners, and appropriate clinical care on improving health outcomes at a lower cost" (CMS, 2015). In 2015, the American Society of Clinical Oncology released a conceptual framework that was designed to assess the value of new cancer therapies based on clinical benefit (efficacy), toxicity (safety), and cost (efficiency). The framework cited the IOM's *Delivering High-Quality Cancer Care* report and focused heavily on efficacy, safety, efficiency, patient centeredness, timeliness, and equity—elements identified by the IOM as essential to high-quality care.[77]

Cognitive Aging and Dementia

Understanding cognitive aging and preventing cognitive decline and dementia are among the most complex challenges the health care system and health scientists have ever faced. As the U.S. population ages and life expectancy in many countries around the globe increases, it is becoming more pressing to find solutions to these challenges and better understand cognitive aging. By 2030, all of the 73 million baby boomers living in the United States will be over the age of 65 (U.S. Census Bureau, 2019). Although cognitive aging is a normal part of life that comes with both positive and negative experiences, the effects of aging on the brain and cognition vary widely across individuals. In 2015, the IOM released a report called *Cognitive Aging: Progress in Understanding and Opportunities for Action,* which focused on cognitive aging rather than neurodegenerative dementia, such as Alzheimer's disease. The committee, which was chaired by Dan G. Blazer,[78] conducted in-depth assessments to characterize the current knowledge base related to "definitions and terminology, epidemiology and surveillance, prevention and intervention, education of health professionals, and public awareness and education (IOM, 2015i, p. 2)." In its report, the committee offered specific actions for individuals (e.g., remaining active, staying socially engaged, getting enough sleep, reducing cardiovascular risk factors) and health care providers (e.g., identifying risk factors for cognitive decline, reviewing patients' medications, discussing cognitive health concerns). The report also reviewed opportunities to improve public education and engagement and described options for strengthening community-based and public health services designed to support older adults and their families in light of their cognitive aging needs (IOM, 2015i).

In 2016, the IOM reviewed a sometimes-overlooked risk factor in cognitive decline and dementia: hearing loss (NASEM, 2016h). Its report, *Hearing Health Care for Adults: Priorities for Improving Access and Affordability,* considered hearing loss as a public health concern and offered recommendations geared toward "improving hearing and communication abilities for individuals and across the population" (NASEM, 2016i, p. 3). Among other things, the report emphasized the social aspects of hearing loss, from diminished social engagement—a potential risk factor for cognitive decline and dementia—to the social stigma associated with hearing aids. The report was the subject of multiple pieces of legislation introduced in Congress, including a bill called the Over-the-Counter Hearing Aid Act of 2016. The bill was enacted into law in 2017, making hearing aids available over the counter to those with mild to moderate hearing loss.[79]

In 2015, the NIH commissioned a study to evaluate available evidence related to the "effectiveness, comparative effectiveness, and harms of interventions associated with preventing, or delaying the onset" of age-related cognitive decline, cognitive impairment, and dementia (NASEM, 2017g, p. 5). In 2017, the HMD released *Preventing Cognitive Decline and Dementia: A Way Forward.*

---

[77] Impact of IOM Reports (Database), IOM/NAM Records.

[78] Dan G. Blazer was the J.P. Gibbons Professor of Psychiatry Emeritus at the Duke University Medical Center when this report was released.

[79] Impact of IOM Reports (Database), IOM/NAM Records.

Following its evidence review, the committee, which was chaired by Alan I. Leshner,[80] concluded that there was enough "encouraging although inconclusive evidence" to highlight the potential beneficial effects of interventions related to cognitive training, blood pressure management for those with hypertension, and increased physical activity. The committee also identified areas that were ripe for additional research, such as diabetes and depression treatment; interventions related to sleep, diet, and social engagement; and new anti-dementia treatments. In providing its priority research areas, the committee called for high-quality prevention research with improved methodologies that involved "a diverse set of population, with variation across racial and ethnic backgrounds, socioeconomic status, age at the time of intervention initiation, and risk of dementia" (p. 11). In 2018, the HMD released a follow-on letter report called *Considerations for the Design of a Systematic Review of Care Interventions for Individuals with Dementia and Their Caregivers*. The report, which was produced by a committee chaired by NAM member Eric B. Larson,[81] provided guidance for AHRQ's review of evidence for care interventions that addressed behavioral and psychological symptoms, as well as other symptoms, overall functioning, and quality of life. The AHRQ's systematic review process had been used to assess the evidence base for the 2017 report (NASEM, 2018e).

Prior to the release of these consensus studies, the Forum on Neuroscience and Nervous System Disorders, which was established in 2006, also held a number of public meetings that resulted in workshop summaries related to Alzheimer's disease and dementia: *Future Opportunities to Leverage the Alzheimer's Disease Neuroimaging Initiative* (IOM, 2011k), *Alzheimer's Diagnostic Guideline Validation: Exploration of Next Steps* (IOM, 2012q), and *Neurodegeneration: Exploring Commonalities Across Diseases* (IOM, 2013n). In addition to its dementia-specific work, the forum's work more broadly "examines significant—and sometimes contentious—issues concerning scientific needs and opportunities, priority setting, and policies related to neuroscience and nervous system disorders research; the development, regulation, and use of interventions for the nervous system; and related ethical, legal, and social implications" (NASEM, n.d.o).

End-of-Life Care

Another topic that remained a consistent priority on the IOM's agenda was end-of-life and associated palliative care. The IOM long realized that care at the end of life represented a crucial responsibility of the health care system that was often overlooked or delivered too late. Improving care at the end of life is an important component of the continuum of care that also requires equitable access to high-quality, evidence-based care, as well as care for any other type of complex or serious illness. The IOM's interest in end-of-life care dated back to 1984, when it published *Bereavement: Reactions, Consequences, and Care*. The report, which was written by a committee chaired by external volunteer Morris Green,[82] focused on the needs of grieving survivors as part of care for the dying, highlighting another aspect of death that needed to be considered by the health care system (IOM, 1984b).

A little more than a decade later, the IOM released its first major work on end-of-life care— *Approaching Death: Improving Care at the End of Life*. This 1997 report facilitated the introduction of hospice care as an integral part of the U.S. health care system and called on physicians, nurses,

---

[80] Alan I. Leshner was the Chief Executive Officer Emeritus of the American Association for the Advancement of Science at this time.

[81] Eric B. Larson was the Vice President for Research at the Kaiser Foundation Health Plan of Washington and the Executive Director and a Senior Investigator at the Kaiser Permanente Washington Health Research Institute when this report was released.

[82] Morris Green was the Lesh Professor and the Chair of the Department of Pediatrics at the Indiana University School of Medicine at the time.

social workers, and other members of the care team to make a commitment to improving care for dying patients. The committee, which was chaired by NAM member and Councilor (2003–2008) Christine Cassel,[83] stated that death should be "free from avoidable distress and suffering for patients, families, and caregivers; in general accord with patients' and families, wishes; and reasonably consistent with clinical, cultural, and ethical standards" (IOM, 1997b, p. 4). In order to better meet the needs of people approaching death, the committee envisioned a whole-community model, which would require systematic modifications related to the organization and financing of care, the legal aspects of care, and the education and training of health care providers. Better outcomes data and tools would also be required to establish and track accountability associated with the quality of end-of-life care. The report sought to elevate palliative care to a defined medical specialty and area of expertise as another component of "a humane care system that people can trust to serve them well as they die" (IOM, 1997b, p. 13).

In 2001, the IOM reviewed end-of-life care for patients with a terminal cancer diagnosis in its report *Improving Palliative Care for Cancer.* As with the IOM's report on the psychosocial needs of cancer patients, the committee pointed out that palliative care, education, and research were other areas often overlooked in the pursuit of new therapies and potential cures for the various types of cancer. Despite the nearly half million people who died from cancer each year, the committee found that less than 1 percent of the NCI's budget was dedicated to education or research on palliative care (IOM and NRC, 2001). Building on the themes and recommendations from the IOM's 1997 report *Approaching Death,* the committee, which was chaired by NAM member Arnold J. Levine,[84] offered 10 recommendations that were designed to develop and implement more effective palliative care options within cancer care, integrate palliative care as part of high-quality cancer care, improve communication with patients and their families about palliative care options, and enhance data collection and quality measures for end-of-life care for cancer patients (IOM and NRC, 2001). Following the release of the report, the American College of Physicians released new guidelines for end-of-life care, stating that, "end of life care has been identified by the Institute of Medicine as one of the priority areas to improve quality of health care. We hope that these guidelines would benefit physicians taking care of patients with seriously disabling or symptomatic chronic conditions" (ACP, 2008).

The 2003 report, *When Children Die: Improving Palliative and End-of-Life Care for Children and Their Families,* expanded on the IOM's previous work to explore the unique needs of children with life-threatening medical conditions and their families. The report emphasized the crucial roles of health care providers and the health care system in providing "competent, compassionate, and consistent care [that meets the children and families'] physical, emotional, and spiritual needs" (IOM, 2003d). In order to build a more child- and family-centered system, the committee recommended that stakeholders work together to develop clinical guidelines, institutional protocols, and information programs for palliative, end-of-life, and bereavement care. In terms of financing, the committee stated that hospice services for children should be covered by public (e.g., Medicaid) and private insurers, and that eligibility restrictions related to life expectancy should be eliminated. Public and private insurers also needed to amend their reimbursement policies to cover the time needed to explain a child's condition to parents and provide necessary counseling and guidance. Reinforcing the 1997 report's call to promote palliative care as a specialty, the committee, which was chaired by external volunteer Richard E. Behrman,[85] encouraged better training for those who worked with children and families in palliative, end-of-life, and bereavement care (IOM, 2003d).

---

[83] Christine Cassel was the Chair of the Department of Geriatrics and Adult Development at Mount Sinai Medical Center in New York during this time.

[84] Arnold J. Levine was the President of The Rockefeller University in New York when this report was released.

[85] Richard E. Behrman was the Executive Chair of the Federation of Pediatric Organizations, Education Steering Committee, and a Clinical Professor of Pediatrics at Stanford University and the University of California during this time.

The report served as a compelling call to action, received extensive media coverage, and attracted political attention. Most of the newspapers that covered the report led with its primary finding that "too often, children with fatal or potentially fatal conditions and their families fail to receive competent, compassionate and consistent care that meets their physical, emotional, and spiritual needs" (IOM, 2003d, p. 3). In the medical sphere, the *New England Journal of Medicine* lauded the IOM's commitment to explore and publicize end-of-life issues (Faulkner, 2003; McFeatters, 2002; Robernicks, 2002). A few days after the release of the report, Behrman, a distinguished pediatrician, met with NIH staff to discuss the report. He then participated in a congressional briefing in the fall of 2002. In response to the report, Senators Michael DeWine (R-OH) and Chris Dodd (D-CT) and Representatives Deborah Pryce (R-OH) and John Murtha (D-PA) drafted legislation called the Children's Compassionate Care Act that was based on the report's recommendations.[86]

The next installment in the IOM's end-of-life series, *Dying in America: Improving Quality and Honoring Individual Preferences Near the End of Life,* was released in 2014 following a politically charged debate in the country regarding end-of-life care. A provision of the ACA, which had gained some bipartisan support and an endorsement from the AARP, would have authorized Medicare reimbursement for end-of-life counseling, such as discussions with physicians about options for end-of-life care. Opponents of the ACA seized on the provision, with some stating that it would create "death panels" that would allow the federal government to participate in end-of-life decisions. The provision was removed from the final version of the bill to quiet some of the opposition. However, the debate had brought new attention to end-of-life issues and motivated the IOM to launch a study to revisit end-of-life care and assess advances that had been made since its 1997 report (IOM, 2015d).

The report, which was funded by an anonymous donor, elaborated on and reinforced messages from the earlier reports. The committee found that progress had been made since the 1997 report, noting that hospice had become a mainstay in end-of-life care and that palliative care was now a regular part of care in larger hospitals. However, training for health care professionals was lacking, and systematic changes were needed to improve the delivery of care. The committee, which was chaired by NAM member and Councilor (2007–2012) Philip A. Pizzo,[87] called for comprehensive end-of-life care that was seamless, of high quality, accessible around the clock, and consistent with an individual's values and preferences. In its report, the committee noted that palliative care should be delivered by a well-trained, interdisciplinary team that included board-certified hospice and palliative care physicians, nurses, social workers, and chaplains. To ensure high-quality care, new standards were needed for clinician-patient communication that were "measurable, actionable, and evidence-based." The committee also discussed the need for greater public engagement and education about end-of-life planning, care, and decision making (IOM, 2015d). In July 2015, citing the IOM's report, the CMS announced that Medicare would begin to reimburse health care providers to counsel patients about end-of-life care and "advance care planning," a term that was meant to emphasize that individuals should make their own end-of-life wishes known and that those wishes should be revisited at different stages in life.[88]

The end-of-life reports demonstrate how the IOM developed a persistent, action-oriented agenda that not only wove together themes from across the end-of-life reports but also drew upon themes from the IOM's other work. Throughout its history, the IOM delivered reports that were meant to facilitate change across the U.S. health care system in the interest of providing high-quality, evidence-based care that was also person- and family-centered and accessible. The end-of-

---

[86] Impact of IOM Reports (Database), IOM/NAM Records.

[87] Philip A. Pizzo was the Former Dean and David and Susan Heckerman Professor of Pediatrics and of Microbiology and Immunology and the Founding Director, Stanford Distinguished Careers Institute, Stanford University, Stanford, California when this report was released.

[88] Impact of IOM Reports (Database), IOM/NAM Records.

life reports enabled the IOM to speak with a consistent voice in health policy conversations across the United States.

HEALTH CARE REFORM AND UNINSURANCE

Health care reform and equitable access to high-quality health care were long-term priorities for the IOM. Although the topic of health care reform was often politically charged, the IOM approached it through careful review of public, health-related programs and opportunities to improve those programs. Medicare was one such program that the IOM revisited frequently, starting in the IOM's early days when the organization weighed in on questions about expanding Medicare benefits using a disease-by-disease approach (e.g., end-stage renal disease) in the 1970s (see Chapter 2). The IOM continued its review of the Medicare program with a three-part series in the 1990s called *Medicare: A Strategy for Quality Assurance* (see above). In 2000, the IOM released a report called *Extending Medicare Reimbursement in Clinical Trials*,[89] which led to an executive order signed by President Clinton that required Medicare to cover routine medical costs for beneficiaries participating in clinical trials in an effort to encourage expanded clinical trials participation among older adults (IOM, 2000d; White House, 2000). The executive order was followed by a national coverage decision through Medicare that implemented the president's executive order and detailed specific benefits that would be provided through the Medicare program.[90]

The IOM reviewed Medicare provider reimbursements and incentives in its 2007 report, *Rewarding Provider Performance: Aligning Incentives in Medicare* (IOM, 2007m).[91] In many ways, the IOM's body of work offered advice on incremental changes to the Medicare program that could be translated to improvements in the U.S. health care system more broadly. However, many of the IOM's committees highlighted the need for more robust and far-reaching systematic changes and reforms across the health care system, stating that incremental change was not sufficient.

One of the primary goals of health care reform efforts in the United States has been to reduce the number of people living without health care insurance. From 1978 through 1990, the number of uninsured individuals under the age of 65 increased by 14.2 million, growing from 12 percent of the population to 17 percent of the population. For the next 17 years (1990–2007), the uninsurance rate in the United States hovered around 17 percent, with 43.3 million people without insurance in 2007 (CDC, 2009). Despite periods of economic growth and low rates of unemployment, the rates of uninsurance in the United States persisted (IOM, 2004e). Rates of uninsurance vary by socioeconomic factors (e.g., education, employment, income), demographic factors (e.g., race and ethnicity, gender, age), as well as geographic location (IOM, 2001e). The consequences of uninsurance affect individuals, families, communities, states, and the nation as a whole and range from poorer health outcomes to strains on emergency departments and the health care system to financial and economic repercussions across all levels (IOM, 2002b, 2003e, 2009b).

As each U.S. president considered questions of health care reform and options for national health insurance, the IOM stood ready to offer non-partisan advice. For example, the Clinton administration developed a proposal for national health insurance in the early 1990s. Following Clinton's failed attempt at reform, President George W. Bush worked toward the smaller goal of adding prescription drug coverage to Medicare in 2003. Although this achievement provided a much-needed benefit to older adults and individuals with disabilities, it did not provide improvements for the general population. Americans who were not eligible for Medicare or Medicaid or

---

[89] The committee that drafted this report was chaired by Henry J. Aaron, who was at the Brookings Institution in Washington, DC, when this report was released.

[90] Impact of IOM Reports (Database), IOM/NAM Records.

[91] The committee that was responsible for this report was chaired by Steven A. Schroeder, who was a Distinguished Professor of Health and Health Care at the University of California, San Francisco, during this time.

were not covered through employers' health plans continued to face the consequences of living without health insurance. Other access challenges existed for those individuals and families who had some degree of coverage through employer health plans but who could not afford deductibles and copays.

In response to growing concerns about uninsurance in the United States, the IOM, with funding from the RWJF, launched a 3-year effort to examine the consequences of uninsurance at the individual, family, community, and national levels. In conducting its work, the committee was organized into six subcommittees that would each contribute a report to the series between September 2001 and January 2004 (see Box 5-4).

Each report in the series built on the previous reports, with the final report offering the committee's principles and recommendations, along with its vision to have everyone in the United States covered by insurance by 2010. The committee, which was co-chaired by NAM members Mary Sue Coleman[92] and Arthur Kellermann,[93] stated that health care coverage should be universal, continuous, affordable for individuals and families, and affordable and sustainable for society, also noting that coverage should "enhance health and well-being by promoting access to high-quality care that is effective, efficient, safe, timely, patient-centered, and equitable" (IOM, 2004e, p. 9).

BOX 5-4
The Institute of Medicine's Uninsurance Series

- *Coverage Matters: Insurance and Health Care* (IOM, 2001e): The committee's first report evaluated uninsurance in terms of subpopulations and demographics (e.g., age, gender, race, health status), as well as geographic distribution. The committee also considered differences between intermittent and long-term uninsurance.
- *Care Without Coverage: Too Little, Too Late* (IOM, 2002b): The second report evaluated research on the "effects of having or lacking health insurance on a variety of personal health-related outcomes" and offered criteria for reviewing the quality of available data related to insurance status and health outcomes.
- *Health Insurance Is a Family Matter* (IOM, 2002f): The third report assessed the effects of uninsurance on the health, financial, and psychosocial well-being and stability of families and children with an emphasis on childhood development.
- *A Shared Destiny: Community Effects of Uninsurance* (IOM, 2003l): The committee's fourth report looked at the impact of uninsurance on communities and the interactions between uninsurance and factors related to local economies, public health, ethnic composition, and availability of health care resources.
- *Hidden Costs, Value Lost: Uninsurance in America* (IOM, 2003e): The fifth report explored the direct and indirect costs of uninsurance, estimating that annualized costs associated with uninsurance were between $65 and $130 billion due to diminished health and shorter life spans. The committee also described who bears these costs, from out-of-pocket payments covered by families to uncompensated care that is paid for by taxpayers.
- *Insuring America's Health: Principles and Recommendations* (IOM, 2004e): The committee's final report reviewed various insurance models, policies, and programs that could be used to expand health care coverage and eliminate consequences of uninsurance.

---

[92] Mary Sue Coleman was the President of the Iowa Health System and the University of Iowa and the President of the University of Michigan during this time.

[93] Arthur Kellermann was a Professor and the Chair of the Department of Emergency Medicine and the Director of the Center for Injury Control at Emory University in Atlanta when these reports were released. Kellermann served as a member of the NAM Council from 2013 to 2016.

The committee used evidence presented in the previous reports to emphasize the need for universal coverage to eliminate gaps in coverage and costs associated with uninsurance. When the final report was released in January 2004, Executive Officer Susanne Stoiber described the series as the "most comprehensive evidence base yet developed on who is uninsured, why, and what the impact is on individuals, families, communities and the nation."[94]

Five years after the release of the IOM's uninsurance series and without significant political action to reform the health care system or expand health care coverage in the United States, the IOM revisited the topic in 2009, releasing *America's Uninsured Crisis: Consequences for Health and Health Care*. The new report found that rates of insurance coverage continued to decline and that the population of Americans without insurance had reached more than 45 million (more than 17 percent of the population). The committee, which was chaired by external volunteer Lawrence S. Lewin,[95] pointed to "literature on health consequences [that] is more robust than that available to the previous committee—lack of insurance coverage does have health consequences, and there is new literature to confirm an important but previously unanswered question: newly providing coverage to the previously uninsured does in fact improve things" (IOM, 2009b, p. xii). The committee also found that large uninsured populations in communities could undermine the quality and timeliness of care for those with insurance. The report reiterated messages from the uninsurance series, stating that "coverage matters" and that "expanding health coverage to all Americans is essential" (IOM, 2009b, pp. xii, 9). In its single recommendation, the committee called on the President and Congress to work with other stakeholders to achieve universal coverage.

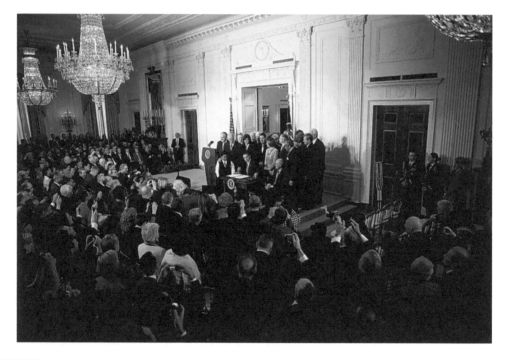

FIGURE 5-2 President Barack Obama signs the Patient Protection and Affordable Care Act into law in the East Room of the White House, March 23, 2010.
SOURCE: Photo by Lawrence Jackson, White House Archives.

[94] Susanne Stoiber to IOM Council, January 12, 2004, IOM/NAM Records.
[95] Lawrence S. Lewin was an executive consultant in Maryland when this report was released.

Essential Benefits and Preventive Health Services for Women

President Obama revived efforts to establish national health insurance coverage, and in spite of much opposition and criticism, Congress passed the ACA in 2010 (see Figure 5-2). The 2010 legislation marked a crucial inflection point in the political debate over expanding access to health care and controlling cost—perpetual areas of concern for the IOM. Not only did the ACA make significant changes to the financing and organization of insurance coverage by expanding Medicaid and individual insurance markets, but it also prompted studies to guide and evaluate the changes that would result from the legislation. For example, HHS called on the IOM to help develop criteria for determining the "essential health benefits" (EHBs), or the minimum set of benefits that health insurance plans had to cover through the state-based "purchasing exchanges."

In response to the HHS request, the IOM released *Essential Health Benefits: Balancing Coverage and Costs* in 2012. The committee, which was chaired by John R. Ball,[96] interpreted its task as "finding the right balance between making coverage available to individuals" and keeping costs at an affordable level for individuals, employers, public funders, and taxpayers. The IOM advised that the essential health benefit package should maximize the number of people with insurance coverage while protecting the most vulnerable. In line with the IOM's previous studies, the components of the essential health benefit package also needed to be safe, effective, and demonstrate improvements in health outcomes. The committee also indicated that future modifications of the EHBs should be transparent, participatory, data driven, and encouraging to innovation (IOM, 2012o). In response to the committee's report, the Essential Health Benefits Coalition, which represents employers from various sectors, advised HHS to adopt the report's first recommendation,[97] which suggested that "the starting point in establishing the initial EHB package should be the scope of benefits and design provided under a typical small employer plan in today's market" (IOM, 2012f, p. 7).

Another study that stemmed from the ACA involved identification of the preventive health services that would be fully covered by health plans without a patient copay. In particular, the HHS asked the IOM "to conduct a review of effective preventive services to ensure women's health and well-being." The IOM's report *Clinical Preventive Services for Women: Closing the Gaps* was released in 2011 and included recommendations for a range of preventive services that should be covered. For example, the committee, which was chaired by NAM member Linda Rosenstock,[98] called for "a fuller range of contraceptive education, counseling, methods, and services" along with improvements in screening for cervical cancer and HIV, counseling related to sexually transmitted infections, and screening and counseling for interpersonal and domestic violence. The committee also highlighted the importance of preventative services for pregnant women (e.g., screening for gestational diabetes) and recommended that at least one comprehensive "well woman" visit be covered annually (IOM, 2011h).

On August 1, 2011, less than 2 weeks after the release of the report, HHS adopted the IOM's recommendations for preventive health services for women that outlined the specific services that should be covered with no out-of-pocket costs under the provision of the ACA. Based on the HHS's adoption of the IOM's recommendations, health plans were required to cover a full range of preventive services for women without cost sharing, including annual well-woman visits, screening for gestational diabetes, breastfeeding support, HPV testing, counseling related to sexually transmitted

---

[96] John R. Ball was the Former Executive Vice President at the American Society for Clinical Pathology when this report was released.

[97] Impact of IOM Reports (Database), IOM/NAM Records.

[98] Linda Rosenstock was the Dean of the School of Public Health at the University of California, Los Angeles, during this time.

infections, HIV screening, contraception methods and counseling, and screening and counseling for interpersonal and domestic violence.[99]

Between 2014 and 2016, when insurance coverage-related provisions of the ACA were implemented, uninsurance rates in the United States dropped by 7 percent—from 17 percent in 2013 (approximately 44.4 million uninsured) to 10 percent in 2016 (approximately 26.7 million uninsured (Tolbert et al., 2020). As provisions of the ACA (including the individual mandate) were challenged in court and the implementation of the law evolved, rates of uninsurance in the United States started increasing again. In 2018, the uninsurance rate stood at 10.4 percent, with approximately 27.9 million people without insurance (Tolbert et al., 2020). In 2015, on the cusp of the 2016 U.S. presidential election, the newly formed NAM launched a major initiative to inform the future reform efforts in terms of the nation's health, health care, and biomedical sciences. The initiative, called Vital Directions for Health and Health Care, was designed "to provide expert guidance on 19 priority issues for U.S. health policy" with "three overarching goals ... better health and well-being; high-value health care; and strong science and technology" (NASEM, n.d.q). The initiative is described in greater detail in Chapter 7.

Prescription Drugs

Continuing the IOM's work to reform the health care system, the NAM partnered with the HMD to take on a pressing challenge for the nation: the cost of prescription drugs. In the first two decades of the 21st century, the increasing cost of prescription drugs became a serious concern for many Americans who struggled to pay for needed medications, some of which had more than doubled in price in a short period of time (e.g., insulin, Epi Pens) (Kodjak, 2019; Rapaport, 2017). The Presidents' Committee of the National Academies of Sciences, Engineering, and Medicine, along with six health foundations and the American College of Physicians, sponsored a study to explore opportunities to make prescriptions more affordable without hindering innovation or the development of new drugs. The resulting report, *Making Medicines Affordable: A National Imperative,* was published in 2018. The report stated that the pharmaceutical industry was "fraught with discordant viewpoints, divergent priorities, and conflicts of interest" (NASEM, 2018d, p. 3). The imperative of "consumer access to effective and affordable medicine" was "not being adequately served by the biophysical sector today" (NASEM, 2018d, p. 4). To resolve some of these concerns, the committee, which was chaired by NAM member Norman Augustine,[100] recommended expanding access to generic drugs and applying more of the government's purchasing power to "improve drug valuation methods" (NASEM, 2018d, p. 6).

One year after the release of the report, Victor Dzau made the price of prescription drugs the topic of the 2018 President's Forum at the NAM's annual meeting. As part of the forum, Dzau invited HHS Secretary Alex M. Azar II to present. In his remarks, Azar argued that people had the right to know a drug's price when it was advertised on television (Pear, 2018). The Secretary's comments were followed by a panel discussion that featured a senator, experts from the pharmaceutical and health care industries, and another official from HHS.

CONCLUSION

In a multitude of ways, the IOM, and subsequently the NAM and the HMD, have played a sustained and essential role in advising the nation, the government, and the health care industry on

---

[99] Impact of IOM Reports (Database), IOM/NAM Records.

[100] Norman Augustine was the Former Chair and the Chief Executive Officer of Lockheed Martin Corporation when this report was released.

how best to improve health care and set health policies designed to ensure equitable access to high-quality, evidence-based health care for all Americans. Throughout its history, the IOM expanded its reach to cover a wide range of topics related to the delivery of health care and improvement of the health care system. Even though modifications to the U.S. health care system have been slow and have come with varying degrees of success, the IOM served as a steady and unbiased voice, consistently calling for change and providing recommendations to guide that change. Although the transition from the IOM to the NAM and the HMD was a historic shift for the organization, its members, and its staff, the transition did not interrupt the focus of the organization or its commitment to achieving better health in the United States through an improved health care system. The creation of the NAM and its action-oriented portfolio of programs augmented the previous work of the IOM and the continuing work of the HMD. The NAM's drive to build stronger collaborations afforded new opportunities to facilitate the implementation of the organization's recommendations and further influence change across the health care system.

6

Advancing the Health of the Public in the United States and Globally

The goal of improving public health was a long-standing cornerstone of the Institute of Medicine (IOM) and was an essential legacy carried forward by the National Academy of Medicine (NAM) and the Health and Medicine Division (HMD). From the beginning, the IOM's founders recognized that health outcomes were influenced by a complex array of social, economic, behavioral, and environmental factors, such as education, income, geography, housing, transportation, and family and social interactions. Over the years, the organization devoted a sizable portion of its portfolio to better understanding the interactions across these factors. "To improve health for all" by "accelerating health equity" was made a part of the NAM's new mission statement in 2018, demonstrating the organization's ongoing commitment to public health and ensuring greater health equity for all populations. As a "national academy with a global scope," the NAM also expanded its reach to facilitate improvements for populations worldwide, acknowledging that the world was becoming more interconnected with each passing decade—a fact that was never more apparent than during the COVID-19 pandemic that swept the globe beginning in 2020. The reports and convening activities described in this chapter were led by staff from the IOM, the NAM, or the HMD with the help of NAM members and expert external volunteers.

DEFINING AND SHAPING PUBLIC HEALTH

Throughout its history, the IOM played a crucial role in defining and shaping the field of public health and public health programs in the United States. For example, in 1988 the IOM released a report called *The Future of Public Health*. The widely cited report defined public health as "what society does collectively to assure the conditions for people to be healthy" and sought to reaffirm the nation's traditional public health mission (IOM, 2003f). The committee, which was chaired by external volunteer Richard D. Remington,[1] recommended "core functions in public health assess-

---

[1] Richard D. Remington was the Vice President for Academic Affairs and the Dean of the Faculties at the University of Iowa at the time.

ment, policy development, and service assurances" that could reinvigorate the U.S. public health system and ensure better responses to ongoing and emerging public health threats (IOM, 1988a).

In 2002, the IOM released a follow-on report that revisited the state of the public health system. *The Future of the Public's Health in the 21st Century* was drafted by a committee co-chaired by Christine K. Cassel[2] and Jo Ivey Boufford,[3] who served as the NAM's Foreign Secretary from 2006 to 2014 and on its Council from 2001 to 2006. The report concluded that the country continued to fall short in terms of population health despite having the largest health expenditures in the world. The report offered a conceptual framework designed to strengthen the public health infrastructure, build partnerships, emphasize accountability and evidence, improve communication, and account for the multiple determinants of health, going beyond factors related to the health care system. It also recommended the formation of a national commission to consider the benefits of a public health accreditation system (IOM, 2003f). As a result of the report, the Robert Wood Johnson Foundation (RWJF) funded the Exploring Accreditation Initiative, which brought together the Association of State and Territorial Health Officials (ASTHO), the National Association of County and City Health Officials, and other organizations to recommend a national framework for the voluntary accreditation of state and local public health departments.[4]

The IOM also explored opportunities to strengthen the public health workforce in its report *Who Will Keep the Public Healthy?: Educating Public Health Professionals for the 21st Century* (IOM, 2003g), and options to integrate public health and primary care in its 2012 report *Primary Care and Public Health: Exploring Integration to Improve Population Health* (IOM, 2012g). This latter report is credited with inspiring the Practical Playbook website launched by the de Beaumont Foundation, Duke Community and Family Medicine, and the Centers for Disease Control and Prevention (CDC) in 2014. The Practical Playbook was designed to improve public health and primary care integration by providing resources for health care providers, including action steps for starting a collaborative project and case studies of successful projects. The website drew on a database of examples from a Primary Care and Public Health Collaborative, which had been established by ASTHO in response to the IOM's report.[5]

Throughout its history, the IOM also played a valuable role in advising the Department of Health and Human Services (HHS) on its national public health priorities through a series of reports focused on health indicators. In 1978, the IOM released a paper that informed the first iteration of *Healthy People* (see Chapter 2), the government's national agenda for improving the public's health. *Healthy People* was updated regularly to set new 10-year objectives for 2000, 2010, and 2020, and the IOM provided input to each of those efforts. For example, the IOM released three reports—*Healthy People 2000: Citizens Chart the Course* (IOM, 1990d), *Leading Health Indicators for Healthy People 2010: Final Report* (IOM, 1999e), and *Leading Health Indicators for Healthy People 2020: Letter Report* (IOM, 2011)—each of which offered a set of health indicators and objectives for HHS to consider for inclusion in *Healthy People*.

The IOM also provided guidance on how communities and the nation could develop and implement quality measures to monitor progress against the leading health indicators in its report *Toward Quality Measures for Population Health and the Leading Health Indicators* (IOM, 2013o). In carrying on the IOM's advisory role to HHS and in preparation for Healthy People 2030, the National Academies released *Criteria for Selecting the Leading Health Indicators for Healthy People 2030* (NASEM, 2019l), and is expected to release a second report that will offer input on

---

[2] Christine K. Cassel was the Dean of the School of Medicine at Oregon Health & Science University when this report was released.

[3] Jo Ivey Boufford was the Professor of Health Policy and Public Service at the Robert F. Wagner Graduate School of Public Service at New York University during this time.

[4] Impact of IOM Reports (Database), IOM/NAM Records.

[5] Ibid.

specific leading health indicators for the 2030 national agenda. The IOM's (and now the HMD's) relationship with HHS exemplifies how the organization has informed the nation's public health priorities over the last half-century.

To expand its role in advising the nation on topics related to public and population health, the IOM launched the Roundtable on Population Health Improvement in 2012. With sponsorship from nearly 20 foundations, government entities, academic institutions, and corporations, the round-table's members envisioned "a strong, healthful, and productive society which cultivates human capital and equal opportunity" (NASEM, n.d.r). Since its inception, the roundtable has created 2 Action Collaboratives, held more than 30 public meetings, and released numerous workshop summaries, commissioned papers, perspectives, and briefing documents. The roundtable's work has explored topics related to the social determinants of health, including education and economic policy; opportunities to improve health equity; and collaboration across health care, education, and public health. The roundtable has continued its work under the auspices of the HMD but has also collaborated with the NAM on programs, such as the DC Public Health Case Challenge, with the intended goal of improving population health across the United States.

RESPONDING TO PUBLIC HEALTH PANDEMICS AND EPIDEMICS

In addition to its role as an advisor on identifying national public health priorities, the IOM and now the NAM and HMD have also delved into public health epidemics the nation and the world have faced throughout the organization's existence. Some pandemics and epidemics are urgent and require an immediate response, including the development of short- and long-term strategies to mitigate the effects, such as the HIV/AIDS epidemic; tuberculosis, Zika, and Ebola outbreaks; the COVID-19 pandemic; and the opioid crisis in the United States (described in Chapter 7). Other epidemics represent persistent public health challenges that require decades of multi-faceted inter-ventions to see shifts in prevalence, such as the tobacco use and violence epidemics. The organiza-tion also identified childhood obesity as an ongoing epidemic that warranted in-depth consideration.

HIV/AIDS Epidemic

During the HIV/AIDS epidemic the IOM demonstrated its ability to provide timely advice and active guidance to inform a national and international response to a novel disease. The IOM's work on HIV/AIDS had a notable impact on public health decisions at the time and became the standard by which future IOM activities would be judged in terms of impact. Throughout its history, the IOM released nearly 30 consensus studies that reviewed various aspects of HIV/AIDS, including prevention, screening, and treatment; research and drug discovery; health policy and financing; and global health issues (see Box 6-1).[6] The IOM's work in the early years of the epidemic set the groundwork for later public health and policy responses to HIV/AIDS.

As the epidemic emerged in the early 1980s and fear among the public spread, Fred Robbins, the IOM's fourth president, identified HIV/AIDS as a public health concern in which the IOM should be involved. In the summer of 1983, the IOM Council discussed possible roles for the IOM in responding to the crisis. The discussion at the time focused on the shortage of health care providers and facilities willing to care for the growing number of patients with AIDS. When Rob-bins contacted the Reagan administration about being part of the national response to the disease in 1983, Ed Brandt, the Assistant Secretary for Health at HHS, said there was little the IOM could or should do. Meanwhile, NAM member Anthony Fauci was appointed as director of the National

---

[6] The IOM's AIDS-related activities are covered more fully in the 1998 history of the IOM authored by Edward Berkowitz (IOM, 1998a, Ch. 6). This section draws on that account.

BOX 6-1
Examples of Institute of Medicine Reports on HIV/AIDS

- *Confronting AIDS: Directions for Public Health, Health Care, and Research* (1986)
- *Confronting AIDS: Update 1988* (1988)
- *Equitable Financing of AIDS and Other HIV-Related Health Care: Summary of a Meeting* (1988)
- *The AIDS Research Program of the National Institutes of Health* (1991)
- *Expanding Access to Investigational Therapies for HIV Infection and AIDS* (1991)
- *HIV Screening of Pregnant Women and Newborns* (1991)
- *AIDS and Behavior: An Integrated Approach* (1994)
- *Government and Industry Collaboration in AIDS Drug Development* (1994)
- *HIV and the Blood Supply: An Analysis of Crisis Decisionmaking* (1995)
- *Preventing HIV Transmission: The Role of Sterile Needles and Bleach* (1995)
- *Reducing the Odds: Preventing Perinatal Transmission of HIV in the United States* (1999)
- *Measuring What Matters: Allocation, Planning, and Quality Assessment for the Ryan White CARE Act* (2004)
- *Scaling Up Treatment for the Global AIDS Pandemic: Challenges and Opportunities* (2005)
- *Healers Abroad: Americans Responding to the Human Resource Crisis in HIV/AIDS* (2005)
- *Public Financing and Delivery of HIV/AIDS Care: Securing the Legacy of Ryan White* (2005)
- *Review of the HIVNET 012 Perinatal HIV Prevention Study* (2005)
- *Preventing HIV Infection Among Injecting Drug Users in High-Risk Countries: An Assessment of the Evidence* (2007)
- *PEPFAR Implementation: Progress and Promise* (2007)
- *Methodological Challenges in Biomedical HIV Prevention Trials* (2008)
- *HIV and Disability: Updating the Social Security Listings* (2010)
- *HIV Screening and Access to Care: Exploring Barriers and Facilitators to Expanded HIV Testing* (2010)
- *Preparing for the Future of HIV/AIDS in Africa: A Shared Responsibility* (2011)
- *HIV Screening and Access to Care: Health Care System Capacity for Increased HIV Testing and Provision of Care* (2011)
- *HIV Screening and Access to Care: Exploring the Impact of Policies on Access to and Provision of HIV Care* (2011)
- *Monitoring HIV Care in the United States: Indicators and Data Systems* (2012)
- *Monitoring HIV Care in the United States: A Strategy for Generating National Estimates of HIV Care and Coverage* (2012)
- *Evaluation of PEPFAR* (2013)

Institute of Allergy and Infectious Diseases in 1984. Addressing a conference hosted by the National Institutes of Health (NIH) that year, Fauci spoke passionately about "the extraordinary advances in the evolution of this syndrome" (Newcott, 2021). By the spring of 1985, the Reagan administration's position on the AIDS epidemic had shifted. James Mason, then the director of the CDC, said that the IOM could work on the issue of school admissions policies for HIV-positive students, as many parents feared that contact with an HIV-positive classmate would put their children at risk. The CDC wanted the IOM to confirm that "casual person-to-person contact" among schoolchildren "appears to carry no risk" (CDC, 1985).[7] Under the direction of Robbins, the IOM dedicated its

---

[7] IOM Council Meeting, Minutes, July 20, 1985, IOM/NAM Records.

1985 annual meeting to the topic of HIV/AIDS. A summary of the annual meeting was published by the Harvard University Press in 1986 under the title *Mobilizing Against AIDS: The Unfinished Story of a Virus*. The publication provided a compendium of HIV/AIDS-related information and represented one of the first publications of this type from a reputable science authority (Nichols, 1986).

When Sam Thier became IOM President in November 1985, he encouraged the IOM's continued engagement in HIV/AIDS work and suggested a collaborative Academy-wide response that included a joint National Academy of Sciences (NAS) and IOM committee. Thier kept Surgeon General C. Everett Koop updated on the committee's work, which helped align the IOM's recommendations with those of the Reagan administration.[8] The committee's report, *Confronting AIDS: Directions for Public Health, Health Care, and Research*, was released by the IOM in October 1986. The committee, which was co-chaired by NAM/NAS member David Baltimore[9] and external volunteer Sheldon M. Wolff,[10] recommended a National Commission on AIDS, a major public health campaign to help prevent the spread of HIV, and a scientific research program with the goals of preventing HIV and treating AIDS (IOM and NRC, 1986).

For the first time in the IOM's history, the release of a report received notable media coverage that included front page stories in *The New York Times* and *The Washington Post* and follow-up stories in the days after the report release. On October 29, all three national television networks led their evening news broadcasts with stories about *Confronting AIDS* (Boffey, 1986; Russell, 1986; Network Television Evening News, 1986). According to *The New York Times*, the report "provided a benchmark by which many members of Congress and analysts judged the effectiveness of the nation's effort to combat AIDS" (Boffey, 1988). The report spurred legislation that nearly doubled federal spending on AIDS. The media attention and political response to the report cemented the IOM's position within the public health and health policy worlds. Following the release of the report, the mainstream media began to report routinely on the organization's activities, and impact became an important internal measure of the efficacy of the organization's work.

In November 1986, the IOM Council endorsed a continuation of the IOM's HIV/AIDS-related work. The IOM held workshops on promoting drug development to treat HIV/AIDS, the epidemiology of HIV/AIDS in an international context, and the development of an HIV vaccine. In the spring of 1987, IOM President Thier and NAS President Frank Press joined forces to convene the NAS-IOM AIDS Activities Oversight Committee. This new committee was tasked with reviewing and updating the 1986 report and also coordinating HIV/AIDS activities across the National Academies. *Confronting AIDS: Update 1988* was released in June 1988 and recommended that the HIV infection "itself should be considered as a disease" (IOM, 1988b, p. 37). The committee, which was chaired by external volunteer Theodore Cooper,[11] also affirmed the view, current at the time, that "virtually all [HIV-]infected individuals] will eventually develop AIDS" (IOM, 1988b, p. 2). The report stressed that "we are no closer now to having a licensed vaccine against HIV than we were two years ago" (p. 20) and that developing treatment options offered "the best hope of slowing the epidemic through research."[12] Meanwhile, a grassroots movement to spur the development of treatments for HIV/AIDS gained momentum (see Figure 6-1).

---

[8] Oral Interview with Samuel Thier, November 2018, NAS-NRC Archives.

[9] David Baltimore was at the Whitehead Institute for Biomedical Research and the Massachusetts Institute of Technology during this time.

[10] Sheldon M. Wolff was at the Tufts University School of Medicine and the New England Medical Center Hospital when this report was released.

[11] Theodore Cooper was with the Upjohn Company in Kalamazoo, Michigan, during this time.

[12] "Panel Cites Remaining Deficiencies in National Effort to Combat AIDS," IOM Press Release, June 1, 1988, IOM/NAM Records.

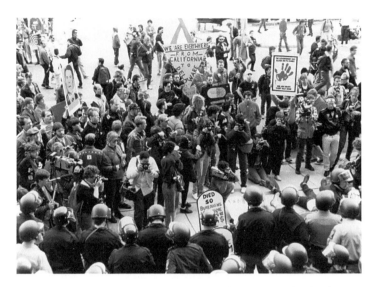

FIGURE 6-1 In 1988 the AIDS Coalition to Unleash Power (ACT-UP) organized a demonstration at the Food and Drug Administration headquarters in Rockville, Maryland, to protest for greater access to investigational drugs to help treat AIDS patients.
SOURCE: Food and Drug Administration.

Like the first iteration of *Confronting AIDS*, the 1988 update garnered a sizable media response. Although the second report did not ultimately have the same level of impact as the original report, the 1988 report led to amendments to the Public Health Service Act that authorized $1.5 billion for HIV/AIDS research, public health programs, and an HIV/AIDS public information campaign. That same year, the IOM and NAS sent a jointly developed white paper to President-elect George H.W. Bush that argued that HIV/AIDS should be a key priority on his administration's health agenda. The paper estimated that AIDS would claim more than 200,000 American lives during Bush's term in office and advised the newly elected president to become involved in "an aggressive, unambiguous education program about behavior changes necessary to avoid HIV infection."[13]

The AIDS Activities Oversight Committee continued its work after the release of the 1988 report by advising the National Academies on activities such as a government-requested evaluation of the NIH's AIDS programs. A separate committee produced a report called *The AIDS Research Program of the National Institutes of Health* that was released in 1991. The report suggested that the NIH should increase its HIV/AIDS research activities in behavioral science, basic science, patient care research, and vaccine development. The committee supported the NIH's organizational approach to its HIV/AIDS research activities, which leveraged a cross-cutting "institute without walls" model rather than creating a new institute (IOM, 1991d).[14] The committee's chair, NAM member William Danforth, testified before Congress indicating that the best way to increase the country's understanding of HIV/AIDS was "to provide support for scientists studying how viruses work" (IOM, 1998a, p. 234).

Before the AIDS Activities Oversight Committee disbanded in June 1991, it advised on activities that involved nearly every board and division across the IOM, and HIV/AIDS became a

---

[13] Frank Press and Samuel Thier to George H.W. Bush, President-Elect of the United States, December 13, 1985, IOM/NAM Records.

[14] William Danforth testimony before the Subcommittee on Human Resources and Intergovernmental Relations of the Committee on Government Relations, March 7, 1991, copy in IOM/NAM Records.

permanent item on the IOM's agenda. For example, in 1989 the IOM established the Roundtable for the Development of Drugs and Vaccines against AIDS, which discussed the potential value of a consortium dedicated to overcoming challenges in developing HIV/AIDS treatments and vaccines such as an "acute shortage" of animals "to test potential preventive and therapeutic activities against AIDS."[15] Other HIV/AIDS-related activities included a collaborative meeting between the IOM and the Russian Academy of Medical Sciences that led to an international information exchange on HIV/AIDS and developed connections between American and Russian scientists.[16] Additionally, the Medical Follow-Up Agency studied a group of HIV-positive servicemen who had previously been lost to follow-up after military discharge. During this timeframe, the NAS also convened its own HIV/AIDS-related activities that contributed to the National Academies' response to the epidemic. For example, in 1987, citing the IOM's "landmark" study, the NAS established the Committee on AIDS Research and the Behavioral, Social, and Statistical Sciences. By February 1989, the committee had developed its report on *AIDS, Sexual Behavior, and Intravenous Drug Use* (NRC, 1989b). In 1990, the NAS released *AIDS: The Second Decade,* which indicated that the disease was nowhere near under control, noting that "morbidity and mortality from HIV infection will continue throughout the 1990s" (NRC, 1990, p. vii).

President's Emergency Plan for AIDS Relief

In the late 1990s and early 2000s—as deaths from AIDS in the United States began to decline and new, more effective treatments for HIV such as antiretroviral drugs became more readily available in the United States—international organizations such as the World Health Organization (WHO) and the United Nations began calling for programs to make these new treatments available globally. In his 2003 State of the Union Address, President George W. Bush proposed the President's Emergency Plan for AIDS Relief (PEPFAR), which was enacted by Congress on May 27, 2003, as part of the United States Leadership against HIV/AIDS, Tuberculosis, and Malaria Act of 2003. PEPFAR was meant to provide "a comprehensive, integrated 5-year strategy to combat global HIV/AIDS" (IOM, 2007g, p. 3). The $15 billion initiative had goals related to preventing transmission of HIV, expanding access to treatment, and improving HIV/AIDS care with an emphasis on 15 countries that were identified as "focus countries."

Around this time, the IOM began to turn its attention to HIV/AIDS outside of the U.S. borders. For example, in April 2005 the IOM released *Healers Abroad: Americans Responding to the Human Resource Crisis in HIV/AIDS,* which indicated that 40 million people across the globe were infected with HIV and that 95 percent of them lived in resource-poor countries, such as the focus countries defined under the PEPFAR initiative (IOM, 2005b). The committee highlighted the critical need for health care professionals in these countries and reviewed options for overseas placement of U.S. health professionals. The committee, which was chaired by NAM member Fitzhugh Mullan,[17] recommended the creation of a United States Global Health Service that would send health care professionals to the PEPFAR countries, functioning somewhat like the Peace Corps but with an emphasis on providing care for individuals with HIV/AIDS. In 2012, the Peace Corps announced a new Global Health Service Partnership (GHSP), which was funded through PEPFAR. The new program would deploy physicians and nurses to serve as faculty members tasked with helping

---

[15] "Roundtable for the Development of Drugs and Vaccines Against AIDS: Meeting Summary," February 7, 1989, June 26, 1990, IOM/NAM Records; "The Potential Value of Research Consortia in the Development of Drugs and Vaccines Against HIV Infection and AIDS: Report of a Workshop," 1989, IOM/NAM Records.

[16] "Summary of the Institute of Medicine U.S.-USSR Aids Symposium, October 4–5, 1989," February 28, 1990, IOM/ NAM Records.

[17] Fitzhugh Mullan was with Health Affairs/Project Hope and the Department of Prevention and Community Health of George Washington University School of Public Health and Health Services in Washington, DC, during this timeframe.

developing countries address health care provider shortages. Mullan advised GHSP Executive Director Vanessa Kerry in developing the program.[18]

Built into the legislation that authorized PEPFAR was a request for the IOM to conduct a short-term evaluation of the initiative 3 years after its launch. To prepare for this evaluation, the IOM released a letter report in October 2005, *Plan for a Short-Term Evaluation of PEPFAR Implementation*, that detailed the approach the committee would use to evaluate the program. The committee's evaluation strategy included 1-week site visits to 13 of the 15 focus countries, which resulted in pre- and post-visit analyses for each country. In its deliberations the committee also reviewed budget and performance data, assessed available literature and documentation, and solicited input and feedback from a range of stakeholders and participants (IOM, 2006c). In 2007, the IOM released *PEPFAR Implementation: Progress and Promise*. The timing of the report release coincided with congressional deliberations related to reauthorization of the initiative. In its report, the committee, which was chaired by NAM member Jaime Sepúlveda,[19] concluded that PEPFAR had "supported the expansion of HIV/AIDS prevention, treatment, and care services in the focus countries" (IOM, 2007g, p. 1). To promote continued progress toward PEPFAR's goals, the committee recommended that the initiative needed to "transition from a focus on emergency relief to an emphasis on the long-term strategic planning and capacity building necessary for sustainability" (IOM, 2007g, p. 1). One year after the release of the IOM's report, Congress reauthorized PEPFAR as part of Tom Lantos (D-CA) and Henry J. Hyde's (R-IL) U.S. Global Leadership Against HIV/AIDS, Tuberculosis, and Malaria Reauthorization Act of 2008. The reauthorization legislation also included a provision requesting the IOM to conduct another evaluation of the initiative with an emphasis on its performance and its impact on health (IOM, 2013i).

On World AIDS Day in 2009, PEPFAR launched an international AIDS strategy for the next 5 years that drew from lessons learned since the program was launched in 2003 and heavily reflected the findings, conclusions, and recommendations of the 2007 IOM report. A press release from the Department of State spelled out the overarching goals for PEPFAR's next phase, many of which were justified in the PEPFAR reauthorization legislation with references to the IOM report:

- Transition from emergency response to promotion of sustainable country programs;
- Strengthen partner government capacity to lead the response to this epidemic and other health demands;
- Expand prevention, care, and treatment in both concentrated and generalized epidemics;
- Integrate and coordinate HIV/AIDS programs with broader global health and development programs to maximize impact on health systems; and
- Invest in innovation and operations research to evaluate impact, improve service delivery and maximize outcomes.

These goals were well aligned with the IOM report's emphasis on the importance of shifting the program's focus from emergency relief to long-term strategic planning and capacity building; strengthening a country's ownership and leadership of its response to the epidemic; and collecting and using data on the precise nature of the epidemic in each country to determine the most appropriate interventions and target them most effectively.[20]

The IOM's second report, *Evaluation of PEPFAR*, was published in February 2013. It noted that the reauthorization of the initiative had shifted priorities toward strengthening local health

---

[18] Impact of IOM Reports (Database), IOM/NAM Records.

[19] Jaime Sepúlveda was the 2007 Presidential Chair and a Visiting Professor at the University of California, San Francisco.

[20] Impact of IOM Reports (Database), IOM/NAM Records.

systems with an emphasis on sustainability, while continuing to scale up services. The committee, which was chaired by NAM member Robert E. Black,[21] concluded that

> PEPFAR's efforts have saved and improved the lives of millions of people by supporting HIV prevention, care, and treatment services; meeting the needs of children affected by the epidemic; building capacity; strengthening systems; engaging with partner country governments and other stakeholders; increasing knowledge about the epidemic in partner countries; and ensuring that attention be paid to vulnerable populations in the response to HIV. (IOM, 2013i, p. 3)

The committee offered recommendations to enhance and strengthen systems, capacity, and leadership in the partner countries in order to ensure sustainability that would allow them to manage their responses to HIV/AIDS (IOM, 2013i).

Tobacco and Marijuana Use

At one time, a high percentage of Americans smoked cigarettes and used other tobacco products (e.g., cigars, pipes, chewing tobacco, snuff), often becoming addicted and unknowingly causing harm to their health. As research demonstrated strong associations and eventually causal relationships between tobacco products and cancer, the evidence persuaded many people to quit using tobacco products and many others not to start in the first place. The prevalence of tobacco use remained high among teenagers and adults, however, and it was characterized as an epidemic by the WHO, the CDC, and public health researchers (CDC, n.d.d; Giovino, 2007; Slade, 1992; WHO, 2019). In the 1970s and 1980s, there was a growing belief among experts that the key to reducing tobacco use was to prevent young people from starting to use tobacco products. Under the direction of IOM President David Hamburg, the IOM began thinking about ways to decrease and prevent tobacco use. One of the IOM's first reports on smoking cessation was released in 1979 as part of the IOM's *Health and Behavior* series (see Chapter 2). Tobacco use was an area in which the IOM not only advised on public health and health policy, but also one in which it became involved in the underlying science with an emphasis on alternative tobacco products. The IOM was one of the few organizations with the necessary credibility and expertise to advise across multiple levels of the national discussion on the tobacco epidemic.

In the early 1990s, the IOM initiated a study focused on preventing addiction in children and youth. In 1994 the IOM released *Growing Up Tobacco Free: Preventing Nicotine Addiction in Children and Youths*. The timing of the report release coincided with the release of a Surgeon General's report on preventing tobacco use among young people (Elders et al., 1994). The Surgeon General's report catalyzed additional public interest and media coverage related to the IOM report, including prominent newspaper articles and television news stories. The report identified tobacco-related deaths as "the leading cause of avoidable death in the United States," resulting in more deaths than the combination of "AIDS, car accidents, alcohol, suicides, homicides, fires and illegal drugs" (IOM, 1994d, p. 1). According to Paul R. Torrens, an external volunteer who chaired the committee,[22] "each year, decisions by more than 1 million youths to become regular smokers" take an average of 15 years off their lives and commit the health care system "to $8.2 billion in extra medical expenditures over their lifetimes" (p. 5). The report concluded that "in the long run, tobacco use can be most efficiently reduced through a youth-centered policy aimed at preventing children and adolescents from initiating tobacco use" (IOM, 1994d, p. 5).

---

[21] Robert E. Black was at Johns Hopkins University in Baltimore, Maryland, when this report was released.

[22] Paul R. Torrens was a Professor of Health Services Administration in the Department of Health Services in the School of Public Health at the University of California, Los Angeles, during this time.

Growing Up Tobacco Free became one of the IOM's best-selling reports of the 1990s.[23] The report was also the first in a series of IOM reports that evaluated the health risks of tobacco and made recommendations to quell tobacco use. In 1998, for example, the National Cancer Policy Board issued its first policy statement on tobacco control, *Taking Action to Reduce Tobacco Use,* which noted that tobacco had joined AIDS as "one of [the] two major growing health threats world-wide" (IOM and NRC, 1998a, p. 30). In a strongly worded statement, the board indicated that "the single most direct and reliable method for reducing consumption is to increase the price of tobacco products" (p. 30). With policy changes and new taxes, the market could aid in promoting public health. Following the release of its policy statement, the board released a summary of evidence related to the efficacy of state tobacco control programs, *State Programs Can Reduce Tobacco Use* (IOM, 2000f). The goal of the publication was to provide examples of successful state-level tobacco control policies and programs that could be implemented in other states.

By the start of the new millennium, it was widely understood that smoking caused cancer, chronic obstructive pulmonary disease, and stroke. Around this timeframe companies began developing alternative tobacco products that might reduce harm. In addition to exploring public health policy actions related to tobacco use and prevention, the IOM also explored the science of tobacco harm reduction. In 2001, the IOM released a report called *Clearing the Smoke: Assessing the Science Base for Tobacco Harm Reduction,* which featured an examination of available literature on products that claimed to "preserve tobacco pleasure while reducing its toxic effects" (e.g., low-yield cigarettes, nicotine patches and gum). The committee, which was chaired by NAM member and Acting President (1991–1992) Stuart Bondurant,[24] concluded that "for many diseases attributable to tobacco use, reducing risk of disease by reducing exposure to tobacco toxicants is feasible" (IOM, 2001f, p. 5). However, the products designed to reduce exposure had not "been evaluated comprehensively enough ... to provide a scientific base to conclude that they reduced the risk of disease" (IOM, 2001f, p. 5). The report found a place for "strengthened federal regulation of all modified tobacco products," including those designed to reduce risk (IOM, 2001f, p. 8).

Continuing its evaluation of public health policy and strategies to reduce tobacco use in the United States, the IOM released *Ending the Tobacco Problem: A Blueprint for the Nation in 2007.* During its deliberations, the committee, which was chaired by Richard J. Bonnie,[25] concluded that while progress had been made in tobacco control, approximately 44.5 million adults in the United States still smoked, with rates of cessation beginning to plateau. Additionally, tobacco-related morbidity and mortality continued to pose large burdens on the health care industry and society as a whole. In its report, the committee presented a blueprint that called for fortifying and expanding state-level control programs and community action, increasing taxes on tobacco products, strengthening bans and restrictions related to smoking, continuing efforts to prevent youth from using tobacco and helping users quit, and granting the Food and Drug Administration (FDA) additional regulatory authority over tobacco products (IOM, 2007h). In 2009, President Obama enabled FDA regulation through the Family Smoking Prevention and Tobacco Control Act, which granted the FDA "broad authority to regulate the manufacturing, distribution, and marketing of tobacco products, including 'modified risk tobacco products'"—fulfilling recommendations from *Clearing the Smoke* (IOM, 2001f) and *Ending the Tobacco Problem* (IOM, 2007h) (IOM, 2012h; see Figure 6-2). In addition, Obama signed additional legislation that increased tobacco taxes by $0.62 per pack—from $0.39 to $1.01—the largest increase in history. The resulting revenue was

---

[23] "IOM Bestsellers," in IOM Council Minutes, January 1997, IOM/NAM Records.

[24] Stuart Bondurant was a Professor in the Department of Medicine at the University of North Carolina at Chapel Hill when this report was released.

[25] Richard J. Bonnie was the John S. Battle Professor of Law and the Director at the Institute of Law, Psychiatry, and Public Policy at the University of Virginia School of Law, Charlottesville, when this report was released.

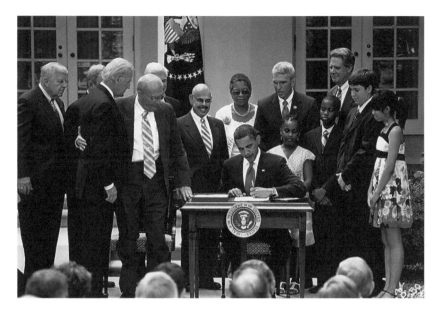

FIGURE 6-2 President Obama signs the Family Smoking Prevention and Tobacco Control Act on June 22, 2009, which vested in FDA oversight of its provisions, including manufacturing standards, labeling, and control of harmful ingredients in tobacco products.
SOURCE: Food and Drug Administration.

used to fund the expansion of the Children's Health Insurance Program.[26] Three years later, the IOM released a report called *Scientific Standards for Studies on Modified Risk Tobacco Products*. This report provided a minimum set of scientific standards that the FDA should use to confirm that a "product has the potential to reduce tobacco related harms as compared to conventional tobacco products" (IOM, 2012i).

In March 2015, prior to the creation of the NAM and the HMD, the IOM released *Public Health Implications of Raising the Age of Legal Access to Tobacco Products*. The committee, which was also chaired by Bonnie,[27] leveraged a strong scientific base, including developmental biology and psychology literature on tobacco use initiation, existing public health policies, and statistical modeling, to conclude that raising the age of legal access to tobacco would "likely lead to a substantial reduction in smoking prevalence" (IOM, 2015e, p. 3). The committee found that 90 percent of daily smokers had their first cigarette before the age of 19 and suggested that raising the nationwide minimum age of legal access to 21 years of age would lead to "approximately 223,000 fewer premature deaths, 50,000 fewer deaths from lung cancer, and 4.2 million fewer years of life lost for those born between 2000 and 2019" (p. 4). Following the release of the report, cities and counties across the nation began changing local laws to increase the legal purchasing age for tobacco products to 21 years of age, which is commensurate with the legal age for buying alcohol.[28]

Following the creation of the NAM and the HMD in 2015, the organization continued its tobacco-related work and its evaluation of the new products that claimed to reduce the harm associated with tobacco use. In the preceding years, companies had begun developing and sell-

---

[26] Impact of IOM Reports (Database), IOM/NAM Records.

[27] Richard J. Bonnie was the Harrison Foundation Professor of Medicine and Law, the Professor of Psychiatry and Neurobehavioral Sciences, and the Director of the Institute of Law, Psychiatry, and Public Policy at the University of Virginia during this time.

[28] Impact of IOM Reports (Database), IOM/NAM Records.

ing electronic cigarettes (also known as e-cigarettes and vaping pens) despite contentious legal battles at the state and federal levels (CASAA, n.d.). The products quickly grew in popularity. However, safety evaluations and data on health effects were lacking. In 2018, the HMD weighed in on the debate over the health effects of e-cigarettes with its report *Public Health Consequences of E-Cigarettes*. The report reviewed existing scientific literature and made recommendations to guide future research efforts, identifying gaps and priority areas. Although the committee, which was chaired by NAM member David L. Eaton,[29] concluded that e-cigarettes potentially contained fewer toxicants than traditional combustible cigarettes and might promote cessation of traditional cigarettes, the committee urged caution, noting that the use of these devices was not without risk and the long-term health effects were not yet known. The committee also warned that evidence suggested that youth who began using e-cigarettes might subsequently transition to more harmful combustible cigarettes (NASEM, 2018f). One year after the report was released, the CDC linked an outbreak of severe lung injuries and several deaths to the use of e-cigarettes. The CDC reported that 38 percent of those with lung injuries were under the age of 21 (22 percent between the ages of 18 and 21; 16 percent under the age of 18). Preliminary findings from the outbreak indicated a potential association with marijuana-containing products that had been used in e-cigarettes and were possibly contaminated (CDC, n.d.e). The use of e-cigarettes with tobacco- and marijuana-containing products will require continued study to fully understand the risks and long-term health implications for users.

Marijuana

In addition to tobacco use, the IOM also explored the health effects of marijuana. In 1981, the IOM released *Marijuana and Health* in response to a request from the NIH (IOM, 1982). Although the report indicated that the public should be concerned about the health effects of marijuana, the committee, which was chaired by NAM member Arnold S. Relman,[30] also noted that there was currently little evidence that demonstrated that prolonged marijuana use had a permanent impact on the heart or brain. Due to the lack of available data, the committee called for further research and indicated that a definitive statement about the health effects of marijuana could not be made at the time.

Interest in marijuana persisted, and hypotheses about the potential therapeutic value of the drug began to emerge. The prospect of medicinal uses of marijuana was controversial, and political, legal, social, and religious debates often overshadowed available evidence (IOM, 1999d). In 1999, the IOM released *Marijuana and Medicine: Assessing the Science Base*. The purpose of the report, sponsored by the White House Office of National Drug Control Policy, was to review the available evidence on the risks associated with medical marijuana and the potential therapeutic value for conditions such as glaucoma, multiple sclerosis, chronic pain, nausea and vomiting associated with chemotherapy, and wasting associated with AIDS. The committee, which was chaired by NAM members John A. Benson, Jr.,[31] and Stanley J. Watson, Jr.,[32] described the available scientific evidence supporting the therapeutic properties of marijuana but also called for additional research and clinical trials to better understand safety and efficacy.

---

[29] David L. Eaton was the Dean and the Vice Provost of the Graduate School at the University of Washington during this time.

[30] Arnold S. Relman was the Editor of the *New England Journal of Medicine* when this report was released. Relman also served as a member of the NAM Council.

[31] John A. Benson, Jr., was the Dean and a Professor of Medicine Emeritus at the Oregon Health & Science University School of Medicine during this time.

[32] Stanley J. Watson, Jr., was the Co-Director and a Research Scientist at the Mental Health Research Institute of the University of Michigan at the time of the report release.

In 2017, the HMD built on the IOM's previous work with a report titled *The Health Effects of Cannabis and Cannabinoids: The Current State of Evidence and Recommendations for Research*. In its report, the committee highlighted the rapid increase in the use of medical and recreational cannabis products as a result of shifting state laws and policies, with many states decriminalizing or legalizing marijuana use.[33] Despite the increase in use of cannabis products, the committee found that evidence related to the health effects—both harms and benefits—was still lacking. The report presented almost 100 research conclusions that were categorized based on the strength of the supporting data. For example, the committee found conclusive evidence supporting the efficacy of cannabis to treat chronic pain, nausea, and vomiting associated with chemotherapy, and patient-reported spasticity associated with multiple sclerosis. The committee developed four broad recommendations that could be used to fill research gaps, improve the quality of data and data collection efforts, and remove barriers to advancing research (NASEM, 2017f).

Violence

Violence as a broad public health concern became a recognized priority as early as 1979 with the publication of *Healthy People*. Violence is a complex public health challenge that encompasses a range of topics related to family and domestic violence, child abuse and neglect, elder abuse, suicide, and gun violence. Violence can have long-lasting effects on individuals and families and is often intertwined with mental health and/or substance use concerns (described later in this chapter), further complicating treatment and prevention strategies. One of the IOM's early studies related to violence was a joint study with the National Research Council (NRC) that resulted in a report called *Violence in Families: Assessing Prevention and Treatment Programs*. The report was released in 1998 and covered topics such as child abuse, domestic violence, and elder abuse. The report served as a comprehensive review of the successes and shortcomings of interventions designed to eliminate violence in the family. The committee, which was chaired by NAM member and Councilor (1998–2000) Patricia A. King,[34] offered recommendations that provided "new strategies that offer[ed] promising approaches for service providers and researchers and for improving the evaluation of prevention and treatment services" (IOM and NRC, 1998b).

In 2002, the IOM revisited family violence, releasing *Confronting Chronic Neglect: The Education and Training of Health Professionals on Family Violence*. The report concluded that "family violence affects more people than cancer, yet it's an issue that receives far less attention." The committee, which was chaired by NAM member John D. Stobo,[35] highlighted the critical role of health care providers in identifying and treating abuse and neglect but found that there was an overall lack of education and training available. To better equip health care providers, the committee provided a set of recommendations to improve multidisciplinary curricula and training programs and to establish evidence-based core competencies related to family violence. The committee also noted that the recognition, treatment, and prevention of family violence cannot be solely managed by the health care system but rather are societal responsibilities that require a multi-faceted response from numerous stakeholders (IOM, 2002g).

Continuing its partnership with the NRC, the IOM released another joint report in 2014 called *New Directions in Child Abuse and Neglect Research*. This new report served as an update to a 1993 NRC report called *Understanding Child Abuse and Neglect*. Research indicated that the psychosocial and economic effects of child abuse and neglect could have long-term impacts on the

---

[33] By 2019, only 11 states in the United States maintained laws that kept marijuana strictly illegal, while all of the other states allowed medical marijuana, had decriminalized marijuana, or had fully legalized it for recreational and medical purposes (Lopez, 2019).

[34] Patricia A. King was at the Georgetown University Law Center when this report was released.

[35] John D. Stobo was at the University of Texas Medical Branch at Galveston during this time.

individual, family, and societal levels. The report also highlighted the biological and psychological consequences of abuse on childhood development (see Chapter 4). The committee, which was chaired by NAM member Anne C. Petersen,[36] concluded that progress in child abuse and neglect research had been made in the two decades since the first report, but more work was needed. In its report, the committee offered an "actionable framework to guide and support future child abuse and neglect research" and called for the development of a "coordinated, national research infrastructure with high-level federal support" (IOM and NRC, 2014a).

Another form of violence that has long-lasting effects on families is suicide. In 2002, the IOM released *Reducing Suicide: A National Imperative*. The report indicated that suicide was the third leading cause of death in the United States, with more than 30,000 people dying annually and another 650,000 treated for attempted suicides in emergency departments each year (IOM, 2002c). Given that 90 percent of suicides are associated with mental health concerns and/or substance use (discussed below), the committee, which was co-chaired by NAM members William E. Bunney, Jr.,[37] and Arthur M. Kleinman,[38] concluded that more could be done to prevent suicides and treat suicidality. The committee's recommendations focused on expanding research funding, improving data collection and surveillance, providing better training for health care providers, and developing and implementing suicide prevention programs. The committee also recommended legislation to restrict access to common means of suicide, including stricter gun control laws.

Firearm violence contributed to a large proportion of suicides (more than half) and homicides (approximately three-quarters) each year in the United States (IOM and NRC, 2013a). This sensitive topic involves advocates on both sides of the debate surrounding gun control and options for reducing gun violence. The December 2012 shooting at Sandy Hook Elementary School in Newtown, Connecticut, reinvigorated the national discussion about gun control and prompted additional public health research on firearm violence (see Figure 6-3). In 2013, President Obama instructed the CDC to take up research related to firearm injuries after a 17-year hiatus that had resulted from a 1995 amendment, known as the Dickey Amendment, which eliminated CDC funding related to firearm violence as a public health concern (Kaplan, 2018).[39] To help set its research agenda, the CDC commissioned an IOM report. The IOM released its fast-track consensus study in June 2013: *Priorities to Reduce the Threat of Firearm-Related Violence*. The research agenda set forth by the committee, which was chaired by NAM member Alan I. Leshner,[40] included priorities related to "the characteristics of firearm violence, risk and protective factors, interventions and strategies, the impact of gun safety technology, and the influence of video games and other media" (IOM and NRC, 2013a).

Following the release of the report, the NIH announced new funding opportunities for research on violence, particularly firearm violence, citing the IOM's call for research investment.[41] However, the CDC's research agenda remained stalled by the prevailing interpretation of the Dickey Amendment until fiscal year 2020, when a congressional appropriations bill included $25 million to fund gun violence research at the CDC and various NIH institutes (Weir, 2021). The funding was timely, as gun sales spiked during the COVID-19 pandemic (Tavernise, 2021) and the United

---

[36] Anne C. Petersen was a Research Professor at the Center for Human Growth and Development at the University of Michigan in Ann Arbor during this time.

[37] William E. Bunney, Jr., was at the University of California, Irvine, when this report was published.

[38] Arthur M. Kleinman was at Harvard University in Cambridge, Massachusetts, at this time.

[39] Judith Salerno to IOM Council, January 22, 2013, IOM/NAM Records; IOM Council Minutes, February 6, 2013, IOM/NAM Records; Judith Salerno to IOM Council, June 28, 2013, IOM/NAM Records.

[40] Alan I. Leshner was at the American Association for the Advancement of Science in Washington, DC, when this report was published.

[41] Impact of IOM Reports (Database), IOM/NAM Records.

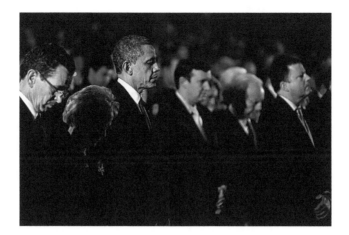

FIGURE 6-3 President Barack Obama attends a Sandy Hook interfaith vigil at Newtown High School in Newtown, Connecticut, on December 16, 2012.
SOURCE: Photo by Pete Souza, White House Archives.

States experienced a surge in mass shootings. In 2020, firearms surpassed vehicle accidents as the leading cause of death for children in the United States (Bendix, 2022).[42]

In 2019, the HMD followed up on the IOM's firearm violence report with a workshop summary called *Health Systems Interventions to Prevent Firearm Injuries and Death: Proceedings of a Workshop*. The standalone workshop, which was organized by a planning committee chaired by NAM member George J. Isham,[43] evaluated the potential role of the health care system and health care professionals in preventing injuries and death associated with firearm violence. Workshop presenters and panelists considered the impact of firearm violence on individuals and communities, including the psychological and social burdens (NASEM, 2019i). The workshop participants also reviewed existing interventions and research related to identifying individuals at a higher risk of firearm violence, the prevention of firearm violence, the role of the health care industry, and developing a culture of health care professionals serving as interveners.

To address violence as an ongoing global public health epidemic, the IOM launched the Forum on Global Violence Prevention in 2010. With an overarching goal "to reduce violence worldwide by promoting research on both protective and risk factors and encouraging evidence-based prevention efforts" (NASEM, n.d.s), the forum provided experts and stakeholders from across the globe with "an ongoing, regular, evidence-based, impartial, scientific setting for the multidisciplinary exchange of information and ideas" (NASEM, n.d.s). The forum held 15 public meetings and workshops, released 14 publications, and engaged more than 1,400 individuals from 37 countries as contributors to its work. Through its work, the forum tackled topics such as violence against children and women, intimate partner violence, elder abuse, the social and economic costs of violence, and the neurocognitive and psychosocial impact of violence.

---

[42] In Spring 2022, two major mass shooting incidents again called attention to the crisis of gun violence in the United States: in Buffalo, New York, 10 people were killed while shopping at a grocery store in an incident motivated by anti-Black racism; and in Uvalde, Texas, 19 students and 3 teachers were killed at an elementary school (see https://nam.edu/statement-by-nam-president-victor-j-dzau-in-response-to-multiple-mass-shootings-in-may-2022).

[43] George J. Isham was a Senior Fellow at the HealthPartners Institute when this stand-alone workshop was held.

RESPONDING TO CHRONIC CONDITIONS

Over the past two centuries, advances in science, health care services, and public health have reshaped the health profiles of people across the globe. People are living longer, and diseases that were once fatal are now chronic conditions that can be managed (e.g., diabetes, heart disease, epilepsy). In the United States, nearly 70 percent of deaths are related to chronic conditions and almost a quarter of people live with more than one chronic condition (IOM, 2012i). In 2012 the IOM released *Living Well with Chronic Illness: A Call for Public Health Action,* which stated that "chronic disease has now emerged as a major public health problem and it threatens not only population health, but our social and economic welfare" (IOM, 2012i, p. 2). The report laid out "public health actions that can help reduce disability and improve functioning and quality of life" (p. 2) related to chronic conditions in the United States. *Living Well* was not the IOM's first report to review topics related to chronic conditions; throughout its history, the organization recognized chronic conditions as serious public health concerns and reviewed topics related to cardiovascular diseases, epilepsy, obesity, mental health, and substance use either as standalone reports or in the context of broader issues related to the health care system, health care research, or public health in general.

Cardiovascular Disease

Cardiovascular disease (CVD) represents a set of chronic conditions (e.g., heart failure, coronary artery disease, vascular disease) that are risk factors for acute cardiovascular events such as myocardial infarction/heart attack, cardiac arrest, and stroke. Prevention and treatment of CVD were long-standing topics of concern for the IOM that were carried forward by the NAM and the HMD. Even before the creation of the IOM, the Board on Medicine, under the direction of Walsh McDermott, dedicated its first report in 1968 to the subject of heart transplants, indicating that the procedure was neither safe enough nor studied enough to play a major part in treating heart disease (see Chapter 1).

The IOM explored many risk factors related to CVD over the years, including three that the IOM studied as public health concerns in their own right: obesity, smoking, and oral health. Obesity, one of the largest risk factors associated with CVD, is discussed in the next section of this chapter. In addition to the IOM's work related to primary tobacco use (e.g., smoking) (described above), the IOM also released a report in 2010 that connected secondhand smoke with CVD risks for nonsmokers. The report, *Secondhand Smoke Exposure and Cardiovascular Effects: Making Sense of the Evidence,* indicated that there was a 25–30 percent increase in the risk of CVD that could be associated with exposure to secondhand smoke. The committee, which was chaired by NAM member and Councilor (2013–2019) Lynn R. Goldman,[44] identified gaps in existing data and provided research recommendations to better understand the health effects of secondhand smoke (IOM, 2010h). The IOM also released two reports in 2011 on oral health that highlighted possible connections between periodontal disease and heart disease and the need for better access to oral health services: *Advancing Oral Health in America* (IOM, 2011m) and *Improving Access to Oral Health Care for Vulnerable and Underserved Populations* (IOM and NRC, 2011b).

As obesity and smoking are risk factors for CVD, CVD is an underlying risk for sudden cardiac arrest—the focus of the final report that was released under the IOM brand in 2015. The report, *Strategies to Improve Cardiac Arrest Survival: A Time to Act,* noted that CVD, including coronary artery disease and structural heart disease, were more common risk factors in men than women in

---

[44] Lynn R. Goldman was at the Johns Hopkins Bloomberg School of Public Health at Johns Hopkins University in Baltimore, Maryland, when this report was published.

terms of cardiac arrest. In its report, the committee, which was chaired by NAM member Robert Graham,[45] stressed the importance of educating the public about recognizing and immediately responding to cardiac arrest, as well as differentiating cardiac arrest from heart attacks (e.g., myocardial infraction) and other types of cardiovascular events that might be associated with CVD (IOM, 2015j).

In terms of health care services and treatment related to CVD, the IOM's portfolio on health disparities often identified CVD as a serious concern. For example, the IOM's 2003 report *Unequal Treatment: Confronting Racial and Ethnic Disparities in Health Care* stated that "some of the strongest and most consistent evidence for the existence of racial and ethnic disparities in care is found in studies of cardiovascular care," noting that "differences in treatment are not due to factors such as racial differences in the severity of coronary disease" (IOM, 2003b, pp. 39–42). While not specific to CVD, the IOM's goal to eliminate health disparities and the NAM's continued work on health equity provided many opportunities to ensure equitable access to high-quality preventative, diagnostic, and treatment services for CVD.

Although CVD has long been considered a concern for industrialized nations, it has also been identified as an emerging public health concern on a global level, with increasing burdens in developing countries. In considering CVD from a global perspective, the IOM released *Control of Cardiovascular Diseases in Developing Countries in 1998* (IOM, 1998c), which was followed by a 2010 report called *Promoting Cardiovascular Health in the Developing World: A Critical Challenge to Achieve Global Health*. The 2010 report found that 30 percent of deaths in low- and middle-income countries were associated with CVD. Given the large burden of CVD in these countries, the committee, which was chaired by NAM member Valentín Fuster,[46] recommended that progress be made in two areas: "creating environments that promote heart healthy lifestyle choices" and "building public health infrastructure and health systems" that can effectively identify and manage CVD while also reducing risk factors associated with CVD. The committee concluded that "without better efforts to promote cardiovascular health, global health as a whole will be undermined" (IOM, 2010d). Following the release of the report, *Barrio Sésamo*, the Spanish version of Sesame Street, announced that it would feature a new character based on Fuster. "Dr. Valentine Ruster" was a Muppet doctor who promoted healthy eating, physical activity, and cardiovascular health to children.[47]

Epilepsy

Epilepsy was the fourth most prevalent neurologic condition in the United States in the first decade of the 21st century, yet it remains one of the most misunderstood and misrepresented chronic health conditions across the globe. With more than 40 variants, epilepsy is a "complex spectrum of disorders … characterized by unpredictable seizures that differ in type, cause, and severity" (IOM, 2012j). Although the seizures can be managed with medication and other types of therapies for approximately two-thirds of people with epilepsy, living with the condition involves many challenges beyond the seizures, including those related to medication side effects, comorbid conditions (e.g., depression, CVD, migraine, sleep disorders), education and employment, driving and transportation, and family and social considerations. In 2010, 24 federal agencies and non-profit organizations came together to commission an IOM report on the public health dimensions of epilepsy with an emphasis on surveillance and data collection; population and public health research; health care, human services, health policy; and education for health care professionals, the public, and people with epilepsy and their families.

---

[45] Robert Graham was at the Milken Institute School of Public Health at The George Washington University in Washington, DC, during this time period.

[46] Valentín Fuster was at Mount Sinai Heart during this time.

[47] Impact of IOM Reports (Database), IOM/NAM Records.

In 2012, the IOM released *Epilepsy Across the Spectrum: Promoting Health and Understanding*. In its report, the committee estimated that the medical costs associated with epilepsy care exceeded $9 billion per year, which did not capture the costs associated with community-based services, loss of productivity, decrements in quality of life, or higher rates of mortality for people with epilepsy. The committee, which was chaired by external volunteer Mary Jane England,[48] presented a vision and a list of research priorities. It also made 13 recommendations to encourage "a better understanding of the public health dimensions of the epilepsies and for promoting health and understanding" that resonated "with broad goals of chronic disease management" (IOM, 2012j, pp. 3–4). One year after the release of the report, the IOM hosted a meeting that allowed the sponsors of the report and other stakeholders to discuss progress and updates that had been made as a result of the report's recommendations as well as plans for the future. Following the release of the report, the CDC also used the "IOM's recommendations to guide research, program activities, and services in collaboration with partners such as nonprofit organizations, academic researchers, and communities" (CDC, 2017) and tracked progress made against the report's recommendations for many years after its release. The National Institute of Neurological Disorders and Stroke (NINDS); the National Heart, Lung, and Blood Institute (NHLBI); and the CDC began work toward a sudden death registry that included a category for sudden unexpected death in epilepsy.[49]

Obesity and Nutrition

Nutrition, and later obesity, were two major public health topics for which the IOM became known throughout its history. The IOM's Food and Nutrition Board (FNB)—established just before World War II as part of the NRC and then transferred to the IOM in 1988—spearheaded the IOM's efforts related to nutrient intake requirements, military nutrition, food safety (see Box 6-2), and childhood obesity. In the summary of the FNB's 80th anniversary symposium, organizers noted that the board "studies issues of national and global importance on the safety and adequacy of the U.S. food supply; establishes principles and guidelines for good nutrition; and provides authoritative judgment on the relationships among food intake, nutrition, and health maintenance and disease prevention."[50]

BOX 6-2
Examples of Reports from the Food and Nutrition Board on Food Safety

- *Seafood Safety* (1991)
- *Ensuring Safe Food: From Production to Consumption* (1998)
- *Escherichia coli O157:H7 in Ground Beef: Review of a Draft Risk Assessment* (2002)
- *Dioxins and Dioxin-Like Compounds in the Food Supply: Strategies to Decrease Exposure* (2003)
- *Scientific Criteria to Ensure Safe Food* (2003)
- *Infant Formula: Evaluating the Safety of New Ingredients* (2004)
- *Safety of Genetically Engineered Foods: Approaches to Assessing Unintended Health Effects* (2004)
- *Seafood Choices: Balancing Benefits and Risks* (2007)
- *Enhancing Food Safety: The Role of the Food and Drug Administration* (2010)
- *Stronger Food and Drug Regulatory Systems Abroad* (2020)

---

[48] Mary Jane England was at Boston University in Massachusetts when this report was published.
[49] Impact of IOM Reports (Database), IOM/NAM Records.
[50] Food and Nutrition Board: 80th Anniversary Symposium (IOM/NAM Records).

In 1989, the FNB produced a report called *Diet and Health: Implications for Reducing Chronic Disease Risk* that explored the connections between nutrition and chronic diseases (NRC, 1989a). In its report, the committee, which was chaired by NAM member and past Councilor Arno G. Motulsky,[51] concluded that diet represented a risk factor for several noncommunicable and chronic conditions, including CVD and hypertension, some forms of cancer, chronic liver disease, obesity, and diabetes. Much of the FNB's subsequent work considered the role of food and nutrition in chronic conditions including relationships between obesity and comorbid conditions connected with obesity, particularly CVD and diabetes. The IOM also provided advice on pregnancy weight gain and nutrition for women and children, which have direct linkages to childhood development and health over the lifespan.

Although the following sections emphasize the FNB's work as it relates to nutrition, obesity, and chronic health conditions—topics selected to highlight prominent, ongoing public health challenges in the United States and in many other countries around the world in recent decades—the FNB also produced an extensive body of work that has contributed to broader food and nutrition policies and science across the globe during its 80-year history. One example of the breadth of the board's work is the Food Forum, which was established in 1993 "to allow selected science and technology leaders in the food industry, top administrators in the federal government, representatives from consumer interest groups, and academicians to periodically discuss and debate food and food related issues openly and in a neutral setting" (NASEM, n.d.t). Since its launch nearly three decades ago, the Food Forum has become one of the National Academies' longest running forums and engaged a diverse cross section of representatives from large, international corporations, such as Coca-Cola, ConAgra Foods, and Mars, Inc., along with representatives from U.S. federal agencies and non-profit organizations, such as the FDA, the NIH, the Department of Agriculture, the American Heart Association, the American Society for Nutrition, among many others. Through its work, the Food Forum has hosted numerous public meetings, fostered ongoing and open dialog across relevant stakeholders and interested parties, and produced a range of workshop summaries and publications that explored topics including sustainable diets, food safety, food literacy, food waste, nutrigenomics, nutrition and aging, and food technology.

One important and specialized area that the FNB explored during the second half of its history was military nutrition and health. The military's physical fitness and performance requirements along with the sometimes extreme environments in which the military operates often necessitate nutritional considerations and guidance that may differ from those available for the general population. In 1982, the Assistant Surgeon General of the U.S. Army called on the National Academies, through the FNB, to establish a committee to advise the military on nutritional research and guidance for military personnel. The Committee on Military Nutrition Research was charged with "identifying nutritional factors that could critically influence the physical and mental performance of military personnel under environmental extremes, with identifying deficiencies in the existing relevant data base, with recommending approaches for studying the relationship of diet to physical and mental performance, and with reviewing and advising on nutritional standards for military feeding systems" (IOM, 1994e, p. 3). Over the years, the Committee on Military Nutrition Research, along the other consensus committees, provided the military with recommendations to meet the unique nutritional needs of military personnel so that they are ready for deployment and can fulfill military requirements (see Box 6-3).

Dietary Reference Intakes

The FNB has a long history in advising the nation on dietary intake recommendations that date back to its origins. In 1941, the FNB defined the first Recommended Dietary Allowances (RDAs) with the goal of providing advice for WWII food relief efforts and to recommend "allowances

---

[51] Arno G. Motulsky was at the Center for Inherited Diseases at the University of Washington in Seattle at this time.

BOX 6-3
Examples of Institute of Medicine Reports on Military Nutrition

- *Food Components to Enhance Performance: An Evaluation of Potential Performance-Enhancing Food Components for Operational Rations* (1994)
- *Committee on Military Nutrition Research: Activity Report 1992–1994* (1994)
- *Not Eating Enough: Overcoming Underconsumption of Military Operational Rations* (1995)
- *Nutritional Needs in Cold and High-Altitude Environments: Applications for Military Personnel in Field Operations* (1996)
- *Emerging Technologies for Nutrition Research: Potential for Assessing Military Performance Capability* (1997)
- *Assessing Readiness in Military Women: The Relationship of Body, Composition, Nutrition, and Health* (1998)
- *Committee on Military Nutrition Research: Activity Report 1994–1999* (1999)
- *Military Strategies for Sustainment of Nutrition and Immune Function in the Field* (1999)
- *The Role of Protein and Amino Acids in Sustaining and Enhancing Performance* (1999)
- *Caffeine for the Sustainment of Mental Task Performance: Formulations for Military Operations* (2001)
- *Weight Management: State of the Science and Opportunities for Military Programs* (2003)
- *Monitoring Metabolic Status: Predicting Decrements in Physiological and Cognitive Performance* (2004)
- *Mineral Requirements for Military Personnel: Levels Needed for Cognitive and Physical Performance During Garrison Training* (2006)
- *Nutrient Composition of Rations for Short-Term, High-Intensity Combat Operations* (2006)
- *Use of Dietary Supplements by Military Personnel* (2008)
- *Nutrition and Traumatic Brain Injury: Improving Acute and Subacute Health Outcomes in Military Personnel* (2011)

sufficiently liberal to be suitable for maintenance of good nutritional status" (Yaktine and Ross, 2019). The RDAs, reviewed and occasionally updated, served as a source for dietary guidance in the United States for the next 40 years, bringing "together the concepts of a healthy diet while meeting essential nutritional requirements."[52] As the American diet evolved and rates of obesity and chronic diseases associated with obesity increased, the nutritional health challenges shifted (Yaktine and Ross, 2019). In the mid-1990s, Dietary Reference Intakes (DRIs), established by committees that worked under the auspices of the IOM, replaced the RDAs. The DRIs are a set of reference values that cover 40 nutrient substances that, "when adhered to, predict a low probability of nutrient inadequacy or excessive intake" (NASEM, n.d.u; Yaktine and Ross, 2019). Box 6-4 provides a list of the organization's DRI reports released from 1997 through 2019. The DRI series contributed to the scientific basis for the 2005 *Dietary Guidelines for Americans*—the U.S. government's nutrition policy document. As of 2019, the IOM's DRI framework had been adopted by the governments of the Netherlands and China, the Australia-New Zealand Food Authority, and nutrition societies in Germany, Austria, and Switzerland.[53]

The 2002/2005 report *Dietary Reference Intakes for Energy, Carbohydrate, Fiber, Fat, Fatty Acids, Cholesterol, Protein, and Amino Acids* (IOM, 2005e) contributed to a 2003 decision by the FDA to require manufacturers to list trans fat on the Nutrition Facts Panel for foods and some

[52] Food and Nutrition Board: 80th Anniversary Symposium (IOM/NAM Records).
[53] Impact of IOM Reports (Database), IOM/NAM Records.

BOX 6-4
Institute of Medicine and Health and Medicine Division
Reports on Dietary Reference Intakes

- *Dietary Reference Intakes for Calcium, Phosphorus, Magnesium, Vitamin D, and Fluoride* (1997)
- *Dietary Reference Intakes: A Risk Assessment Model for Establishing Upper Intake Levels for Nutrients* (1998)
- *Dietary Reference Intakes: Proposed Definition and Plan for Review of Dietary Antioxidants and Related Compounds* (1998)
- *Dietary Reference Intakes for Thiamin, Riboflavin, Niacin, Vitamin B_6, Folate, Vitamin B_{12}, Pantothenic Acid, Biotin, and Choline* (1998)
- *Dietary Reference Intakes for Vitamin C, Vitamin E, Selenium, and Carotenoids* (2000)
- *Dietary Reference Intakes: Applications in Dietary Assessment* (2000)
- *Dietary Reference Intakes for Vitamin A, Vitamin K, Arsenic, Boron, Chromium, Copper, Iodine, Iron, Manganese, Molybdenum, Nickel, Silicon, Vanadium, and Zinc* (2001)
- *Dietary Reference Intakes: Proposed Definition of Dietary Fiber* (2001)
- *Dietary Reference Intakes: Guiding Principles for Nutrition Labeling and Fortification* (2003)
- *Dietary Reference Intakes: Applications in Dietary Planning* (2003)
- *Dietary Reference Intakes for Water, Potassium, Sodium, Chloride, and Sulfate* (2005)
- *Dietary Reference Intakes for Energy, Carbohydrate, Fiber, Fat, Fatty Acids, Cholesterol, Protein, and Amino Acids* (2005)
- *Dietary Reference Intakes: The Essential Guide to Nutrient Requirements* (2006)
- *Dietary Reference Intakes for Calcium and Vitamin D* (2011)
- *Guiding Principles for Developing Dietary Reference Intakes Based on Chronic Disease* (2017)
- *Dietary Reference Intakes for Sodium and Potassium* (2019)

---

dietary supplements. The FDA estimated that removing trans fats from foods would prevent up to 1,200 cases of coronary heart disease and up to 500 deaths annually. In 2004, food manufacturers Frito Lay and Kraft Foods announced efforts to eliminate trans fats from their products, and in 2007, New York City banned the use of trans fats in restaurants—all three citing the IOM report as the basis for action. The report continued to have an impact more than a decade later, when the FDA, citing the IOM report, ruled that partially hydrogenated oils (PHOs)—the primary source of artificial trans fat in processed foods—were not safe for human consumption and ordered manufacturers to remove PHOs from their products within 3 years.[54]

Over the years, the IOM and subsequently the HMD updated the DRIs based on the availability of new research and also modified its process for reviewing the nutrients. For example, nutrients were no longer grouped together, as was the approach in the beginning. In 2011, the IOM released *Dietary Reference Intakes for Calcium and Vitamin D*, which updated the calcium and vitamin D information originally found in its 1997 DRI report, *Dietary Reference Intakes for Calcium, Phosphorus, Magnesium, Vitamin D, and Fluoride* (IOM, 1997d, 2011n). In 2019, the HMD released *Dietary Reference Intakes for Sodium and Potassium*, which updated a portion of the IOM's 2005 report, *Dietary Reference Intakes for Water, Potassium, Sodium, Chloride, and Sulfate* (IOM, 2005f; NASEM, 2019l).

One of the DRI nutrients that the IOM returned to study frequently was sodium. Prior research, such as that undertaken by Board on Medicine member Irvine Page, had identified linkages between high sodium intake and elevated blood pressure, which increased the risks associated with chronic

---

[54] Ibid.

illnesses and acute illnesses such as heart disease, congestive heart failure, stroke, and kidney disease. In 2010, the IOM released *Strategies to Reduce Sodium Intake in the United States*. The committee, which was chaired by NAM member, Home Secretary (2014–2020), and former FDA Commissioner Jane E. Henney,[55] concluded that sodium intake from processed foods and foods served in restaurants remained high, despite 40 years of initiatives and public health efforts to lower sodium intake. The committee called for "mandatory national standards for the sodium content of foods," with an emphasis on strategies to reduce sodium in the food supply (e.g., pre-packaged and processed foods, food sold in restaurants) (IOM, 2010i). Following the release of the report, Walmart, a major food distributor, announced an effort to reduce the sodium content of the items on its shelves.[56] In 2011, Subway, the fast food restaurant chain, also committed to reducing the amount of sodium in its "Fresh Fit" sandwiches by 28 percent.[57]

In 2013, the IOM released a second report focused on sodium called *Sodium Intake in Populations: Assessment of Evidence*. In its report, the committee conducted a review of available evidence related to sodium intake and the possible benefits and harms of reducing dietary sodium, with a focus on the design, methodologies, and conclusions of relevant research. Based on its review, the committee, which was chaired by NAM member Brian L. Strom,[58] reaffirmed connections between high sodium intake and risks for CVD but stated it could not find evidence to support further lowering sodium intake below 2,300 mg per day—the current recommended maximum—for the general population (IOM, 2013j).

Of all the public health topics covered by the IOM, the FNB reports arguably garnered the most public interest. For example, when the IOM released *Dietary Reference Intakes for Calcium and Vitamin D* in November 2010, more than 31,000 people visited the website (IOM, 2011o). As many as 5,000 of these visitors arrived via a link from *The New York Times* website, which included extensive coverage of the report. A few days later, content from the report became a question in *The New York Times* "Weekly Health Quiz"—an opportunity to reinforce the report's message that Americans typically received adequate amounts of vitamin D without the need for supplements.[59]

Nutritional Guidelines for Women and Children

In addition to providing nutritional guidance for the military and the general population, the IOM and the FNB also recognized the unique nutritional needs of women and children. In 1970, the FNB produced a report under the NRC called *Maternal Nutrition and the Course of Pregnancy* that served as a benchmark in pre- and perinatal nutrition. Twenty years later, the IOM revisited topics covered in the 1970 report when it released reports focused on the nutritional needs of pregnant and lactating women. For example, in 1990 the IOM issued *Nutrition During Pregnancy: Part I: Weight Gain, Part II: Nutrient Supplements*. Part I of the report called for a review and update to guidelines related to weight gain during pregnancy, and Part II focused on guidance related to nutritional supplements needed during pregnancy (e.g., folate, iron), as well as the effects of caffeine, tobacco, alcohol, and other drugs on maternal nutrition (IOM, 1990c). In 1991, the IOM released *Nutrition During Lactation*, which reviewed available data and examined how maternal nutrition affects milk composition and infant nutrition (IOM, 1991e).

Nearly two decades after the release of *Nutrition During Pregnancy,* the health and weight profile of women of childbearing age in the United States had changed (e.g., increased maternal

---

[55] Jane E. Henney was at the College of Medicine at the University of Cincinnati, Ohio, when this report was published.

[56] Impact of IOM Reports, January–March 2011 in IOM Council Minutes, April 11, 2011, IOM/NAM Records.

[57] Impact of IOM Reports (Database), IOM/NAM Records.

[58] Brian L. Strom was the George S. Pepper Professor of Public Health at the University of Pennsylvania Perelman School of Medicine in Philadelphia when this report was released.

[59] Judith Salerno to IOM Council, "Overview of IOM Program Activity, September 10, 2011, IOM/NAM Records.

age, rates of chronic conditions, rates of maternal obesity), requiring modifications to the pregnancy weight guidelines the IOM had put forth in 1990. *Weight Gain During Pregnancy: Reexamining the Guidelines* was released in 2009. The committee, which was chaired by external volunteer Kathleen M. Rasmussen,[60] reviewed new data and research that had become available since the previous report and "updated target ranges for weight gain during pregnancy and guidelines for proper measurement," adding guidelines for women with obesity (IOM and NRC, 2009c). When the report was released, the IOM created an online toolkit designed to provide information about healthy weight gain directly to pregnant women and women considering pregnancy. In 2013, the IOM, in coordination with the NRC, held a workshop to discuss strategies to promote behavior change aligned with the updated guidelines (IOM and NRC, 2013b). At this time, the IOM and the NRC jointly released two supplemental publications that synthesized the information from the 2009 report into consumer-friendly formats: *Guidelines on Weight Gain* and *Pregnancy and Implementing Guidelines on Weight Gain and Pregnancy* (IOM and NRC, 2013c,d).

Beyond pre- and perinatal nutritional guidelines for women, the IOM and the FNB also offered policy guidance for the Supplemental Nutrition Program for Women, Infants, and Children (WIC), which was established to provide "specific supplemental foods, nutrition education, and social service and health care referrals to low-income pregnant, breastfeeding, and postpartum women, infants, and children up to age 5 years" (IOM, 1996d, p. 1). Over the course of the IOM's history, the organization provided guidance on nutritional risk assessment and eligibility requirements for the program (e.g., *WIC Nutrition Risk Criteria: A Scientific Assessment* [IOM, 1996d], *Dietary Risk Assessment in the WIC Program* [IOM, 2002h]) and also offered recommendations to update the WIC food packages—the allowable foods and beverages that could be obtained through the program (e.g., infant formula, fruits and vegetables, meat, dairy products). The IOM's 2006 report, *WIC Food Packages: Time for a Change,* which was drafted by a committee chaired by NAM member Suzanne P. Murphy,[61] offered recommendations to fulfill the goal of improving the "quality of the diet of WIC participants while also promoting a healthy body weight that will reduce the risk of chronic diseases" (IOM, 2006d). As a result of the committee's recommendations, the WIC program was modified to align with the government's *Dietary Guidelines for Americans* and applicable *Healthy People 2020* goals and objectives (NASEM, 2017i). To fulfill a new congressional mandate to review the WIC food packages every 10 years, the HMD released an updated report in 2017 called *Review of WIC Food Packages: Improving Balance and Choice: Final Report,* which provided recommendations to encourage breastfeeding and offer greater variety and choice in the food packages (NASEM, 2017j).

Childhood Obesity

In 2002, the transition year between IOM Presidents Ken Shine and Harvey Fineberg, Congress charged the IOM with developing a prevention strategy to decrease obesity among children and youth in the United States. In 2004, the IOM released *Preventing Childhood Obesity: Health in the Balance,* which indicated that approximately 9 million children between the ages of 6 and 11 were obese. The report stated that the rate of obesity was approaching epidemic levels and constituted a critical public health threat, noting that obesity increased risks for a range of chronic illnesses such as diabetes, hypertension, and CVD. The committee, which was chaired by NAM

---

[60] Kathleen M. Rasmussen was a Professor of Nutrition in the Division of Nutritional Sciences at Cornell University in Ithaca, New York, during this time.

[61] Suzanne P. Murphy was at the Cancer Research Center of Hawaii at the University of Hawaii in Honolulu when this report was released.

member and Councilor (2003–2008) Jeffrey P. Koplan,[62] developed a range of recommendations that highlighted actions for federal policy makers, private industry, states and local communities, schools, and parents, all with the goal of improving children's diets and increasing physical activity (IOM, 2005c).[63]

In 2007, the IOM released a follow-up report called *Progress in Preventing Childhood Obesity: How Do We Measure Up?*, which assessed progress since the release of the 2004 report. The committee found that although numerous initiatives and programs had been launched, they "generally remain[ed] fragmented and [were] small in scale" (IOM, 2007i). The committee, which was also chaired by Koplan, encouraged continued efforts with an emphasis on evaluating the initiatives, sharing best practices, and scaling up promising programs. In 2011, the IOM revisited childhood obesity with a focus on children under the age of 5 in its report *Early Childhood Obesity Prevention Policies*. The committee, chaired by external volunteer Leann L. Birch,[64] stressed that "the first years of life are important to health and well-being throughout the life span," offering recommendations to health care professionals, parents, and child care providers to keep young children active, provide healthy diets, minimize screen time, and ensure that children get enough sleep (IOM, 2011p, p. 1).

In addition to high-level examinations of the childhood obesity epidemic, the IOM released targeted reports that were meant to provide guidance in specific areas. For example, the IOM released a report in 2006 called *Food Marketing to Children and Youth: Threat or Opportunity?*, which evaluated how current food marketing practices affected the nutritional status of children and youth and how marketing could be leveraged to promote healthier choices and diets. When the committee began its work in 2004, it found that products heavily marketed to children had low nutritional value and were high in calories, sugar, salt, and fat. The committee, which was chaired by NAM member and Leonard D. Schaeffer Executive Officer (2016–) J. Michael McGinnis,[65] concluded that "sustained, multisectoral, and integrated efforts" would be required to improve the diets of children and youth. In its recommendations, the committee called on companies in the food and beverage industry along with restaurants to use the resources and ingenuity they put into advertising to promote healthy diets in children. The committee also indicated that television networks, the federal government, and state and local education authorities should also be involved in promoting healthy foods and beverages for children (IOM, 2006e).

The release of this report was followed by a series of events that demonstrated the report's reach and impact. One tangible sign of impact was a March 2006 letter signed by 10 Democratic senators and addressed to HHS Secretary Mike Leavitt. The senators cited the IOM report as proof of "scientific evidence that food marketing to children has a significant impact on children's food preferences." The senators agreed with the report's call for the federal government to assume the lead role in solving the problem. They therefore urged Secretary Leavitt to take the necessary steps to begin monitoring progress toward the IOM's recommendations.[66] The television industry also took immediate notice; between 2006 and 2007, Disney, Nickelodeon, and the Cartoon Network announced that they would no longer allow the use of their characters to market unhealthy food to children. Additionally, the British broadcast regulator Ofcom issued a ban on all junk food advertising in children's programming. Major food and beverage companies including Burger King

---

[62] Jeffrey P. Koplan was at the Woodruff Health Sciences Center of Emory University in Atlanta, Georgia, when this report was released.

[63] Board Briefs, Food and Nutrition Board, IOM Council Minutes, July 11, 2011, IOM/NAM Records.

[64] Leann L. Birch was a Professor and the Director of the Center for Childhood Obesity Research at The Pennsylvania State University in University Park during this timeframe.

[65] J. Michael McGinnis was at the IOM when this report was released.

[66] Tom Harkin, Dick Durban, Ted Kennedy, Patty Murray, Chuck Schumer, and Hillary Rodham Clinton to Mike Leavitt, March 3, 2006, IOM/NAM Records.

and ConAgra also made commitments to promote healthier food to children. In line with a recommendation from the report, the Patient Protection and Affordable Care Act (ACA) required that all restaurants with 20 or more locations post the calorie content of their foods.[67]

In 2009, the IOM provided specific guidance to community leaders in its report *Local Government Actions to Prevent Childhood Obesity*. The committee, which was chaired by external volunteer Eduardo J. Sanchez,[68] highlighted the important role that communities and local governments play in creating healthy environments for children—from grocery stores that offer healthy food options, such as fresh fruits and vegetables, to safe playgrounds where children can be physically active. The committee offered a set of strategies to improve diet and physical activity that could be implemented at the community level by mayors, city councils and managers, and country commissioners and boards (TRB et al., 2009).

In addition to providing recommendations related to food marketing and actions communities could take, the IOM also directed recommendations to schools in an effort to guide their food and physical activity policies. In 2007, the IOM released *Nutrition Standards for Foods in Schools: Leading the Way Toward Healthier Youth,* which stated that many children spend the majority of their day in school and the food consumed in schools can represent a large portion of children's diets. The committee—chaired by NAM member Virginia A. Stallings[69]—laid out "a set of guiding principles to support the creation of a healthful eating environment for children in U.S. schools" (IOM, 2007j, p. 2). The committee also organized foods and beverages that were offered outside of the federally reimbursable nutrition programs into two tiers to help schools develop policies regarding foods offered in vending machines, school stores, and concession stands. In 2010, the IOM released a complementary report called *School Meals: Building Blocks for Healthy Children* that was drafted by a committee also chaired by Stallings. The report evaluated nutritional standards and requirements for the School Breakfast Program and the National School Lunch Program (IOM, 2010e). Together, these two reports examined the various types of food and beverages offered in schools and provided recommendations "to better meet the nutritional needs of children, foster healthy eating habits, and safeguard children's health" (IOM, 2010e, p. 2).

Many actions took place at the community, state, and national levels as a result of these reports. In 2010, President Obama signed into law the Healthy, Hunger-Free Kids Act, which directed the Secretary of Agriculture to propose updated regulations for nutrition standards for school breakfasts and lunches based on the School Meals report. Two years later, First Lady Michelle Obama and Secretary of Agriculture Tom Vilsack announced improved nutrition standards for school meals, including daily fruits and vegetables; fat-free or low-fat milk; whole grains; and less saturated fat, trans fat, and sodium—the first health-focused updates in 15 years (see Figure 6-4). School food service companies ARAMARK, Sodexo, and Chartwells also announced efforts to meet the IOM's recommendations for fat, sugar, sodium, and whole grains within 5–10 years.[70]

The IOM also considered physical activity in schools as another opportunity to prevent obesity and promote healthier lifestyles for children. In its 2013 report, *Educating the Student Body: Taking Physical Activity and Physical Education to School,* the IOM highlighted associations between physical inactivity and risks for chronic conditions such as diabetes, elevated blood pressure, CVD, certain types of cancers, osteoporosis, anxiety, and depression. As with healthy eating habits, habits related to physical activity are formed at a young age and affect health across the lifespan. The

---

[67] Impact of IOM Reports (Database), IOM/NAM Records.

[68] Eduardo J. Sanchez was the Vice President and the Chief Medical Officer of Blue Cross and Blue Shield of Texas at the time.

[69] Virginia A. Stallings was at the Joseph Stokes Jr. Research Institute of the Children's Hospital at the University of Pennsylvania Perelman School of Medicine in Philadelphia when this report was published.

[70] Impact of IOM Reports (Database), IOM/NAM Records.

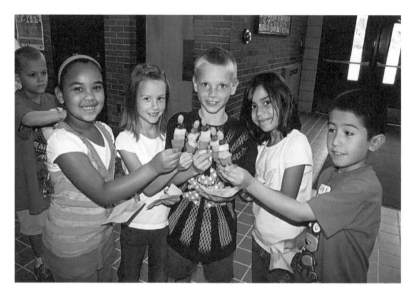

FIGURE 6-4 Waterford, Michigan, students learned how to make "Smart Snacks" (fruit kabobs) and the nutrition benefits of each fruit as part of Michelle Obama's Let's Move Campaign.
SOURCE: FioRito, K. 2014. Moving Forward … Healthy Choices for Michigan Kids! Let's Move Blog. White House Archives. https://letsmove.obamawhitehouse.archives.gov/blog/2014/08/22/moving-forwardhealthy-choices-michigan-kids (accessed July 11, 2022).

committee, which was chaired by external volunteer Howard W. Kohl III,[71] made recommendations that were designed to strengthen and improve physical activity policies and programs in schools (IOM, 2013k).

In 2012 the IOM once again revisited obesity and reviewed national progress since the release of its previous reports. In its report, *Accelerating Progress in Obesity Prevention: Solving the Weight of the Nation* (IOM, 2012l), the committee concluded that while "many aspects of the obesity problem have been identified and discussed … there has not been complete agreement on what needs to be done to accelerate progress" (NASEM, n.d.d1). To drive progress, the committee—chaired by external volunteer Daniel R. Glickman[72]—stated that broad societal changes using a systems approach would be required. According to the committee, there were five critical environments to address: physical activity, food and beverage, message, health care and work, and school. The committee developed goals that corresponded to these areas—for example, making "physical activity an integral and routine part of life" and making "schools the national focal point" for obesity prevention. Through its recommendations, the committee's goal was to reshape the environments in which individuals and families "work, learn, eat, and play" (IOM, 2012k).

To further expand the reach of its work in obesity, the IOM entered into a collaboration with the CDC, the NIH, and HBO Documentary Films to produce a film series on the obesity epidemic under the title of *The Weight of the Nation*. The RWJF supported the project, and the Michael & Susan Dell Foundation and Kaiser Permanente contributed an additional $10 million. HBO made the films available to subscribers and non-subscribers alike, offering wide availability to anyone who

---

[71] Howard W. Kohl III was a Professor of Epidemiology and Kinesiology at the School of Public Health at the University of Texas Health Science Center-Houston and the Department of Kinesiology and Health Education at The University of Texas at Austin during this time.

[72] Daniel R. Glickman was the Executive Director of Congressional Programs at The Aspen Institute in Washington, DC, when this report was released.

might be interested.[73] The reviews of the documentary were mixed, but generally acknowledged the importance of the topic and the content presented (Fryhofer, 2012; Lowry, 2012; Umstead, 2012). One review stated that the series "cast a very sobering light on the state of America's health and the consequences of the continual expansion of our waistlines" (Umstead, 2012). As part of this series, the children's film *The Weight of the Nation for Kids: Quiz Ed!* was nominated for a 2013 Emmy Award in the Outstanding Children's Program category.

To continue its obesity work and create platforms to facilitate ongoing discussion, the IOM established the Standing Committee on Childhood Obesity Prevention in 2008 and the Roundtable on Obesity Solutions in 2014. The standing committee, which was sponsored by the RWJF, was designed to bring together leaders from government, academia, and corporate entities to have ongoing policy discussions and guide the selection of topics for future IOM workshops and consensus studies. Between 2009 and 2013, the standing committee held six meetings and workshops that covered topics related to food marketing, legal strategies, parents and children, and health equity in the prevention of childhood obesity. After the disbandment of the standing committee, the FNB formed the Roundtable on Obesity Solutions as a means of continuing the work of the standing committee (NASEM, n.d.v). With more than 30 sponsors and 50 members, the Roundtable on Obesity Solutions brought together leaders and stakeholders from multiple sectors in order to "view the problem of obesity from a systems perspective; achiev[e] health equity through focused action and research; develop and us[e] effective communication strategies; identify innovative financing mechanisms; and foster evaluation." The roundtable worked toward fulfilling its mission by hosting workshops and public meetings, commissioning background papers, and operating four innovation collaboratives. Since its launch, the roundtable has released 20 publications that have reviewed topics such as the global obesity pandemic, obesity in the military, physical activity, and cross-sector responses to obesity.

Mental Health and Substance Use

Dating back to the IOM presidency of psychiatrist David Hamburg, mental health and substance use became ongoing priorities within the IOM's portfolio and remained so for both the HMD and the NAM. During the IOM's existence, the organization released an assortment of reports that covered topics related to preventing mental health disorders, quality of care, specific mental health needs of parents and children (see Chapter 4), substance use and addiction, and the mental health needs and concerns of military personnel and veterans. When the NAM was established in 2015, the NAM leadership carried forward the IOM's legacy in mental health and substance use by elevating the U.S. opioid crisis to one of the organization's top focus areas. The NAM identified the crisis as an urgent public health need that required a timely, united national response (see Chapter 7). While coordinating with and supporting the NAM's opioid work, the HMD also continued the IOM's mental health portfolio with work that cut across many of its boards and activities.

Approaching its 25-year anniversary, the IOM explored the possibility of preventing mental health disorders in a 1994 report called *Reducing Risks for Mental Disorders: Frontiers for Preventive Intervention Research*. The congressionally mandated study examined prevention as a possible mechanism to reduce the immense economic and social burdens of mental health disorders on individuals, families, and communities. The committee—chaired by NAM member and Councilor Robert J. Haggerty[74]—estimated that approximately 20 percent of the U.S. population had one or more mental health or substance use condition (IOM, 1994f). Throughout its delibera-

---

[73] The story of the HBO documentary can be followed through IOM Council Minutes, January 11, 2010, IOM Council Minutes, October 16, 2010, and Judith Salerno to IOM Council, February 8, 2012, all in IOM/NAM Records.

[74] Robert J. Haggerty was a Professor of Pediatrics Emeritus at the University of Rochester School of Medicine and Dentistry in Rochester, New York, during this time.

tions, the committee members considered successful public health prevention strategies that had been implemented to prevent CVD, injuries, and smoking, and they evaluated risk factors associated with mental health disorders such as Alzheimer's disease, schizophrenia, alcohol use and addiction, depressive disorders, and conduct disorders (IOM, 1994f). The committee developed a research agenda and recommendations that focused on "develop[ing] effective intervention programs, creat[ing] a cadre of prevention researchers, and improv[ing] coordination among federal agencies" (NASEM, n.d.e1).

In 2005, as part of the IOM's Quality Chasm Series (see Chapter 5), the organization took a special interest in the quality of care for individuals living with mental health and substance use conditions. *Improving the Quality of Health Care for Mental and Substance-Use Conditions,* which was authored by a committee chaired by Mary Jane England,[75] concluded that while effective treatments were available, care for mental health and substance use conditions was often fragmented, placing considerable burdens on individuals, families, and society (IOM, 2006h). In 2015, the IOM released a complementary study called *Psychosocial Interventions for Mental and Substance Use Disorders: A Framework for Establishing Evidence-Based Standards.* More than two decades after the IOM's 1994 report on prevention, this committee, which was also chaired by England,[76] reiterated that 20 percent of the population lived with one or more mental health conditions. The new report developed a framework that could be employed to ensure that available care was high-quality and evidence-based. The committee also offered recommendations to strengthen the evidence base and develop quality measures relevant to psychosocial programs and interventions (IOM, 2015f).

Recognizing the need for long-term, collaborative discussions regarding mental health and substance use conditions, the HMD established the Forum on Mental Health and Substance Use Disorders in 2019. With more than 20 sponsors and 30 members, the forum held its inaugural workshop in October 2019. Picking up on themes from previous IOM work, including the 2005 Quality Chasm report, the workshop focused on "key policy challenges to improve care for people with mental health and substance abuse disorders." Speakers and panelists considered opportunities to promote person-centered care, better define adequate care, apply knowledge to practice, and encourage innovation and coordination across health care systems and the health care workforce (NASEM, n.d.w).

Substance Use and Addiction

Under the umbrella of mental health, the IOM and HMD also focused on topics related to substance use and addiction. The organization evaluated substance abuse in broad terms (e.g., *Treating Drug Problems* [Volume 1: IOM, 1990e; Volume 2: IOM, 1992c], *Pathways of Addiction* [IOM, 1996h]) and also evaluated specific topics related to the use of alcohol, opioids, tobacco, and marijuana. The organization reviewed evidence and provided recommendations related to quality of care, treatment and prevention options, and health care workforce needs. Box 6-5 provides a list of examples of the organization's reports on substance use and addiction.

One of the subtopics the organization explored over the years was alcohol use. In 2003, the IOM investigated alcohol use among youth in its report *Reducing Underage Drinking: A Collective Responsibility.* The committee, which was chaired by Richard J. Bonnie,[77] identified underage drinking as a serious public health concern due to risks associated with "traffic fatalities, violence, unsafe sex, suicide, educational failure, and other problem behaviors." In an effort to curb underage drinking and attempt to prevent it altogether, the committee described strategies that could be

---

[75] Mary Jane England was President of Regis College in Weston, Massachusetts, when this report was released.

[76] Mary Jane England was a Professor of Health Policy and Management at the School of Public Health at Boston University when this report was published.

[77] Richard J. Bonnie was at the School of Law at the University of Virginia during this time.

BOX 6-5
Examples of Reports Related to Substance Use and Addiction

- *Mental Health, Substance Use, and Wellbeing in Higher Education: Supporting the Whole Student* (2021)
- *Measuring Success in Substance Use Grant Programs: Outcomes and Metrics for Improvement* (2020)
- *Medications for Opioid Use Disorder Save Lives* (2019)
- *Getting to Zero Alcohol-Impaired Driving Fatalities: A Comprehensive Approach to a Persistent Problem* (2018)
- *Pain Management and the Opioid Epidemic: Balancing Societal and Individual Benefits and Risks of Prescription Opioid Use* (2017)
- *Psychosocial Interventions for Mental and Substance Use Disorders: A Framework for Establishing Evidence-Based Standards* (2015)
- *Substance Use Disorders in the U.S. Armed Forces* (2013)
- *The Mental Health and Substance Use Workforce for Older Adults: In Whose Hands?* (2012)
- *Preventing HIV Infection Among Injecting Drug Users in High-Risk Countries: An Assessment of the Evidence* (2007)
- *Improving the Quality of Health Care for Mental and Substance-Use Conditions: Quality Chasm Series* (2006)
- *Reducing Underage Drinking: A Collective Responsibility* (2004)
- *New Partnerships for a Changing Environment: Why Drug and Alcohol Treatment Providers and Researchers Need to Collaborate* (1999)
- *Bridging the Gap Between Practice and Research: Forging Partnerships with Community-Based Drug and Alcohol Treatment* (1998)
- *Dispelling the Myths About Addiction: Strategies to Increase Understanding and Strengthen Research* (1997)
- *Pathways of Addiction: Opportunities in Drug Abuse Research* (1996)
- *Fetal Alcohol Syndrome: Diagnosis, Epidemiology, Prevention, and Treatment* (1996)
- *Treating Drug Problems: Volume 2* (1992)
- *Treating Drug Problems: Volume 1* (1990)
- *Broadening the Base of Treatment for Alcohol Problems* (1990)

---

implemented and expanded such as building partnerships with the alcohol and entertainment industries, modifying marketing practices, and enhancing the effectiveness of underage drinking laws by ensuring compliance and enforcement at the state level (NRC and IOM, 2004). In 2005, the Sober Truth on Preventing (STOP) Underage Drinking Act became the first major national legislation to address underage drinking. Based on the IOM's 2003 report, the legislation called for investment in prevention coalitions, public marketing, and additional research. HHS Secretary Mike Leavitt launched a public service announcement campaign targeting parents and encouraging them to talk to their kids about drinking. Nickelodeon and the Century Council (financed by a number of distilling companies) (now known as the Foundation for Advancing Alcohol Responsibility) also created a $2 million ad campaign discouraging children from drinking.[78]

In 2018, the HMD examined alcohol-impaired driving and opportunities to prevent injury and death in its report *Getting to Zero Alcohol-Impaired Driving Fatalities: A Comprehensive Approach to a Persistent Problem*. The report, which was produced by a committee chaired by external

---

[78] Impact of IOM Reports (Database), IOM/NAM Records.

volunteer Steven M. Teutsch,[79] included recommendations related to "increasing alcohol excise taxes, lowering state per se laws for alcohol-impaired driving to 0.05% blood alcohol concentration (BAC), preventing illegal alcohol sales to underage persons and to already-intoxicated adults, strengthening regulation of alcohol marketing, and implementing policies to reduce the physical availability of alcohol" (NASEM, 2018g, p. 1).

Mental Health and Substance Use Care in Military and Veteran Populations

Military and veterans' health constituted another area of focus for the IOM and subsequently the HMD (see also Chapter 4). Through its work, the organization recognized the specific needs and challenges for these populations in terms of mental health—including posttraumatic stress disorder (PTSD) (see Box 6-6)—and substance use prevention and treatment. In 2010, after nearly a decade of war in Iraq and Afghanistan, the IOM released a report called *Provision of Mental Health Counseling Services Under TRICARE,* which assessed the mental health care needs of TRICARE[80] beneficiaries, including active duty personnel, reservists, military family members, and retirees. The committee—chaired by George J. Isham[81]—reviewed counseling options, TRICARE requirements, and determinants of high-quality care. In its report, the committee recommended that TRICARE

BOX 6-6
IOM Reports on Posttraumatic Stress Disorder
(PTSD) in Military and Veteran Populations

- *Posttraumatic Stress Disorder: Diagnosis and Assessment* (IOM, 2006f): a brief report that responded to a set of specific questions from the Department of Veterans Affairs (VA), concluding that "health professionals should be aware that veterans, especially those who have served in war theaters, are at risk for the development of PTSD, but might present with physical or psychiatric complaints that are symptomatic of substance use disorder or other psychiatric conditions."
- *PTSD Compensation and Military Service* (IOM and NRC, 2007b): the report's recommendations were designed to "[enact] changes that would improve the fairness, consistency, and scientific foundation of [how the VA evaluates veterans with possible PTSD]."
- *Treatment of Posttraumatic Stress Disorder: An Assessment of the Evidence* (IOM, 2008d): this report provided a comprehensive evaluation of the existing literature and research on the treatment of PTSD. The committee "found the evidence inadequate to determine the efficacy of most treatment modalities," suggesting an urgent need for additional research to produce high-quality data.
- *Treatment for Posttraumatic Stress Disorder in Military and Veteran Populations: Final Assessment* (IOM, 2014f): following an initial assessment released in 2012, the final report concluded that the Department of Defense and the VA had made sustained commitments to the treatment and management of PTSD, but also highlighted deficiencies related to standards, reporting, and evaluation and called for additional process and infrastructure improvements.

---

[79] Steven M. Teutsch was an Adjunct Professor at the University of California, Los Angeles, Fielding School of Public Health; a Senior Fellow at the Public Health Institute; and a Senior Fellow at the Leonard D. Schaeffer Center for Health Policy and Economics at the University of Southern California when this report was released.

[80] TRICARE is the Department of Defense's health insurance program, which provides coverage for more than 9.4 million active duty military personnel, reservists, retired members of the military, family members, and other select individuals with military connections (Health.mil, n.d.).

[81] George J. Isham was the Medical Director and the Chief Health Officer at Health Partners, Inc., in Bloomington, Minnesota during this time.

update its policies to allow autonomous practice for mental health counselors, removing the requirement that all counselors must practice under the supervision of a physician (IOM, 2010f).

The IOM followed up on the 2010 TRICARE report with a pair of reports in 2013 and 2014 that responded to the physical and psychosocial needs of military personnel returning from wars in Afghanistan and Iraq, as well as the needs of their families: *Returning Home from Iraq and Afghanistan: Assessment of Readjustment Needs of Veterans, Service Members, and Their Families*[82] (2013) and *Preventing Psychological Disorders in Service Members and Their Families: An Assessment of Programs*[83] (2014). In terms of mental health, the first report focused on the Department of Defense's (DOD's) and the Department of Veterans Affairs' (VA's) screening and treatment programs, whereas the latter report focused on prevention (IOM, 2014c). Specifically, the 2014 report evaluated the DOD's "reintegration programs and prevention strategies for PTSD, depression, recovery support, and prevention of substance abuse, suicide, and interpersonal violence." Together the reports made recommendations for the implementation of strategies at the "individual, interpersonal, institutional, community, and societal" levels to provide better support and mental health care to more than one million service members who were living with one or more psychological disorders and their families (IOM, 2014c).

The HMD produced a complementary report in 2018 called *Evaluation of the Department of Veterans Affairs Mental Health Services*. During its deliberations, the committee—chaired by NAM member Alicia L. Carriquiry[84]—identified "a substantial unmet need for mental health services" among military personnel who had served in Afghanistan and Iraq. Although many veterans received high-quality mental health services through the VA, the committee identified a need to expand that care across all facilities and veteran populations. The report urged the VA to set "a goal of becoming a high-reliability provider of high-quality mental health services" within 5 years (NASEM, 2018h, p. 5). In doing so, the VA would have to adopt strategies to "engage veterans, expand outreach efforts …, and improve its transitional services" (NASEM, 2018h, p. 6).

Throughout its history, the VA has been the subject of intense public scrutiny that was often triggered by feedback from veterans and their encounters with the system—not limited to mental health services. For example, in 2014 the VA launched an investigation of the Phoenix VA health care system in response to concerns regarding serious scheduling problems and wait times. The investigation revealed that 1,700 veterans who needed care had not been included on the mandatory electronic waiting list, and 40 veterans who had been included on the list died while waiting for an appointment. In response to these findings, the VA asked the IOM to conduct a study and make recommendations to improve scheduling and access to the VA health system and throughout the U.S health care system more broadly. The IOM released its fast-track study—*Transforming Health Care Scheduling and Access: Getting to Now*—in 2015. The study examined systems-based engineering methods and various scheduling models, such as leaving openings in the schedule for same-day appointments. The committee, which was chaired by NAM member Gary Kaplan,[85] recommended that the VA and other health systems employ innovations such as queue streamlining and leverage non-physician clinicians and technology-based consultations in order to alleviate long wait times and improve access to needed care (IOM, 2015g).

---

[82] George W. Rutherford chaired this committee. At the time, he was the Salvatore Pablo Lucia Professor, the Vice Chair of the Department of Epidemiology and Biostatistics, and the Director of the Prevention and Public Health Group at the University of California, San Francisco.

[83] Kenneth E. Warner chaired the committee that drafted this report. During this time he was the Avedis Donabedian Distinguished University Professor of Public Health at the University of Michigan School of Public Health in Ann Arbor, Michigan.

[84] Alicia L. Carriquiry was at Iowa State University when this report was published.

[85] Gary Kaplan was the Chair and the Chief Executive Officer at the Virginia Mason Health System during this time.

In addition to the IOM's work on mental health concerns among military and veteran populations, the organization also reviewed topics related to substance use in these populations. For example, in 2009, the IOM released a report called *Combating Tobacco in Military and Veteran Populations*. In its report, the committee, chaired by Stuart Bondurant,[86] concluded that the short- and long-term health and economic costs of tobacco use warranted DOD and VA investment in comprehensive tobacco-control programs that would encourage cessation and prevent initiation of tobacco use (IOM, 2009c). The committee recommended that the DOD take specific actions toward realizing its goal of becoming a tobacco-free military, including banning tobacco use on military installations and eliminating the sale of tobacco in commissaries. In 2013, the IOM conducted a broader review of substance use in the military with its report *Substance Use Disorders in the U.S. Armed Forces*. The report reviewed alcohol and other drug use, such as the misuse of prescription drugs including opioids, and concluded that substance use in the military was a public health crisis that threatened the readiness and psychological fitness of military personnel (IOM, 2013l). To reduce substance use and misuse, the committee, which was chaired by NAM member Charles P. O'Brien,[87] urged the DOD "to consistently implement evidence-based prevention, screening, diagnosis, and treatment services and take leadership for ensuring that these services expand and improve" (IOM, 2014d, p. 4).

U.S. overdose deaths saw a 30 percent increase during 2020, exacerbated by the opioid epidemic as well as the physical distancing restrictions and extreme stress imposed by the COVID-19 pandemic (CDC, n.d.f). Mental health concerns among adults and children also rose during the pandemic, and combating the overdose epidemic as well as ensuring the mental health and well-being of people across the globe was of critical importance (Panchal et al., 2021). In 2018, the NAM established an Action Collaborative on Countering the U.S. Opioid Epidemic (see Chapter 7).

Neglected Health Concerns and Chronic Conditions in Developing Countries

In addition to the IOM's work on cardiovascular diseases globally, the organization also explored the impact of often neglected health concerns and chronic conditions, such as women's health, brain disorders, and cancer in developing countries. For example, in 1996 the IOM released a report called *In Her Lifetime: Female Morbidity and Mortality in Sub-Saharan Africa,* which cut across a variety of neglected health concerns and chronic conditions. In sub-Saharan Africa, women's health had largely been neglected due in large part to competing public health and social priorities. In its report, the committee, which was chaired by external volunteer Maureen Law,[88] reviewed the impact of specific diseases and conditions, such as HIV/AIDS, cancer, CVD, and mental health conditions, as well as broader concerns related to nutrition and obstetric care, on female populations. Highlighting the important role of women in the global economy, especially in sub-Saharan Africa, the report offered an agenda to promote research and health policies to improve women's health in developing nations (IOM, 1996e).

In 2001, the IOM reviewed brain disorders and mental health challenges in developing nations in its report *Neurological, Psychiatric, and Developmental Disorders: Meeting the Challenge in the Developing World*. Focusing on developmental disabilities, epilepsy, schizophrenia, bipolar disorder, depression, and stroke, the committee highlighted "negative attitudes, prejudice, and stigma"

---

[86] Stuart Bondurant was a Professor of Medicine and the Dean Emeritus at the University of North Carolina at Chapel Hill when this report was released.

[87] Charles P. O'Brien was the Kenneth E. Appel Professor of Psychiatry, the Vice-Chair of Psychiatry, and the Director of the Center for Studies of Addiction at the University of Pennsylvania Perelman School of Medicine in Philadelphia during this time.

[88] Maureen Law was the Director General of the Health Sciences Division at the International Development Research Centre in Ottawa, Ontario, Canada, when this report was published.

as barriers to ensuring adequate diagnosis, treatment, and care for these often neglected conditions. The committee, which was co-chaired by external volunteers Assen Jablensky[89] and Richard Johnson,[90] proposed specific strategies to reduce the burden of brain disorders and mental health, emphasizing the need for increased awareness among health care providers and the public (IOM, 2001g). In 2003, the Fogarty International Center of the NIH announced a new research program called *Brain Disorders in the Developing World: Research Across the Lifespan*. The program was designed to support international collaborations to study brain disorders in developing countries, and in its first decade, the program "awarded more than 150 grants totaling about $85 million" (Fogarty International Center, 2014).

Cancer—another often-neglected health concern in developing countries—was reviewed in the IOM's 2007 report, *Cancer Control Opportunities in Low- and Middle-Income Countries*. In its review, the committee concluded that "more people die from cancer in [low- and middle-income] countries than from AIDS and malaria combined" and that cancer is often overlooked as a health concern by foundations, international health organization, and government aid agencies (IOM, 2007k). In the report, the committee, which was chaired by NAM member and Councilor (1990–1992) Frank A. Sloan,[91] described opportunities to improve screening and treatment efforts for highly curable types of cancers such as leukemias, lymphomas, and retinoblastoma, which often occur in childhood. It also underscored the need for palliative care and reviewed options to prevent cancer in developing countries, such as suppressing increasing rates of smoking and increasing vaccination rates for hepatitis B and human papillomavirus.

ENVIRONMENTAL HEALTH

As defined by the American Public Health Association, environmental health is a broad subdiscipline within public health that considers the connections and interactions between humans and their environment. Programs and policies in environmental health are typically dedicated "to reduc[ing] chemical and other environmental exposures in air, water, soil and food to protect people and provid[ing] communities with healthier environments" (APHA, n.d.). Throughout its existence, the IOM recognized the importance of environmental health in ensuring and improving the health of populations in the United States and across the globe. Over the years, the organization studied topics related to occupational health and safety, including advising the military on hazardous exposures and advising the National Institute of Occupational Safety and Health on personal protective equipment (see Chapter 4). The IOM also examined lead in the environment, indoor air quality, environmental risk factors for cancer, climate change, and natural disasters.

In the early 1990s, the Board on International Health (later renamed the Board on Global Health) proposed an international symposium and series of workshops to examine lead in the environment and possible health risks in the Americas. Lead was selected as the area of focus because at the time lead poisoning was "thought to be one of the most serious diseases of environmental and occupational origin because of its high prevalence, environmental pervasiveness, and persistence of toxicity in affected populations" and it "is also an entirely preventable disease" (IOM, 1996f, p. 15). This topic was also selected, in part, due to increasing trade between the United States and Mexico and associated concerns related to transport of goods and waste across borders. The IOM came together with the National Institute of Public Health of Mexico to plan and execute work-

---

[89] Assen Jablensky was a Professor in the Department of Psychiatry at the University of Western Australia, Perth, when this report was published.

[90] Richard Johnson was a Professor in the Department of Neurology and the Co-Chair of the Department of Microbiology and Neurosciences at the John Hopkins University School of Medicine in Baltimore, Maryland, during this time.

[91] Frank A. Sloan was at the Center for Health Policy, Law & Management at Duke University in Durham, North Carolina, when this report was released.

shops in 1994 and 1995. The resulting workshop report, *Lead in the Americas: A Call for Action,* noted that symposium participants concluded that "for many populations in the Americas, human exposure to lead is excessive, produces disease, and must be reduced" (IOM, 1996f, p. 23). The report also provided a nine-step action plan and a series of recommendations designed to achieve primary prevention of lead poisoning wherever possible (e.g., removing lead from gasoline, limiting/eliminating workplace exposures), emphasize sustainable solutions, and implement surveillance strategies to monitor progress.

The IOM, and subsequently the HMD, also took an interest in how indoor air quality affected health due to the effects of allergens, microbes, and other chemical and biological substances that are found in indoor environments. In 2000, the IOM released *Clearing the Air: Asthma and Indoor Air Exposures.* Highlighting overall increases in the prevalence of asthma and asthma-related hospitalizations and deaths during the previous decades, the committee, which was chaired by NAM member Richard B. Johnston, Jr.,[92] reviewed the possible influence of indoor exposure to irritants on asthma, including pests (e.g., dust mites, cockroaches), mold and moisture, pet dander, secondhand smoke (e.g., cigarettes), and other biological and chemical pollutants (IOM, 2000e). Indicating that "asthma mortality is disproportionately high among African Americans and in urban areas that are characterized by high levels of poverty and minority populations" (p. 1), the committee indicated that "identifying effective means to address prevalent exposure" (IOM, 2000e, p. 17) for these vulnerable populations should be a top priority.

In 2004 the IOM followed up on *Clearing the Air* with a related report called *Damp Indoor Spaces and Health.* The report included a comprehensive literature review that confirmed that there was sufficient evidence to support a linkage between "damp indoor environments and some upper respiratory tract symptoms, coughing, wheezing, and asthma symptoms" in sensitive populations (IOM, 2004f). The committee, which was chaired by external volunteer Noreen M. Clark,[93] called for additional research on limiting moisture and eliminating mold in indoor environments in order to aid in developing standardized assessment methods and a better understanding of potential impacts on health outcomes (IOM, 2004f). Following the release of the IOM's report, the WHO issued a new public health guidelines document called *Guidelines for Indoor Air Quality: Dampness and Mould,* which heavily cited the IOM report and adopted the IOM committee's health classification scheme (WHO, 2004).

Continuing its work on indoor air and indoor environments, the IOM released a report in 2011 called *Climate Change, the Indoor Environment, and Health.* In the report, the committee investigated how climate change could potentially reshape indoor environments and how those alterations could, in turn, affect human health. The committee, which was chaired by external volunteer John D. Spengler,[94] concluded that climate change could exacerbate existing indoor environmental concerns (e.g., air quality, dampness and moisture, thermal stress, ventilation, energy consumption, weatherization, existence of infectious agents and pests) and could also introduce new challenges (IOM, 2011i). The report urged the Environmental Protection Agency (EPA) and other government stakeholders to establish building codes that account for climate charge; to update testing standards for emissions from building materials and furnishings; and to better educate the public, health care providers, and building professionals on potential risks and how to mitigate them. In response, the

---

[92] Richard B. Johnston, Jr., was a Professor in the Department of Pediatrics at the University of Colorado School of Medicine and the National Jewish Medical and Research Center in Denver when this report was released.

[93] Noreen M. Clark was the Dean, the Marshall H. Becker Professor of Public Health, and a Professor of Pediatrics at the University of Michigan in Ann Arbor when this report was released.

[94] John D. Spengler was the Akira Yamaguchi Professor of Environmental Health and Human Habitation in the Department of Environmental Health at the Harvard T.H. Chan School of Public Health in Boston, Massachusetts, during this timeframe.

EPA issued a new request for applications for research addressing climate change, indoor environments, and health.[95]

Following the creation of the NAM and the HMD in 2015, the HMD was involved in a report called *Microbiomes of the Built Environment: A Research Agenda for Indoor Microbiology, Human Health, and Buildings* in 2017. The study, which was chaired by NAS member Joan Wennstrom Bennett,[96] was a collaborative effort across the National Academies that included several divisions and boards. The report estimated that people living in developed countries spend upward of 90 percent of their time indoors—from homes to cars and public transportation to workplaces and places of entertainment (e.g., restaurants, movie theaters, stores). Ever present in these environments are microorganisms (e.g., viruses, bacteria, fungi) that are spread by humans and animals, which contribute to indoor microbiomes. However, the committee concluded that little is known about how these microbiomes affect health, what constitutes a healthy indoor environment, or how improvements can be made to these environments (e.g., modifications to ventilation, building materials, furnishings) to ensure health (NASEM, 2017k). The report presented a 12-part research agenda to help better understand interactions across humans, microbiomes, and indoor environments and to help realize the committee's "vision in which these interactions can be predicated and managed so as to design, operate, and maintain more healthful buildings" (NASEM, 2017l, p. 4).

In addition to its work on indoor environments, the IOM also considered how environmental factors can contribute to cancer risks. In May 2001, the IOM's Roundtable on Environmental Health Sciences, Research, and Medicine (described below) held a workshop that resulted in a publication called *Cancer and the Environment: Gene–Environment Interaction* (IOM, 2002a). During the workshop, presenters and attendees examined how environmental factors such as chemicals, radiation and sun exposure, pollutants, and diet interact with an individual's genes to determine their cancer risk profile. In 2012, the IOM followed up with a consensus study called *Breast Cancer and the Environment: A Life Course Approach,* which reviewed evidence related to specific environmental risk factors for breast cancer (e.g., radiation, smoking and alcohol use, postmenopausal hormone replacement therapy, weight gain, exposure to pesticides and other chemicals) over the life course (IOM, 2012b). The committee, chaired by external volunteer Irva Hertz-Picciotto,[97] presented 13 research-oriented recommendations that, if implemented, could lead to a better understanding of the underlying environmental risk factors for breast cancer and how these risk factors might be mitigated. As a result of the report, the Susan G. Komen organization announced $4.5 million in new research grants to examine environmental exposures and links to breast cancer.[98]

In 1998, the IOM's launch of the Roundtable on Environmental Health Sciences, Research, and Medicine created a long-term home for ongoing environmental health discussions among researchers, policy makers, government officials, industry partners, health care professionals, and other interested stakeholders. During its two decades of operation, the roundtable held nearly 70 meetings and released almost 30 publications with a recurring theme of sustainability and climate change. Through its work, the roundtable also responded to emergent environmental concerns (NASEM, n.d.x). For example, 2 months after Hurricane Katrina devastated New Orleans and the Gulf Coast region, the roundtable hosted a workshop to review the "status of the recovery effort …, consider the ongoing challenges in the midst of a disaster …, and facilitate scientific dialogue to understand the impacts of Hurricane Katrina on people's health" (IOM, 2007l, pp. xi, 68; see Figure 6-5). The workshop resulted in a 2007 publication called *Environmental Public Health Impacts of Disasters:*

---

[95] Impact of IOM Reports (Database), IOM/NAM Records.

[96] Joan Wennstrom Bennett was a member of the National Academy of Sciences who was affiliated with Rutgers University at the time.

[97] Irva Hertz-Picciotto was a Professor and the Chief of the Division of Environmental and Occupational Health at the University of California, Davis, when this report was published.

[98] Impact of IOM Reports (Database), IOM/NAM Records.

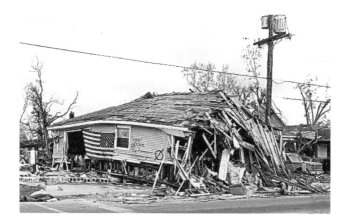

FIGURE 6-5 Barber shop located in Ninth Ward, New Orleans, Louisiana, damaged by Hurricane Katrina in 2005.
SOURCE: Library of Congress.

Hurricane Katrina: Workshop Summary. As the roundtable evolved, the focus of its work became more global, and included discussions related to "nanotechnology, the interrelationship between trade and health, and corporate social responsibility in environmental health" (NASEM, n.d.x).

In 2020, the effects of climate change on human health became a priority focus area for the NAM through its Grand Challenge on Climate Change and Human Health (see Chapter 7).

PROTECTING HEALTH IN AN INTERCONNECTED WORLD

The IOM's early interest in population and public health beyond the borders of the United States led IOM President David Hamburg to include a Board on International Health in his operating structure for the IOM in 1978 (see Chapter 2). Despite intermittent funding challenges and varying levels of commitment across administrations—for example, the board, which was eventually renamed the Board on Global Health, was temporarily dissolved in 1987 and then reinstated in 1989—global health eventually became a mainstay within the IOM's portfolio and was carried forward as part of the NAM's mission in 2015. During a 2001 review of the Board on Global Health, Hamburg, who served on the review committee, noted that "the globalization of the economy, science, popular culture and other domains" reinforced the "importance of thinking about human health from a global perspective."[99] The committee tasked with reviewing the board recommended that global health be infused throughout the work of all of the IOM boards and that the Board on Global Health be reconfigured to include expertise in infectious disease, vaccines for developing countries, and general global health.[100]

U.S. Leadership and Investment in Global Health

One of the roles the Board on Global Health fulfilled over the years was developing reports to advise the federal government on the role of the United States and its investment strategies in global health. The first time the board stepped into this advisory function was during the Carter administration, when Congress requested an IOM study "to determine opportunities, if any, for broadened programs in areas of international health." The board's first report, *Strengthening U.S.*

[99] "Report of the Visiting Committee on Global Health," April 9, 2001, IOM/NAM Records.
[100] Board on International Health Meeting, Minutes, January 17–18, 1989, Yordy Files, IOM/NAM Records.

Programs to Improve Health in Developing Countries, was released in 1978. The report concluded that "the current base of knowledge and experience provides the possibility of ameliorating many [health] problems by commitments of realistic amounts of resources by both developing countries and economically advanced countries" (IOM, 1978).

Nearly two decades later the IOM released *America's Vital Interest in Global Health: Protecting Our People, Enhancing Our Economy, and Advancing Our International Interests* in 1997. In its report, the committee, which was co-chaired by NAM/NAS member and Councilor (1993–1998) Barry R. Bloom[101] and future IOM President and NAM member Harvey V. Fineberg,[102] concluded that the world was becoming more interconnected and that "distinctions between domestic and international health problems are losing their usefulness and are often misleading" (IOM, 1997c). Because diseases and health issues transcend borders, collaborative, international actions were needed. The committee recommended decisive action from the United States to promote global health. The committee indicated that supporting global health was necessary in order to sustain the population health, economic status, and security of the United States in the long term.

With a new administration arriving in the White House, the IOM released *The U.S. Commitment to Global Health: Recommendations for the New Administration* in 2009. The report was expressly developed to advise the Obama administration and Congress on future U.S. investments in global health. The committee, which was co-chaired by external volunteer Thomas R. Pickering[103] and NAM/NAS member Harold Varmus,[104] called on the administration to "highlight health as a pillar of U.S. foreign policy" and urged Congress to double funding for global health initiatives (IOM, 2009f). Following briefings from committee members, the Obama administration's 2010 global health initiative strategy document reflected close adherence to the report's recommendations.[105] In 2014, the IOM assessed U.S. investments in health systems abroad in a report called *Investing in Global Health Systems: Sustaining Gains, Transforming Lives.* In its review, the committee, which was co-chaired by external volunteers John E. Lange[106] and E. Anne Peterson,[107] concluded that "prompt and judicious investment in the management, financing, and infrastructure that support health could have a transformative effect on the lives of the world's billion poorest people and build a more stable world for everyone" (IOM, 2014e). Through its recommendations, the committee outlined "an effective donor strategy for health."

Continuing its tradition of providing guidance to incoming presidents, the IOM released *Global Health and the Future Role of the United States* as the Trump administration was set to take office in 2017. The report noted the benefits of international travel and trade, such as expanded access to goods, but also provided words of caution related to the spread of infectious diseases on a global scale. In light of the current global health landscape and the identified challenges, the committee, which was co-chaired by external volunteer Jendayi E. Frazer[108] and NAM member Valentín Fuster,[109] described four priority areas that offered the greatest potential for improving global

---

[101] Barry R. Bloom was at the Howard Hughes Medical Institute of the Albert Einstein College of Medicine during this time.

[102] Harvey V. Fineberg was the Dean of the faculty of public health at Harvard University at the time.

[103] Thomas R. Pickering was the Vice Chair of Hills & Company, International Consultants in Washington, DC, at the time.

[104] Harold Varmus was the President and the Chief Executive Officer of Memorial Sloan Kettering Cancer Center in New York when this report was released.

[105] Impact of IOM Reports (Database), IOM/NAM Records.

[106] John E. Lange was a retired U.S. Ambassador and a Senior Fellow for Global Health Diplomacy at the United Nations Foundation at this time.

[107] E. Anne Peterson was the Director of the Public Health Program at the Ponce School of Medicine and Health Sciences when this report was released.

[108] Jendayi E. Frazer was with the Council on Foreign Relations in Washington, DC, during this time.

[109] Valentín Fuster was at the Mount Sinai Medical Center in New York when this report was published.

health: achieve global health security, maintain a sustained response to the continuous threats of communicable diseases, save and improve the lives of women and children, and promote cardiovascular health and prevent cancer (NASEM, 2017n).

During the first year of the COVID-19 pandemic, policies under the Trump administration limited international cooperation and ran counter to the recommendations of the studies described in this section, prompting NAM members and leadership to speak out more boldly on behalf of U.S. leadership in global health than they had in the past (see Chapter 7).

The Safety of Food and Medical Products

As global trade expanded, concerns regarding the safety of food and medical products that are imported into the United States increased. For example, much of the seafood consumed in the United States originates in Southeast Asian countries, and many of the active ingredients found in American medications come from other countries. Less stringent regulatory systems outside of the United States, combined with limitations in inspecting these products as they are imported, pose ongoing risks to U.S. consumers (IOM, 2012l). In 2012, the IOM released *Ensuring Safe Foods and Medical Products Through Stronger Regulatory Systems Abroad,* which was developed to help the FDA navigate these challenges. In its report, the committee, which was chaired by NAM member Jim E. Riviere,[110] offered strategies and recommendations to bolster regulatory environments globally and ensure safer foods and medical products in the United States and worldwide. It encouraged the FDA to be a global leader "in the development and adoption of international standards for food and medical products" (IOM, 2012l, p. 238).

The IOM continued its review of medication safety in an interconnected world in its 2013 report, *Countering the Problem of Falsified and Substandard Drugs.* Substandard and falsified drugs can be sold in any country, but low- and middle-income countries with limited regulatory and safety standards and oversight are most vulnerable. The committee, which was chaired by NAM member Lawrence O. Gostin,[111] stated that "eradicating falsified and substandard drugs from the market will require strong national regulation and international cooperation." The report provided a dozen recommendations for the United States to provide leadership in areas such as building global partnerships, adopting agreed-upon definitions, and establishing a code of practice; strengthening surveillance and detection efforts, including use of detection technologies; and ensuring compliance with international standards for manufacturing and quality control (IOM, 2013q). Implementing one of the recommendations from the report, the FDA launched an initiative in Ghana in 2013 to expand the availability of a handheld device used to detect falsified malaria drugs (CBS News, 2013).[112]

Infectious Diseases and Emerging Health Threats

The global spread of infectious disease has been a topic of interest for the IOM and many other international health organizations for decades. This threat has been amplified in recent years with the increasing prevalence of international travel; concerns regarding drug-resistant diseases (e.g., tuberculosis [TB], malaria); and outbreaks, epidemics, and pandemics of emerging infectious diseases without well-defined, effective treatments (e.g., Ebola, Zika, COVID-19). In the past 25 years,

---

[110] Jim E. Riviere was the Burroughs Wellcome Fund Distinguished Professor of Pharmacology and the Director of the Center for Chemical Toxicology Research and Pharmacokinetics at the College of Veterinary Medicine at North Carolina State University in Raleigh during this time.

[111] Lawrence O. Gostin was the Linda and Timothy O'Neill Professor of Global Health Law and the Director of the World Health Organization Collaborating Centre on Public Health Law and Human Rights at the Georgetown University Law Center in Washington, DC, when this report was released.

[112] IOM Council Minutes, July 8, 2013, IOM/NAM Records.

the IOM, and subsequently the NAM and the HMD, leveraged its reputation for providing reliable evidence-based advice and expanded its presence in global health policy by focusing a subsection of its work on preventing and responding to these emerging health threats in a timely manner.

In 1989, the IOM initiated a study to "assess the interactions between etiologic agents, environmental effects on disease, and host defenses to understand factors related to emergence of microbial disease."[113] In 1992, the resulting report, *Emerging Infections: Microbial Threats to Health in the United States,* was released (IOM, 1992b). It explored the spread of infectious diseases such as HIV/AIDS, Lyme disease, malaria, TB, and dengue in context of "human demographics and behavior, technology and industry, economic development and land use, international travel and commerce" (IOM, 1992b). The committee, which was co-chaired by NAS member Joshua Lederberg[114] and external volunteer Robert E. Shope,[115] cautioned against complacency and provided recommendations related to "disease surveillance; vaccine, drug, and pesticide development; vector control; public education and behavioral change; research and training; and strengthening of the U.S. public health system" (NASEM, n.d.f1).

The release of the report was met with considerable media attention, in part, due the fear-based messaging associated with the report. In conjunction with the report's release, the IOM hosted a press conference, and the co-chairs and members of the committee participated in numerous interviews with the media to communicate the report's findings and recommendations, indicating that microbial "threat[s] will continue and may even intensify in coming years" (IOM, 1992b, p. 1). A feature article in *The New Yorker* called the IOM report "frightening," noting that "new diseases will emerge, although it is impossible to predict their individual emergence in time and place" (Preston, 1992). A *New York Times* article called the report a "wake up call" and highlighted the inadequacy of public health surveillance systems "to detect threats from new diseases and the reemergence of old ones" (Altman, 1992).

The 1992 report ultimately led to the establishment of a new section within the U.S. military's Armed Forces Health Surveillance Branch called the Department of Defense–Global Emerging Infections Surveillance. In a 1996 directive announcing the new section, President Bill Clinton stated that "the mission of the DoD will be expanded to include support of global surveillance, training, research, and response to emerging infectious disease threats. DoD will strengthen its global disease reduction efforts through: centralized coordination, improved preventive health programs and epidemiologic capabilities; and enhanced involvement with military treatment facilities and overseas laboratories" (IOM, 2001h, p. 2). Several years later, the IOM, through its Medical Follow-up Agency (see Chapter 4), was asked to conduct a review of the program. In response, the IOM released a report in 2001, *Perspectives on the Department of Defense Global Emerging Infections Surveillance and Response System: A Program Review,* which concluded that "substantial progress has been made toward achieving system goals" (IOM, 2001h).

In 2003, nearly a decade after the release of the first *Microbial Threats* report, the IOM released a follow-up report titled *Microbial Threats to Health: Emergence, Detection, and Response.* Reassessing the state of research and international policy, the report described a recent SARS outbreak to illustrate the potential hazards of the global transmission of infectious diseases. The committee, which was co-chaired by NAM member and Foreign Secretary (2014–2020) Margaret A.

---

[113] Board on Health Sciences Policy, "Microbial Threats to Health," September 12, 1989, IOM/NAM Records.

[114] Joshua Lederberg was a University Professor and a Sackler Foundation Scholar at The Rockefeller University in New York during this time.

[115] Robert E. Shope was a Professor of Epidemiology and the Director of the Yale Arbovirus Research Unit at the Yale University School of Medicine in New Haven, Connecticut, when this report was published.

Hamburg[116] and Joshua Lederberg,[117] offered recommendations designed to enhance the global capacity to detect and respond to threats. Reinforcing recommendations from previous reports, the committee called for the development of new vaccines and treatments for infectious diseases and emphasized the need to strengthen the domestic public health and surveillance infrastructure (IOM, 2003i). Shining a light on another form of microbial threat, the IOM released a report called *Sustaining Global Surveillance and Response to Emerging Zoonotic Diseases* in 2009. Zoonotic diseases—those that can be transmitted between animals and humans (e.g., SARS, HIV/AIDS, H1N1 [swine flu], mad cow disease)—present unique challenges as they are generally "novel and unpredictable," they can "emerge anywhere and spread rapidly," and they tend to have a "major economic toll" (IOM and NRC, 2009b). In its report, the committee, which was co-chaired by NAM member Gerald T. Keusch[118] and external volunteer Marguerite Pappaioanou,[119] reviewed existing surveillance systems that could detect zoonotic diseases and provided recommendations to improve early identification and response, while encouraging greater collaboration and coordination across human and animal health researchers and policy makers. The report was cited as an influence for a new Emerging Pandemic Threats program that was launched by the U.S. Agency for International Development program in 2009.[120]

Following the release of the IOM's 1992 *Microbial Threats* report, the IOM launched the Forum on Emerging Infections in 1996 (later renamed the Forum on Microbial Threats) at the request of the CDC and the NIH. The forum was established "to provide a structured opportunity for discussion and scrutiny of critical, and possibly contentious, scientific and policy issues related to research on and the prevention, detection, surveillance, and responses to emerging and reemerging infectious diseases in humans, plants, and animals, as well as the microbiome in health and disease." With the support of its nearly 20 sponsors, the Forum on Microbial Threats held more than 45 public meetings and workshops on a wide variety of topics that built on the themes and recommendations from the previous reports. In 2008, for example, the forum hosted a workshop on "Infectious Disease Movement in a Borderless World." Because of the ongoing nature of the forum and its ability to set its own agendas, the forum was also able to respond to emerging global concerns in a timely manner. For example, the forum hosted a discussion meeting and workshop on the H1N1 influenza pandemic in 2009 and a workshop on the Ebola epidemic in West Africa in 2015 (NASEM, 2016j). In 2015, the forum collaborated with the NAM to host a workshop that resulted in a summary called *Global Health Risk Framework: Governance for Global Health: Workshop Summary* (NASEM, 2016l), which contributed to the NAM's Global Health Risk Framework Program (see Chapter 7).

In addition to its broad review of infectious diseases and emerging global health threats, the IOM also concentrated a segment of its work on specific mosquito-borne diseases such as malaria and Zika, and other infectious diseases, such as TB. The evolution and transmission of drug-resistant variants of these diseases have complicated global public health strategies to contain and treat them. In 1991, the IOM released its first report on malaria—*Malaria: Obstacles and Opportunities*—which described a resurgence of the disease with cases identified in more than 100 countries. The report indicated that malaria had become the top health challenge for sub-Saharan Africa, with more than 1 million deaths per year and rapidly increasing rates of drug-resistant cases. The com-

---

[116] Margaret A. Hamburg was the Vice President for Biological Programs at the Nuclear Threat Initiative during this time.
[117] Joshua Lederberg was a Professor Emeritus and a Sackler Foundation Scholar at The Rockefeller University when this report was released.
[118] Gerald T. Keusch was at Boston University at the time.
[119] Marguerite Pappaioanou was at the Association of American Veterinary Medical Colleges in Washington, DC, at the time this report was published.
[120] Impact of IOM Reports (Database), IOM/NAM Records.

mittee, which was chaired by external volunteer Charles C. J. Carpenter,[121] provided a comprehensive review of the state of malaria research, prevention, and control efforts, highlighting concerns with increasing rates of drug-resistant strains of the parasites that cause malaria (*P. falciparum* and *P. vivax*) and insecticide-resistant strains of mosquitoes. The committee recommended increased support for research and surveillance, and urged expanded collaboration to develop vaccines, new treatments, and better control options (IOM, 1991c). A 1996 IOM report, *Vaccines Against Malaria*, reiterated the urgent need for a malaria vaccine, stating that the successful development and widespread application of a vaccine that can prevent the illness and death of malaria could be one of the most important advances in medicine, with the potential for improving the lives of hundreds of millions of people (IOM, 1996g).

Nearly a decade later, the IOM released a follow-up report in 2004 called *Saving Lives, Buying Time: The Economics of Malaria Drugs in an Age of Resistance,* which made recommendations to expand access to new, more effective combination treatments in countries where the disease was endemic. In its report, the committee, which was chaired by NAS member Kenneth J. Arrow,[122] concluded that without funding to supply these new treatments, "malaria mortality could double over the next 10–20 years and transmission will intensify" (IOM, 2004g). The report's central recommendation became a reality in 2009, when private and public donors, including the Bill & Melinda Gates Foundation and the World Bank, collaborated to establish the Affordable Medicines Facility-malaria, which is managed through the Global Fund to Fight AIDS, Tuberculosis and Malaria. The Affordable Medicines Facility-malaria was developed as a financing program with an initial budget of $225 million to expand access to affordable and high-quality therapies.[123] Through its African Science Academy Development Initiative (see Chapter 4), the IOM was also able to support other countries in improving their responses to malaria; one example of this was the Cameroon Academy of Sciences' 2004 report *Drug Resistance to Anti-Malaria Drugs in Cameroon: Strategies for Control.*[124]

In addition to malaria, the IOM also considered the global impact of drug-resistant TB. For example, the IOM's Forum on Drug Discovery, Development, and Translation examined the threat of drug-resistant variants of TB and possible responses in a series of six workshop summaries. As part of its series, which was released between 2009 and 2014 (see Box 6-7), the forum collaborated with the academies of sciences in South Africa, Russia, India, and China to host workshops in each of those countries. Through its joint workshops, the forum estimated that TB killed about 4,500 people every day, making TB the leading cause of death worldwide (IOM, 2009d). The presenters and participants at these international workshops discussed a range of topics that included the "increasing burden of drug-resistant tuberculosis," the "new challenges to traditional TB control and treatment programs" that drug-resistant TB presented, and the urgent need for "the global health community to collaborate and share scientific information in new and different ways," as well as country-specific experiences and needs in managing drug-resistant TB locally (IOM, 2012p, p. 129).

Following the rapid transmission of the Zika virus—a mosquito-borne illness associated with a specific mosquito species (*Ae. aegypti* and *Ae. albopictus*)—across 26 countries in the Americas, HHS called on the National Academies in 2015 to help define "future research that could be conducted under real-world conditions ... that would provide ... additional accurate information about virus transmission, mitigation of health risks, and appropriate measures to prevent the spread

---

[121] Charles C.J. Carpenter was a Professor of Medicine at Brown University and the Physician-in-Chief at the Miriam Hospital in Providence, Rhode Island, when this report was released.

[122] Kenneth J. Arrow was a Professor Emeritus in the Department of Economics at Stanford University in Stanford, California, during this time.

[123] Impact of IOM Reports (Database), IOM/NAM Records.

[124] IOM Council Minutes, October 21, 2014, IOM/NAM Records.

BOX 6-7
Forum on Drug Discovery, Development, and Translation's
Series on Drug-Resistant Tuberculous

- *The Global Crisis of Drug-Resistant Tuberculosis and Leadership of China and the BRICS: Challenges and Opportunities* (2014)
- *Developing and Strengthening the Global Supply Chain for Second-Line Drugs for Multidrug-Resistant Tuberculosis* (2013)
- *Facing the Reality of Drug-Resistant Tuberculosis in India: Challenges and Potential Solutions* (2012)
- *The New Profile of Drug-Resistant Tuberculosis in Russia: A Global and Local Perspective* (2011)
- *The Emerging Threat of Drug-Resistant Tuberculosis in Southern Africa: Global and Local Challenges and Solutions* (2011)
- *Addressing the Threat of Drug-Resistant Tuberculosis: A Realistic Assessment of the Challenge* (2009)

NOTE: Publications in this list are workshop summaries.

---

of disease" (NASEM, 2016k; see Figure 6-7). In response, the HMD hosted a fast-track, 1-day workshop in February 2016 that brought together experts and stakeholders to discuss factors that could reduce the risk of transmission in the United States, knowledge gaps related to prevention strategies, specific high-priority research questions, and opportunities to improve evidence-based communication regarding risk factors, transmission mechanisms, prevention measures, and health consequences (NASEM, 2016k). HMD published a workshop in brief that summarized the key points of discussion, reinforcing the National Academies' ability to respond to emerging public health threats while maintaining its commitment to providing evidence-based advice.

Disaster Preparedness and Response

As with infectious diseases and emerging health threats, terrorism and natural disasters often have a global reach that requires varying degrees of international response and preparedness. Following the terrorist attacks of September 11, 2001, the IOM along with many government agencies and interested stakeholders, began reevaluating disaster preparedness plans. Weighing in on medical response plans, the IOM released *Preparing for Terrorism: Tools for Evaluating the Metropolitan Medical Response System Program* in 2002. HHS commissioned this study to help formulate mechanisms to evaluate the efficacy of HHS's Metropolitan Medical Response System program, which provided large U.S. cities with assistance "in develop[ing] plans for coping with the health and medical consequences of a terrorist attack with chemical, biological, or radiological … agents" (IOM, 2002d). In its report, the committee, which was chaired by NAM member Lewis Goldfrank,[125] provided a set of program assessment tools that corresponded to a three-part evaluation strategy and preparedness indicators for specific response capabilities. The following year, the IOM released *Preparing for the Psychological Consequences of Terrorism: A Public Health Strategy.* The report considered the degree to which the U.S. public health infrastructure was adequately prepared to respond to the nation's psychological needs following an attack. The committee, which was also chaired by Goldfrank, offered an array of recommendations that spoke to "the training

---

[125] Lewis Goldfrank was the Director of Emergency Medicine at the New York University Medical Center and Bellevue Hospital Center in New York when this report was released.

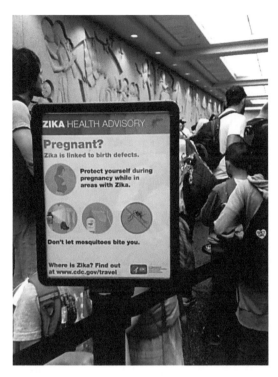

FIGURE 6-7 A CDC Zika health advisory for travelers posted at the Honolulu airport in 2016.
SOURCE: Mayra Morales, CDC/CDC Connects.

and education of service providers, ensuring appropriate guidelines for the protection of service providers, and developing public health surveillance for pre-event, event, and post-event factors related to psychological consequences" (IOM, 2003j, p. 5).

During this timeframe, the IOM also considered preparedness and response plans for potential bioterrorism attacks, focusing on threats from agents such as smallpox and anthrax. In 2005, the IOM released *The Smallpox Vaccination Program: Public Health in an Age of Terrorism*, which was the culmination of 2 years of work and encompassed seven letter reports to the Director of the CDC. The purpose of the committee's work, which was chaired by Brian Strom,[126] was to advise the CDC as it planned and implemented a national smallpox vaccination program that would be designed to "vaccinate people against a disease that does not exist with a vaccine that poses some well-known risks" in a "low-likelihood, high-consequence" bioterrorism attack scenario (IOM, 2005d, p. 1). Following the 2001 anthrax mailing attacks, the IOM also reviewed the safety of the currently available anthrax vaccine for wide-scale use in the military and possible public use in its 2002 report *The Anthrax Vaccine: Is It Safe?* (see Chapter 4). Because wide-scale implementation and use of the anthrax vaccine was not recommended or practical—in part because "it require[d] multiple initial doses followed by annual boosters"—preparedness and response plans for an anthrax attack also required plans to quickly deliver antibiotics to potentially large populations of exposed people. In 2012, the IOM released *Prepositioning Antibiotics for Anthrax,* which considered "the use of prepositioning strategies to complement current plans for distributing and dispensing anthrax antibiotics" (IOM, 2012m, p. 1). The committee, which was chaired by external

---

[126] Brian Strom was the George S. Pepper Professor of Public Health and Preventive Medicine and a Professor of Biostatistics and Epidemiology, Medicine, and Pharmacology at the University of Pennsylvania Perelman School of Medicine in Philadelphia when this report was released.

volunteer Robert R. Bass,[127] provided a framework and seven recommendations to aid state and local policy makers and public health officials to determine what, if any, prepositioning strategies would be advantageous for their specific populations and communities.

Seeing the need for a permanent convening body to host ongoing discussions related to preparedness and response, the IOM established the Forum on Medical and Public Health Preparedness for Disasters and Emergencies in 2007. The forum's stated mission was to "improve the nation's preparedness for, response to, and recovery from disasters, public health emergencies, and emerging threats" (NASEM, n.d.z). Its wide focus included such topics as how emergency medical services should respond to a multisite terrorist attack and which strategies should be used to mitigate the Zika virus. Over the years, the forum hosted workshops related to rural mass casualty response, the distribution of antiviral medications, data priority needs in the wake of Hurricane Sandy, and the preparedness impacts of the ACA. As with other forums and roundtables, the goal of the forum was to provide a neutral space in which interested parties could come together to discuss timely issues with a dedicated focus on how best to prepare the country for medical and public health emergencies and disasters.

In 2009, the IOM launched a series of reports and workshop summaries that explored crisis standards of care that could be applied in disaster situations such as pandemics, natural disasters, and terrorist attacks—scenarios "in which thousands, tens of thousands, or even hundreds of thousands of people suddenly require and seek medical care in communities across the United States" (IOM, 2009e). The first report in the series was a letter report titled *Guidance for Establishing Crisis Standards of Care for Use in Disaster Situations: Letter Report*. In this report, the committee, which was chaired by Lawrence O. Gostin,[128] laid out its vision for crisis standards of care, including application of fairness; equitable processes; community and provider engagement, education, and communication; and the rule of law (IOM, 2009e). The IOM's next two reports were released in 2012 and 2013 and were called *Crisis Standards of Care: A Systems Framework for Catastrophic Disaster Response* (2012) and *Crisis Standards of Care: A Toolkit for Indicators and Triggers* (2013). The 2012 report, which was produced by a committee also chaired by Gostin, consisted of seven volumes that provided detailed functions and tasks for various groups that would be engaged in crisis standards of care following a disaster (e.g., state and local governments, hospitals, first responders) (IOM, 2012n). The 2013 report—drafted by a committee co-chaired by external volunteers Dan Hanfling[129] and John L. Hick[130]—explored possible indicators and triggers that could "help guide operational decision making about providing care during public health and medical emergencies and disasters" (IOM, 2013m). The Forum on Medical and Public Health Preparedness for Disasters and Emergencies continued the conversation about crisis standards of care with a parallel effort that included three workshops that featured discussions related to medical surge capacity and barriers to integrating crisis standards into international disaster response plans. Together, these publications were designed to guide policy makers, governments, health care systems, and other stakeholders in planning for disasters in which it "is necessary to provide the best possible health care during a crisis and, if needed, equitably allocate scarce resources" (IOM, 2013m).

The IOM's series on crisis standards for care examined how communities could provide health care and social services during a crisis, but questions about what happens after a crisis and how communities and health systems recover and restore services required additional study. In 2015, the IOM released a report called *Healthy, Resilient, and Sustainable Communities After Disasters*. Not-

---

[127] Robert R. Bass was with the Maryland Institute for Emergency Medical Services Systems when this report was published.

[128] Lawrence O. Gostin was at Georgetown University Law Center, Washington, DC during this timeframe.

[129] Dan Hanfling was with the Inova Health System in Falls Church, Virginia, when this report was released.

[130] John L. Hick was at Hennepin County Medical Center in Minneapolis, Minnesota, at the time.

ing that pre-disaster socioeconomic and health conditions in communities are not often optimal, the committee, which was chaired by NAM member Reed V. Tuckson,[131] described disaster recovery as an opportunity to "advance the long-term health, resilience, and sustainability of communities—thereby better preparing them for future challenges" (IOM, 2015h). The committee also argued that ensuring health and well-being should be at the forefront of all disaster planning and recovery efforts. The committee's report proposed a conceptual framework and 12 recommendations that provided operational guidance for stakeholders involved in disaster planning, such establishing a post-disaster vision for healthy communities and coordinating and leveraging available recovery resources to promote health.

CONCLUSION

From its earliest days, the IOM was committed to improving public health both within the United States and internationally. The organization played a key role in defining the field and mission of public health, as well as outlining the investments and infrastructure necessary for its successful practice. Advice from the IOM—and later the NAM and HMD—guided the national and global response to many of the most significant public health threats of the 20th and 21st centuries—including setting the initial research agenda for HIV/AIDS and later driving the expansion of PEPFAR, a historically impactful program that expanded access to HIV/AIDS prevention and treatment internationally. The IOM was also influential in promoting recognition of the global burden of chronic conditions such as cardiovascular disease and mental health and substance use disorders. Confronting the obesity epidemic in the United States was a particularly important area of focus for the IOM, and its recommendations were impactful, leading in particular to increased access to healthy foods (and decreased marketing of unhealthy foods) to children. Finally, the IOM, the NAM, and the HMD, arguing for the fundamental interconnectedness of health across borders, countries, and nations, were stalwart proponents of U.S. leadership and investment in global health—a position that gained new importance amid the COVID-19 pandemic and drove an related focus on environmental health and climate change, which threatened to increase the spread of novel infectious diseases.

Over five decades, the IOM, the NAM, and the HMD produced a sweeping body of work in the area of public health—with subjects ranging from individual infectious disease outbreaks to the worldwide burden of chronic illness, from recommendations for the implementation of specific U.S. programs to broader guidance about the future of public health and the necessity of international collaboration and coordination. Equity was a common theme across this work, as studies emphasized the importance of attention to health disparities and extending research and services to underserved populations. In sum, the organization made its mark both in the United States and internationally as a dedicated proponent of public health and an advocate for support of populations in need—building on the vision of its founders more than 50 years earlier.

---

[131] Reed. V. Tuckson was the Managing Director at Tuckson Health Connections, LLC, in Sandy Springs, Georgia, when this report was released.

Part III

A New Era: The Early Years of the National Academy of Medicine

The years after the establishment of the National Academy of Medicine (NAM) in 2015 were marked by unprecedented crises in the United States and abroad, including the COVID-19 pandemic and other pandemic infectious diseases, climate change, racial injustice, and an erosion of trust in government and science. The following chapters describe how the NAM advanced new strategic priorities and developed program models to achieve impact amid a challenging and rapidly evolving landscape—ushering in a dynamic new era for the organization.

7

Responding to National and Global Crises, 2015–2021

As fate would have it, the early years of the National Academy of Medicine (NAM) coincided with a period of great upheaval in U.S. politics and society, as well as the most damaging global public health crisis in a century—the COVID-19 pandemic. The NAM's new strategic focus on proactivity and flexibility, as well as its readiness to speak out on issues of concern to its leaders and members, proved ideally suited to respond to the dramatic societal challenges that emerged between 2015 and 2021. The NAM quickly established itself as an organization capable of effecting change at the highest levels through innovative and nimble program models designed to drive collective action and collaborative solutions—while staying rooted in the scientific rigor that formed the core of its credibility and influence.

In 2017, following 2 years of intensive consultation with NAM members, volunteers, sponsors, and other stakeholders, the NAM published its "Strategic Plan 2018–2023: Goalposts for a Healthier Future" (described in Chapter 3) (NAM, 2017d). The plan laid out three overarching strategic goals: (1) identify and address critical issues; and lead and inspire action; (2) diversify and activate the membership of the NAM; and engage emerging leaders and scholars; and (3) build leadership capacity across diverse disciplines. This chapter describes the NAM's programs and impact between 2015 and 2021 within the context of this strategic framework.

IDENTIFYING, ADDRESSING, AND INSPIRING ACTION IN RESPONSE TO CRITICAL ISSUES (STRATEGIC GOAL 1)

The first overarching goal in the NAM's strategic plan dictated that it proactively identify and respond rapidly to address the most urgent challenges that present a threat to the health of people worldwide. This approach was in contrast to the early decades of the Institute of Medicine, when the organization developed programs only in response to a request from an external sponsor. This strategic goal also looked beyond the confines of the NAM's own programmatic response and called for it to catalyze collective action among diverse stakeholders. As described below, the NAM applied this proactive and collaborative orientation in response to global infectious disease outbreaks, the national crisis of health worker burnout, the U.S. opioid epidemic, health system transformation, and structural racism.

The Ebola Crisis in West Africa

In 2014–2016, the emergence of Ebola in West Africa became the first major issue the NAM took on as a new Academy. The outbreak was the largest of its kind in history, ultimately infecting nearly 30,000 people and killing more than 11,000 (CDC, n.d.f; see Figure 7-1). In Spring 2015, Victor Dzau[1] met with Jim Yong Kim, an NAM member who was then president of the World Bank Group, to discuss the unfolding crisis. The two leaders agreed that the global response to the outbreak appeared slow, uncoordinated, and largely uninformed by scientific evidence. Kim encouraged Dzau to mount a response through the IOM that would be seen as independent and authoritative by the international community.

The Commission on a Global Health Risk Framework for the Future (GHRF), which launched in July 2015, the same month the IOM became the NAM, leveraged the NAM's position as a neutral advisor and convener to lead a formal assessment of the global response to Ebola and develop a framework to guide the response to future pandemics (NAM, n.d.d). The GHRF project developed a novel program model that would become a staple of the NAM's work in ensuing years: the International Commission. The NAM appointed an oversight board with responsibility for guiding the initiative and a commission to carry out the assessment and author an independent report. The commission consisted of 17 members from diverse geographic regions with expertise in finance, governance, research and development, health systems, and social science. To inform its report, the commission hosted information-gathering workshops across 4 continents and received input from more than 250 experts and stakeholders (NAM, 2015).

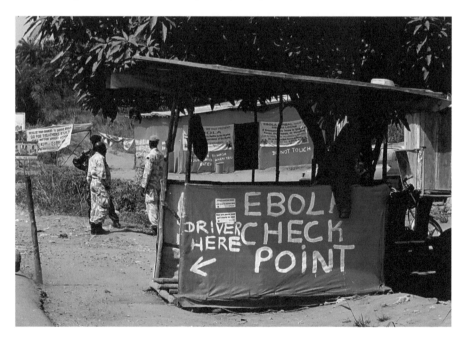

FIGURE 7-1 An Ebola checkpoint in Sierra Leone, 2016.
SOURCE: Rebecca Myers, CDC/CDC Connects.

---

[1] As this event preceded the July 2015 transition of the Institute of Medicine (IOM) to the National Academy of Medicine, Dzau was then president of the IOM.

The Neglected Dimension of Global Security: A Framework to Counter Infectious Disease Crises, published in January 2016, noted that Ebola and other outbreaks "revealed gaping holes in preparedness, serious weaknesses in response, and a range of failures of global and local leaders" (NAM, 2016a, p. v). Despite the potential of infectious diseases to produce a catastrophic loss of life and an estimated $60 billion in annualized expected losses, nations devoted only a small fraction of the money they spent on national security to pandemic preparedness (NAM, 2016a). The commission urged world leaders to look at health security as a "global public good" and to commit to the creation and maintenance of a "comprehensive global framework to counter infectious disease crises" (NAM, 2016a, p. 1).

The GHRF report was among the first major publications to make a strong case for investment in global health security. It recommended a three-pronged approach that included strengthening public health systems, improving global and regional coordination and capabilities, and accelerating research and development of tools such as diagnostics and vaccines (NAM, 2016a). In the months and years immediately following its publication, a number of new international organizations were formed to take action in these areas. In May 2016, the World Health Organization (WHO) announced the creation of a new Health Emergencies Programme "designed to deliver rapid, predictable, and comprehensive support to countries and communities as they prepare for, face or recover from emergencies caused by any type of hazard to human health" (Bahuguna, 2016). The following year, the Coalition for Epidemic Preparedness Innovations (CEPI), was founded "as the result of a consensus that a coordinated, international, and intergovernmental plan was needed to develop and deploy new vaccines to prevent future epidemics" (CEPI, n.d.a). In 2018, the WHO and the World Bank Group launched the Global Preparedness Monitoring Board (GPMB) to "[bring] together political leaders, heads of United Nations agencies and health experts to strengthen global health security through stringent independent monitoring and regular reporting" (UN, 2018). Dzau served on CEPI's interim board of directors as well as the GPMB board, alongside GHRF Commission members Jeremy Farrar (Wellcome Trust) and Chris Elias (Bill & Melinda Gates Foundation) (CEPI, n.d.b; GPMB, n.d.a, n.d.b).[2]

The COVID-19 Pandemic

The lessons of the GHRF report proved prescient as SARS-CoV-2 (the virus that caused COVID-19) emerged in early 2020 (see Figure 7-2). Following declarations of U.S. and global public health emergencies, the staff of the NAM and the National Academies of Sciences, Engineering, and Medicine (the National Academies) were asked to work remotely for an initial period of 3 weeks beginning on March 16, 2020. The remote work period was eventually extended for more than 2 years. Despite challenges in adjusting to working from home, especially for parents of young children, the NAM quickly pivoted its operations and programmatic priorities to focus on the response to COVID-19. "The COVID-19 pandemic brings the National Academies' mission into stark relief," Dzau wrote in a letter to NAM members on April 7, 2020.

> We were chartered to provide scientific leadership to the nation and the world and advance evidence-based solutions for the most urgent and complex challenges facing humanity. As we witness the most significant pandemic for a century unfold across international borders—and as misinformation threatens the lives of thousands—there is no question of our fundamental obligation to act.[3]

---

[2] Dzau served on the interim board of CEPI. As of January 2022, Farrar served on the boards of CEPI and GPMB, and Elias served on the board of CEPI.

[3] Victor Dzau to NAM Members, "Fourth Update on NAM/NASEM Response to COVID-19," April 7, 2020, IOM/NAM Records.

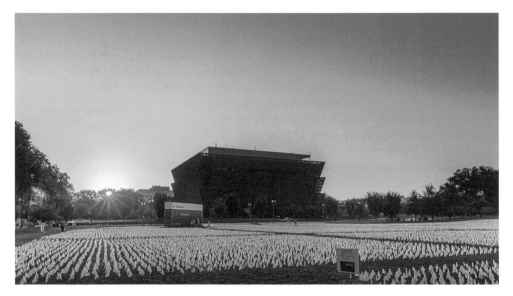

FIGURE 7-2 The "In America: Remember" COVID-19 memorial art installation on the National Mall in Washington, DC, featured a white flag for each of the nearly 700,000 Americans who had died from COVID-19 by September 2021.
SOURCE: Photograph by Hal Chen, iStock.

Dzau himself quickly assumed a prominent role in the international COVID-19 response, helping to initiate a Coronavirus Global Response Pledging Conference hosted by the European Commission on May 4, 2020. "This is about solidarity—we cannot let the poorest and most affected countries struggle alone," said Dzau in remarks at the event. "Infectious disease outbreaks like COVID-19 are among the most complex challenges we face as a global society. We need to work together to accelerate the development of vaccines and treatments and ensure that they will be available to everyone" (NAM, 2020j). Dzau also served on the boards of the Global Preparedness Monitoring Board and Access to COVID-19 Tools (ACT) Accelerator (ACT-A), which supported equitable global access to COVID-19 vaccines through its COVAX facility (Gavi, n.d.).

Providing Scientific Advice in the Early Days of the Pandemic

Dzau also spearheaded a comprehensive response to COVID-19 at the NAM and supported a coordinated effort across the National Academies. One of the NAM's first actions in response to the pandemic was to launch the "COVID-19 Conversations" webinar series in partnership with the American Public Health Association (APHA) (APHA and NAM, n.d.). Designed to disseminate reliable scientific information during a time of uncertainty and amid conflicting information from government sources, the series was hosted by Dzau and APHA executive officer Georges Benjamin. The series' advisory committee was co-chaired by NAM members Carlos del Rio of Emory University and Nicole Lurie, who served as the Assistant Secretary for Preparedness and Response under the Obama administration.[4] The first webinar of the series, titled "The Science of Social Distancing," was hosted on March 25, 2020, and attracted more than 10,000 participants—record attendance for the NAM. Webinars were hosted every 2 weeks in the early months of the crisis, amounting to a total of 21 events by August 2021. The series provided rapid scientific analysis of

---

[4] Carlos del Rio was NAM International Secretary at the time. Nicole Lurie was affiliated with the Coalition for Epidemic Preparedness Innovations.

topics that were top of mind for health leaders, policy makers, and the public, ranging from testing and treatment to the reopening of K–12 schools and universities to vaccines, virus variants, and impacts on health equity.

The NAM-APHA series ran in parallel to the work of the National Academies' Standing Committee on Emerging Infectious Diseases and 21st Century Health Threats (SCEID), launched on February 28, 2020, at the request of the White House Office of Science and Technology Policy. Chaired by former IOM President Harvey Fineberg,[5] and with the participation of multiple NAM members, the SCIED produced evidence-based rapid expert consultations (RECs) and consensus reports on topics such as the seasonality of SARS-CoV-2, the effectiveness of face coverings, and crisis standards of care, among many others. By the end of 2021, SCEID had produced 15 RECs and 2 consensus studies, and Fineberg had appeared frequently on national news channels to report on the committee's findings.

Guidance on COVID-19 Vaccine Allocation and Acceptance

In August 2020, in anticipation of the imminent availability of one or more COVID-19 vaccines, the NAM and the National Academies launched a study at the request of the National Institutes of Health (NIH) and the Centers for Disease Control and Prevention to recommend a framework for equitable allocation of vaccine in the United States and globally. One month prior, NIH director Francis Collins had, in testimony before Congress, called for a "group of big thinkers who [can] take a high-level view of this and lay out a foundation of principles that could then be utilized … when the moment comes to actually turn that into an implementation plan" (U.S. Congress, Senate, 2020). The study committee was co-chaired by NAM members William H. Foege,[6] former director of the Centers for Disease Control and Prevention (CDC), and Helene Gayle,[7] former Chief Executive Officer of the international humanitarian organization CARE. In anticipation of a limited initial supply of vaccine, the committee was charged with determining which groups (e.g., health care workers, older adults, people with serious illnesses, etc.) should be eligible for vaccination first. The study also prioritized the promotion of health equity, given the much higher rates of infection and death among people of color, and of strategies to mitigate vaccine hesitancy. Given the high stakes of this issue, the committee prioritized transparency and the collection of diverse public input. Nearly 1,500 public comments were analyzed and incorporated into the final study, *Framework for Equitable Allocation of COVID-19 Vaccine*, which was released on October 2, 2020 (NASEM, 2020b).

The report recommended a four-phased allocation framework founded on broadly accepted ethical principles and guided by evidence to maximize the reduction of morbidity and mortality from transmission of the virus. Additional recommendations included the adaptation of existing public health systems and structures for vaccine distribution; measures to ensure that the vaccine would be free of charge; and a CDC-led vaccine risk communication and community engagement program. Finally, the report recommended that the United States take a leadership role in the equitable distribution of vaccine globally. Following publication, several states incorporated principles from the report into their individual vaccine allocation frameworks along with recommendations from the CDC's Advisory Committee on Immunization Practices.

Shortly thereafter, as pharmaceutical companies Pfizer and Moderna prepared applications for Emergency Use Authorization (EUA) of their COVID-19 vaccines, alarm among public health leaders ran high that misinformation and mistrust could imperil the success of a COVID-19 vac-

---

[5] Harvey Fineberg was President of the Gordon and Betty Moore Foundation at the time.

[6] William H. Foege was affiliated with the Rollins School of Public Health at Emory University at the time.

[7] Helene Gayle was affiliated with the Chicago Community Trust at the time.

cination campaign (Darrough and Adib, 2020). Widespread mistrust among health care workers, who were first in line to receive the vaccine, was particularly concerning, given that this group was both at the highest risk for contracting the virus and highly influential in advising the general public about the safety of the vaccine. As it had in the 1990s, the federal government reached out to the NAM for help in mitigating concerns about vaccine safety. At the request of CDC and the Food and Drug Administration (FDA), Dzau hosted a private "NAM Town Hall on the COVID-19 Vaccine for Health Care Leaders" on December 5, 2020. CDC, FDA, and NIH leaders delivered remarks before about 100 executive-level health care leaders about the trustworthiness of the COVID-19 vaccine development process, despite its unprecedented speed.

By March 2021, vaccines had become readily available to most people in the United States, but remained very scarce in other areas of the globe. Dzau, Gayle, and Foege wrote an open letter urging the U.S. government to immediately allocate a portion of the U.S. supply to nations in need. Such an action "would send an important signal to other nations that investment in global health equity must be part of first-line pandemic response, not an afterthought," they wrote (NAM, 2021d). In June 2021, the Biden administration announced its plan to share at least 80 million doses internationally by the end of that month, 25 percent of which would support direct surge capacity in other countries (The White House, 2021a). The remainder would be allocated through the COVAX program co-administered by Gavi: The Vaccine Alliance, CEPI, and the WHO as part of ACT-A (Gavi, n.d.). By late 2021, the United States had donated approximately 140 million doses to at least 93 countries, with the largest quantities going to Pakistan, Bangladesh, the Philippines, Columbia, South Africa, Vietnam, Indonesia, Guatemala, Uzbekistan, and Nigeria (KFF, 2021).

Strengthening the U.S. Health System After COVID-19

NAM programs that pre-existed the COVID-19 pandemic also rallied to offer guidance within their specific areas of focus. The Action Collaborative on Clinician Well-Being and Resilience (CWB Collaborative), for example, provided a list of resources to support caregivers, which became one of the NAM's top five most visited webpages in 2020 (NAM, n.d.b). Dzau and CWB Collaborative Co-Chairs Darrell Kirch[8] and Thomas Nasca[9] published a perspective article in the *New England Journal of Medicine* in which they called COVID-19's impact on clinician well-being a "parallel pandemic" that required a federal response akin to that after the September 11 terrorist attacks (Dzau et al., 2020). In a follow-up op-ed in the *Los Angeles Times*, Dzau called for a "national strategy, not only to help healthcare workers recover from the pandemic, but also to mitigate preexisting drivers of burnout" (Dzau, 2021). The NAM's Action Collaborative on Countering the U.S. Opioid Epidemic (Opioid Collaborative) and the Culture of Health Program (COHP), in turn, provided resources for other populations hard hit by the pandemic, including individuals with substance use disorder and populations experiencing health inequities that predated the pandemic (NAM, n.d.e, n.d.f).

Attention also turned to rebuilding crucial health systems on the basis of lessons learned from COVID-19. The NAM Leadership Consortium: Collaboration for a Value & Science-Driven Health System undertook a comprehensive review of nine sectors of the U.S. health care system called *Emerging Stronger from COVID-19: Priorities for Health System Transformation*. The initiative produced assessments of (1) public health; (2) care systems; (3) research; (4) health payers; (5) clinicians; (6) quality, safety, and standards organizations; (7) health product manufacturers and innovators; (8) patients, families, and communities; and (9) digital health (NAM, 2021g). Each

---

[8] Darrell Kirch, an NAM member, was the President Emeritus of the Association of American Medical Colleges.

[9] Thomas Nasca was the President and the Chief Executive Officer of the Accreditation Council for Graduate Medical Education.

assessment identified weakness that existed prior to COVID-19, explored how the given sector had responded to the pandemic, and highlighted opportunities for strengthening and transforming the delivery of health care after COVID-19. The sector assessments were delivered to members of Congress, federal agencies including the Office of the Assistant Secretary for Health and the Office of Science and Technology Policy, and organizations such as the Patient-Centered Outcomes Research Institute to inform their strategic planning.

The NAM also established a Working Group on Urgent Priorities for Science, Medicine, and Public Health After COVID-19, which delivered a letter detailing nine recommended actions to the White House Office of Science and Technology Policy in March 2021 (NAM, 2021l).

Pandemic Prevention, Preparedness, and Response

The COVID-19 pandemic lent a new urgency to the issue of global pandemic prevention, preparedness, and response. In January 2020, as a member of GPMB, Dzau had co-signed a statement recommending "urgent global action" in response to the COVID-19 outbreak and expressing grave concern that many countries were unprepared to respond to the virus—a concern that unfortunately proved justified (NAM, 2020i).

In 2021, Dzau arranged for the NAM to serve as Administrative Secretariat (alongside the Wellcome Trust) of a G20 High Level Independent Panel on Financing the Global Commons for Pandemic Preparedness and Response. The panel's report called for new international funding totaling $74 billion over 5 years to adequately prepare for the next global pandemic (G20, 2021a). "It is our obligation to prepare for future pandemics with a global mindset," Dzau said in a news release. "This report makes major requests of many countries, but we know that the financial impact of a future pandemic would be much greater than the investments the Panel has identified" (NAM, 2021e).[10]

In addition to these activities, with funding from the Office of Global Affairs in the Department of Health and Human Services (HHS), the NAM launched a fast-track initiative to enhance pandemic and seasonal influenza vaccine preparedness and response, drawing on lessons from the COVID-19 pandemic (NAM, n.d.g). The initiative acknowledged that a future influenza pandemic could be even more devastating than COVID-19, as demonstrated by the 1918 pandemic, which killed at least 50 million people worldwide (CDC, n.d.h). The NAM leveraged its International Commission model to explore the current state of the art and recommend improvements to influenza vaccine research and development; vaccine distribution and supply chains; public health interventions and countermeasures; and global coordination, partnerships, and financing. Four consensus studies and an overarching summary were published in November 2021. An overview of the series stated that "the world must learn from [the COVID-19 pandemic] to avoid circumstances similar to or worse than COVID-19, and to finally see preparedness as a muscle that we must strengthen, rather than neglect, during interpandemic times" (NAM, 2021f).

Epidemic of Clinician Burnout

Years before the COVID-19 pandemic, the issue of clinician well-being became a core focus area for the NAM and the subject of one of its inaugural programs. By 2016, a series of high-profile deaths by suicide of medical students and residents had highlighted a disturbing and growing trend among physicians and trainees (Bond, 2017). Yet, the problem went far beyond these groups, with

---

[10] On June 30, 2022, the World Bank approved a proposal to establish a Pandemic Prevention, Preparedness, and Response Financial Intermediary Fund (see https://www.worldbank.org/en/news/speech/2022/07/15/remarks-by-world-bank-group-president-david-malpass-to-g20-finance-ministers-and-central-bank-governors-on-the-global-ec).

serious impacts on clinicians of all types. The crisis of burnout touched every sector of health professional training and care systems, but evidence on prevalence, causes, and interventions was thin, and progress was hampered by lack of awareness. With encouragement from Nasca and Kirch, Dzau established the CWB Collaborative in January 2017.

The CWB Collaborative announced its intention to pursue three major goals within its initial term of 2 years (which would later be extended twice to 2022): (1) to raise the visibility of clinician anxiety, burnout, depression, stress, and suicide; (2) to improve the baseline understanding of challenges to clinician well-being; and (3) to advance evidence-based, multidisciplinary solutions to improve patient care by caring for the caregiver (NAM, n.d.b). More than 60 organizations signed on to the CWB Collaborative as inaugural sponsors, each designating a representative to participate in dynamic working groups on subjects including organizational culture, stigma, workload, technology, measurement, and more.

Among the CWB Collaborative's first outputs was a comprehensive conceptual model illustrating factors affecting clinician well-being and resilience (see Figure 7-3), which served as a blueprint for the program's strategic planning. In January 2018, the CWB Collaborative issued a call for formal commitments from organizations working to mitigate burnout at the systems level, receiving more than 200 public statements by mid-2021 (NAM, 2018a). The CWB Collaborative next launched a comprehensive online Knowledge Hub to compile and disseminate the evidence base on causes, effects, solutions, and measurement instruments for clinician burnout (NAM, n.d.h).

At the end of the CWB Collaborative's second year, its co-chairs began promoting the idea that an NAM consensus report could galvanize policy, organizational, and cultural change. Thirty-one sponsors signed on to support the new study, including universities, foundations, and health care organizations. The Board on Health Care Services within the National Academies' Health and Medicine Division (HMD) partnered with the NAM to administer the study. *Taking Action Against Clinician Burnout: A Systems Approach to Professional Well-Being* was published in October 2019

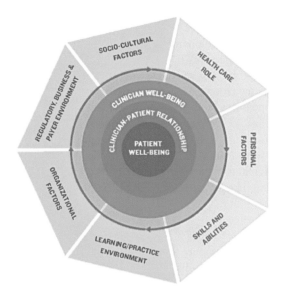

FIGURE 7-3 Conceptual model of factors affecting clinician well-being and resilience.
SOURCE: Brigham, T., C. Barden, A. L. Dopp, A. Hengerer, J. Kaplan, B. Malone, C. Martin, M. McHugh, and L. M. Nora. 2018. A Journey to Construct an All-Encompassing Conceptual Model of Factors Affecting Clinician Well-Being and Resilience. *NAM Perspectives*. Discussion Paper, National Academy of Medicine, Washington, DC. https://doi.org/10.31478/201801b.

and garnered immediate, widespread attention in the media. "Imagine a health-care system in which doctors and nurses are so exhausted and beaten down that many of them work like zombies—error-prone, apathetic toward patients and at times trying to blunt their own pain with alcohol or even suicide attempts," read a story in *The Washington Post.* "That is what America's broken health care system is doing to its health workers" (Wan, 2019).

Speaking on the occasion of the report's release, Dzau emphasized the link between physician burnout and patient safety. "Twenty years ago ... *To Err Is Human* and *Crossing the Quality Chasm* revealed a crisis in patient safety and led to a focus on quality that has revolutionized the U.S. health care system," he noted. "Today, the same type of transformative change is needed to support clinician well-being, which is linked inextricably to the quality of care" (NAM, 2019a).

To drive solutions, the study committee stressed the importance of collective, coordinated action across the entire health care system—with recommendations targeted at health care organizations, health professions educational institutions, policy makers, regulators, health information technology companies, clinician and patient organizations, standard-setting entities, and the research community. At a system level, the report called for actions to create positive work and learning environments, reduce administrative burden, enable technology solutions, support learners and clinicians by eliminating barriers to care, and investing in further research.

As noted earlier in this chapter, the COVID-19 pandemic became a galvanizing event for the CWB Collaborative in 2020. Excessive work hours, lack of personal protective equipment, and fear of infection at the height of the pandemic exacerbated the already high levels of burnout among U.S. clinicians (Dzau et al., 2020). In April 2020, Lorna Breen, a physician who supervised the emergency room at New York-Presbyterian Allen Hospital in New York City, died by suicide. She had contracted COVID-19 and become severely depressed as a result of what she perceived to be her inability to cope with the demands of responding to the pandemic (Knoll et al., 2020). Breen's death was headline news, and her family reached out to the CWB Collaborative for help in sharing her story and preventing other tragic deaths. In July 2020, the Dr. Lorna Breen Health Care Provider Protection Act was introduced in the U.S. Senate.[11] The bill sought to establish well-being programs for health workers, a national campaign to encourage workers to seek support and treatment, grants to support mental health services for workers caring for COVID-19 patients, and a federal study into the mental health of health workers (ACEP, 2020).

"We have the opportunity now to build a better health care system after COVID-19," Nasca noted in a press release announcing the program's extension until 2022. "If this pandemic refocuses us on our moral mission to provide care to others, it will have invigorated the profession as much as it has challenged it" (NAM, 2021a). In June 2021, as a signal of the national imperative to protect clinician well-being, 21st U.S. Surgeon General Vivek Murthy signed on as a co-chair of the CWB Collaborative. "I am hopeful about the Collaborative not only in developing a strategy to advance clinician well-being through and beyond COVID-19, but also in bringing policymakers, the private sector, and the public together around action on this priority. We can emerge even stronger than before the pandemic—for the sake of our clinicians and patients," Murthy said (NAM, 2021n).[12]

Murthy's role as a co-chair of the CWB Collaborative was an example of a novel approach to partnerships spearheaded by Dzau as part of the NAM's orientation toward collective action. By engaging leaders in the public and private sectors as substantive contributors to the NAM's work, Dzau achieved their early buy-in and paved the way for quick and efficient implementation

---

[11] The Dr. Lorna Breen Health Care Provider Protection Act (H.R. 1667) was signed into law on March 18, 2022 (see https://www.aha.org/news/news/2022-03-18-dr-lorna-breen-health-care-provider-protection-act-signed-law [accessed September 8, 2022]).

[12] In 2022, the NAM released a National Plan for Health Workforce Well-Being, which outlined specific actions to strengthen workers' well-being and ensure the health of the nation (see https://nam.edu/initiatives/clinician-resilience-and-well-being/national-plan-for-health-workforce-well-being [accessed September 8, 2022]).

of NAM-facilitated solutions. Other examples of this approach, described later in this chapter, included the role of U.S. Assistant Secretary for Health Rachel Levine in Action Collaboratives on the national opioid epidemic and climate change and the engagement of Johnson & Johnson as a partner in the Healthy Longevity Global Competition.

Building a Learning Health System: The National Academy of Medicine Leadership Consortium

The Leadership Consortium, established in 2006 as the IOM Roundtable on Value & Science-Driven Health Care, formed the backbone of the NAM's efforts to improve the U.S. health system (see Chapter 5 for more on the roundtable's work). Leadership Consortium founder J. Michael McGinnis, an NAM member who also served as the NAM's inaugural Leonard D. Schaeffer Executive Officer, established four Action Collaboratives around key foci for health system improvement: evidence mobilization; digital health; value incentives and systems; and culture, inclusion, and equity. With the engagement of field leaders from public and private sectors, these Action Collaboratives fostered dynamic networks for the sharing of best practices and alignment of goals.

In the years immediately following the IOM-NAM reorganization, the Leadership Consortium developed a number of defining Special Publications,[13] including the *Emerging Stronger from COVID-19* collection, described earlier in this chapter. Others focused on topics ranging from effective care for high-need patients, to artificial intelligence in health care, to innovative approaches to data sharing to improve patient care and advance the continuously learning health system. For example:

- *Effective Care for High-Need Patients: Opportunities for Improving Outcomes, Value, and Health* (Long et al., 2017) resulted from three public workshops that explored what is needed to better care for high-need patients (or the 1 percent of patients who accounted for more than 20 percent of existing health care expenditures) within the existing U.S. health care system, and how the health care system can adapt to more effectively and efficiently care for this patient population. The special publication outlined key characteristics of high-need patients, as there was no consistent definition of need prior to this publication; developed a patient taxonomy with associated implications for care delivery to better understand the subsets of high-need patients; explored existing care models that have effectively cared for high-need patients; and outlined policies that must be enacted or changed to allow for the spread and sustainability of these successful care models.
- *Procuring Interoperability: Achieving High-Quality, Connected, and Person-Centered Care* (Pronovost et al., 2018) contended that a major impediment to achieving true interoperability in the nation's health care system was the fragmented and disconnected purchasing of health technology, medical devices, and software applications within medical centers and between medical centers. Hardware that physically could not connect to other hardware stopped interoperability in its tracks—and as hardware was purchased infrequently and was often extremely expensive, further blocked progress in interoperability for years or even decades. This special publication reviewed requirements for interoperable data exchange at three levels: facility-to-facility, intra-facility, and at point-of-care, and outlined progress that could move U.S. health care to the envisioned future state of fully interoperable systems.
- *Artificial Intelligence in Health Care: The Hope, the Hype, the Promise, the Peril* (Matheny et al., 2022), the NAM's most downloaded special publication by 2022, reviewed opportunities to improve patient and team outcomes, reduce health care costs, and impact population health while reinforcing the need to proceed with caution in order to avoid exacerbat-

---

[13] NAM Special Publications are individually authored, peer-reviewed, report-length publications that summarize the state of knowledge on a subject and offer expert analysis and guidance.

ing existing health- and technology-driven disparities. It outlined current and near-term AI solutions; highlighted challenges, limitations, and best practices for AI development, adoption, and maintenance; offered an overview of the legal and regulatory landscape for AI tools designed for health care application; prioritized the need for equity, inclusion, and a human rights lens for this work; and outlined key considerations for moving forward.

- *Sharing Health Data: The Why, the Will, and the Way Forward* (Greene et al., 2021) spotlighted 11 novel data-sharing collaborations to dispel the myth that sharing health data broadly was impossible. The authors contend that sharing health data and information across stakeholders was the bedrock of a learning health system, and as these data were increasingly combined across various sources, their generative value to transform health, health care, and health equity increased significantly. The special publication showed how barriers were addressed and harvested lessons and insights from those on the front lines. The examples suggested how intentional attention to health data sharing could enable unparalleled advances, securing a healthier and more equitable future for all.

Following the COVID-19 pandemic, the Leadership Consortium turned its focus to building on the challenges and opportunities revealed by the crisis to build a more resilient, efficient, and equitable health care system for the future.

Vital Directions for Health and Health Care

Under the auspices of the Leadership Consortium, the NAM also prepared a package of formal advice on health and health care for incoming U.S. presidential administrations in 2017 and 2021. In another example of a novel program model for the NAM, phase one of the Vital Directions initiative commissioned a series of papers by more than 150 of the nation's leading experts to recommend actions for progress around 19 key priorities in support of 3 core goals: better health and well-being, high-value health care, and strong science and technology. The experts' guidance was published across a series of discussion papers in the *NAM Perspectives* periodical, as well as in a companion commentary series in the *Journal of the American Medical Association* and a 2017 NAM special publication titled *Vital Directions for Health and Health Care: Priorities from an NAM Initiative*. This volume defined a vision, core goals, action priorities, and infrastructure needs, and proposed "vital directions" for advancing health, health care, and biomedical sciences in the United States (NAM, 2017c). The complexity and magnitude of the problems called for strategic investment of existing resources and "vigorous leadership from every corner" and across all levels—organizational, local, state, and federal. Although the challenges were great, so were the opportunities. In addition to informing the incoming presidential administrations in 2017 and 2021 (*Health Affairs*, 2021) and exploring state-level policy opportunities in 2019 (NCMJ, 2020), the Vital Directions initiative set a framework for the NAM and its continuing activities.

Commitment to Racial and Health Equity

On May 25, 2020, George Floyd, an unarmed Black man, was suffocated by a police officer during the course of an arrest for a nonviolent crime in Minneapolis, MN (Hill et al., 2020). The murder set off a national reckoning with the violence, discrimination, and systemic racism experienced by Black people in the United States, as well as other people of color. As protests took place around the nation, Dzau published a statement that read, in part:

> I commit to ensuring that all people, and especially people of color, feel safe and supported while working at the NAM, as well as to pursuing racial equity in our organizational policies and procedures. I commit to using our platform to improve the lives of people who experience disproportion-

ate health disparities as a result of socioeconomic inequity, bias and structural racism. I commit to listening, learning, and working with all of you. (NAM, 2020d)

The NAM moved quickly to operationalize this commitment, appointing Ivory Clarke, director of the COHP, as its inaugural Equity and Inclusion Officer. Clarke, alongside NAM Director of Operations and Chief of Staff Morgan Kanarek, established a Staff Committee on Advancing Racial Equity (CARE) to strengthen internal equity, diversity, and inclusion. CARE's vision and mission were to promote a culture that challenged racism openly and honestly through education, training, and self-reflection; dismantle structures and systems that reinforced racial inequity in the NAM's operations; and foster a safe and supportive work environment. Dzau himself supplied a personal donation to enable every member of the NAM staff to contribute to the work of CARE.

Pre-existing CARE was the IOM (later HMD) Committee to Enhance Diversity and Conclusion (CEDI), which launched in 2014 with annual support from Dzau. CEDI was a volunteer staff committee (led by HMD but open to staff from the IOM/NAM) that hosted staff engagement activities and generated strategies for enhancing diversity and inclusion in the organization's culture and processes. In April 2021, the National Academies hired its first Chief Diversity and Inclusion Officer, Laura Castillo-Page, who was tasked with leading the development of an overall diversity, equity, and inclusion strategy for the organization, including advancing diversity among staff, volunteers, and Academy members.

The sharpened focus on racial equity that began in 2020 augmented the NAM's longtime emphasis on health equity. In 2016, the NAM had added "health equity" as a key value in its new mission statement: *To improve health for all by advancing science, accelerating health equity, and providing independent, authoritative, and trusted advice nationally and globally.* "'Health for all'—the notion of combating health disparities—is built into this statement, as well as the notion that we want to improve health not just domestically, but also globally," Dzau said in his annual address to the NAM membership. "We believe that health equity is a foundational value and an important goal, and decided to call it out specifically in our mission statement" (NAM, 2016c). Acknowledging racism and lack of diverse representation in science and medicine as major drivers of health inequities, the NAM also advanced its work on racial and health equity through the COHP, as well as through membership diversification activities (both described later in this chapter).

Culture of Health Program

The COHP was established in 2015 through a $10 million grant from the Robert Wood Johnson Foundation (RWJF) to develop a program that would advance health equity by strengthening the evidence base around social determinants of health. Half of the grant was allocated for program activities over 5 years, while half was directed to the NAM's endowment. "To build a Culture of Health in America, we must find partners capable of providing rigorous, effective, and inclusive programming that addresses our nation's significant gaps in health equity," said Risa J. Lavizzo-Mourey, an NAM member and RWJF president at the time. "This investment will help us to identify organizations and communities that are ready to achieve positive change at a scale that will enable all to live healthier lives, regardless of who they are or where they live."[14]

The COHP established four goals to guide its work: (1) to lead by issuing a series of consensus studies that strengthen the evidence base and bolster efforts to advance health equity; (2) to translate that evidence by facilitating action and implementation; (3) to strengthen capacity in communities; and (4) to sustain progress by fostering a culture that prioritizes health equity. By 2019, the program had produced four consensus studies, in collaboration with HMD, that served as the

---

[14] See https://sites.nationalacademies.org/giving/noteworthynews/index.htm.

foundation for its efforts: *Communities in Action: Pathways to Health Equity* (NASEM, 2017o); *The Promise of Adolescence: Realizing Opportunity for All Youth* (NASEM, 2019f); *Vibrant and Healthy Kids: Aligning Science, Practice, and Policy to Advance Health Equity* (NASEM, 2019d); and *Integrating Social Care into the Delivery of Health Care: Moving Upstream to Improve the Nation's Health* (NASEM, 2019m).

The COHP also developed a network of diverse community organizations to foster uptake of principles from the Communities in Action report. Over the course of the program's first 5 years, NAM staff built strong relationships with these organizations, conducting site visits and convening representatives twice per year in Washington, DC. The COHP utilized insights from the communities' observations and efforts to advance health equity in their own environments and worked closely with each organization to develop "community-driven health equity action plans." The NAM published the communities' plans in 2020 (NAM, n.d.i).

The COHP's goals to translate science and sustain culture change meant the program invested significantly in innovative communications. To engage audiences at the community level and approach the value of health equity from a cultural, rather than academic, lens, program staff invited submissions for a national art show called "Visualize Health Equity" (see Figure 7-4). The project asked people around the country to illustrate, through any media, what health equity looked, felt, and sounded like to them. The show debuted with a pop-up gallery and reception at NAM headquarters and later became a 6-month installation. The NAM also launched a permanent digital gallery and a traveling version of the show that was booked by organizations year-round. Building on the success of this activity, and to align with the COHP consensus reports focused on the health of children and adolescents, the NAM later debuted "Young Leaders Visualize Health Equity," which was limited to submissions from people ages 5 to 26.

In March 2021, the NAM announced that the COHP would be extended until 2024. "This is a critical moment for our nation to confront racist systems and policies in order to ensure that every-

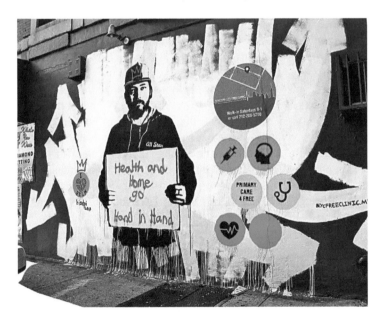

FIGURE 7-4 "Picture of Health" by John Colavito from New York, New York, was part of the NAM's Culture of Health Program's Visualize Health Equity series calling for artists from across the nation to illustrate what health equity looks, sounds, and feels like to them.
SOURCE: Copyright John Colavito.

one in America has a fair and just opportunity for health and well-being. This requires intentionally dismantling discriminatory barriers, including structural racism, because of their negative impacts on the health of people and communities," said Richard Besser, then President and Chief Executive Officer of the RWJF, in a press release announcing the extension (NAM, 2021c).

The U.S. Opioid Epidemic

Another crisis that was exacerbated by the COVID-19 pandemic was the crisis of opioid use disorder in the United States, which became the topic of an NAM Action Collaborative established in 2018. The statistics at the time were alarming. In 2016, 65,000 Americans died from a drug overdose, with nearly two-thirds of recent drug deaths attributed to the misuse of opioids. Half the deaths were related not to drugs bought illegally but rather to drugs obtained by prescription. Nearly two dozen opioid medications were on the market, most used for the treatment of pain. In 2015, about one-third of American adults used prescribed opioids at one time or another, and 2.5 million struggled with opioid-related disorders. Patients with an opioid addiction filled up the emergency departments of hospitals but had trouble gaining access to additional treatment. Opioid addiction surpassed HIV infections and automobile fatalities as a public health problem (NAM, 2017b). The resulting spike in death rates among people ages 25 to 54 contributed, at least in part, to a decrease in life expectancy among middle-aged white men and women in the United States (NAM, 2017b).

Countless community organizations, law enforcement entities, health care organizations, faith communities, researchers, government bodies, and nonprofits dedicated resources to respond to the crisis, but rates of opioid misuse and overdose continued to skyrocket. The NAM recognized the need for a national body to coordinate the response and concentrate efforts around a few key priorities. In July 2018, the NAM announced its intention to form an Action Collaborative on Countering the U.S. Opioid Epidemic (Opioid Collaborative) in partnership with the nonprofit Aspen Institute. "So many organizations are working around the clock to reverse the opioid epidemic, yet progress has been slow," Dzau said in a statement. "The problem is clearly not absence of will, but insufficient alignment and coordination across sectors. The complex drivers of the opioid epidemic make it impossible for any single organization or professional sector to make a significant impact on its own" (NAM, 2018b). By 2021, the Opioid Collaborative had more than 55 participating sponsors and an additional 100 organizations contributing as "network" organizations committed to advancing the goals of the program. Like the CWB Collaborative, the Opioid Collaborative called for and publicly posted statements of commitment from supporting organizations (NAM, 2019b). The program acted as a "one of a kind public-private partnership … to build collective solutions and accelerate the pace of progress" (NAM, 2018b). Members of the collaborative concentrated on four different aspects of the crisis: health professional education and training; pain management guidelines and evidence standards; prevention, treatment, and recovery services; and research, data, and metrics needs.

In early 2021, more than 1 year into the COVID-19 pandemic, there were worrying indications that the U.S. opioid crisis was worsening, with possible drivers including barriers to treatment and the mental health impacts of the pandemic. An analysis by The Commonwealth Fund found that opioid use–related deaths may have exceeded 90,000 in 2020, making it the deadliest of the past 20 years (Baumgartner and Radley, 2021; NCHS, 2020). In April 2021, the Opioid Collaborative announced an extension of its work for another 2 years.

Standing Up for Science

As another indication of the NAM's more proactive strategic orientation, Dzau (as well as other NAM/National Academies leaders) become more vocal in commenting on events and policies with significant impacts on health and where the scientific evidence base offered clear direction. In the years following the IOM-NAM transition, many NAM members believed that respect for the scientific process—by necessity objective and apolitical—was eroding to a dangerous degree. Between 2017 and 2020, at the urging of members, Dzau used the NAM platform to speak out publicly in defense of science more than ever before.

For example, in March 2017, President Donald J. Trump signed an Executive Order preventing citizens of the Muslim-majority countries Iran, Libya, Somalia, Sudan, Syria, and Yemen from entering the United States for a period of 90 days (Siddiqui et al., 2017). In May, the Department of State followed up with a new proposed rule (Department of State, 2017) that would add arduous additional questions to certain foreign visa applications as part of an "extreme vetting" approach promised by President Trump during his campaign (Shear, 2017). Dzau, NAS President Marcia McNutt, and National Academy of Engineering (NAE) President Dan Mote[15] wrote a public letter to the Department of State expressing concern that limiting entry to the United States from certain countries "will have significant negative unintended consequences on the nation's international leadership in research, innovation, and education." The presidents further noted that international collaboration is critical to the advancement of science and that approximately one-quarter of NAM, NAS, and NAE members were born outside the United States (NASEM, 2017m).

In another example, on April 14, 2020, President Trump announced a freeze on funding to the WHO as a reaction to what he characterized as "severely mismanaging and covering up the spread of coronavirus" (Klein and Hansler, 2020). The following day, Dzau expressed his strong disagreement with the decision in a letter to members: "The WHO's work is essential, not only to fight the COVID-19 pandemic, but also to support public health, global development, and international cooperation at all times. To put it bluntly, defunding the WHO will cut off a lifeline for low- and middle-income countries and place hundreds of millions of people at risk."[16] At the urging of Dzau, the NAM, the NAS, and the NAE presidents issued a public statement in support of the WHO the same day (NASEM, 2020d). However, about 6 weeks later, President Trump announced the formal termination of U.S. participation in the WHO (BBC, 2020). The stalemate would last until Joseph Biden took office in January 2021.

Tensions continued, and in September 2020 President Trump suggested that he would oppose the FDA's proposal to enhance approval standards for the emergency use of vaccines against COVID-19. At the urging of NAM and NAS members, Dzau and McNutt went public with a strongly worded statement that read, in part:

> We find ongoing reports and incidents of the politicization of science, particularly the overriding of evidence and advice from public health officials and derision of government scientists, to be alarming. It undermines the credibility of public health agencies and the public's confidence in them when we need it most. Ending the pandemic will require decision-making that is not only based on science but also sufficiently transparent to ensure public trust in, and adherence to, sound public-health instructions. Any efforts to discredit the best science and scientists threaten the health and welfare of us all. (NASEM, 2020e)

The statement, unusually bold coming from an organization accustomed to standing back from the political fray, garnered significant pickup by national media, as well as gratitude and support from the scientific community.

DIVERSIFYING AND ACTIVATING MEMBERS AND ENGAGING EMERGING LEADERS (STRATEGIC GOAL 2)

"Members are the lifeblood of our Academy; without their expert guidance and leadership, our advisory initiatives would not be possible," Dzau wrote in the NAM's 2018 Annual Report (NAM,

---

[15] Mote's term as NAE president ended in June 2019. He was succeeded by John Anderson.

[16] Victor Dzau, "Personal Letter to Members Expressing Support for the WHO," April 15, 2020, IOM/NAM Records.

2018c). As called for in the second overarching goal of the NAM's strategic plan, promoting the engagement and diversity of the membership—in terms of specialty, race, ethnicity, gender, age, and geography—was an early organizational priority, as was the imperative to engage members in the organization's governance.

Member Diversification Initiatives

In 2019, the NAM established a standing membership diversity committee to make recommendations to the NAM Council, monitor progress, and ensure accountability. Members also agreed to a change in the bylaws that would enable the election of 100 new members annually, a 25 percent increase over previous years. In 2020, the NAM elected its most diverse class of members ever in terms of representation of underrepresented minority groups (35 percent) and age (30 percent under age 50). Although proud of these numbers, Dzau acknowledged that "We know that the change we're seeking won't happen overnight and that this will be a continuous journey. But we are committed to advancing diversity, equity, and inclusion in our work, and within our own institution" (NAM, 2020a). The following year, the NAM again broke its record, electing a historical majority of women (52 percent), and the largest ever proportion of underrepresented minority groups (47 percent).[17]

A New Role in Governance

In 2019, members voted for the first time to elect new Officers among the NAM's leadership. Prior to the IOM's reconstitution as the NAM in 2015, IOM Officers were officially appointed by the NAS president (see Chapter 2 for more information about Officers). As an independent Academy, members had the power to elect their own leadership—one of the hallmarks of the new organization.

When Jane Henney completed her first term as Home Secretary (2014–2018), she pursued and won election for a second term, officially becoming the NAM's first elected Officer. Carlos del Rio followed in 2020 as the NAM's first elected International Secretary, and Dzau was elected for a second term as NAM President. "I am truly honored to be elected to a second term and have the privilege of continuing to lead this eminent organization in this new decade, especially on the 50th anniversary of our founding," said Dzau in a press release announcing his election (NAM, 2020g).

NAM members' active role in governance went beyond the election of Officers. Members voted in 2019 to establish a Code of Conduct with clear policies and procedures to hold members accountable to a high standard of personal and professional behavior. "The credibility of the advice from the NAM rests on its reputation and integrity, which depends on the reputation and integrity of its members," the code read (NAM, 2018d). The code prohibited unlawful behavior, prejudicial treatment, harassment, scientific misconduct, professional dishonesty, and concealment of conflict of interest, among other principles. For the first time, the code afforded the NAM a mechanism to take action against members who violated a specific set of principles for ethical behavior.

NAM Member Response to COVID-19

As well as contributing as volunteers to support the NAM's programmatic response to COVID-19, Academy members were on the front lines of the pandemic, driving solutions within their own fields, from laboratory research to clinical care and from national public health leadership to community advocacy. In November 2020, six NAM members were named to President-Elect

---

[17] IOM/NAM Records.

Joseph Biden's COVID-19 task force, including David Kessler (Co-Chair), Ezekiel Emanuel, Atul Gawande, Eric Goosby, and Michael Osterholm (AP, 2020). Several more took on permanent roles in the new administration.

In another prominent example, 60 Black members of the NAM (led by Georges Benjamin and Thomas LaVeist) authored a *New York Times* op-ed encouraging Black Americans to receive the COVID-19 vaccine. "We feel compelled to make the case that all Black Americans should get vaccinated to protect themselves from a pandemic that has disproportionately killed them at a rate 1.5 times as high as white Americans," they wrote in March 2021 (LaVeist and Benjamin, 2021). The op-ed was accompanied by a video for distribution on social media channels (The Skin You're In, 2021). Later that year, more than 20 Latinx NAM members signed a letter "affirming their confidence in the vaccine and urging their community to recognize the debilitating risks of the virus that is 2.3 times as deadly to the Latinx/Latino(a)/Hispanic community as it is to their White peers" (NAM, 2021h,i). The letter was presented alongside video messages in English and Spanish, as well as resources to help people book and obtain transportation to vaccine appointments (NAM, 2021j,k).

Emerging Leaders in Health and Medicine

In addition to cultivating its existing membership, the NAM also devoted attention to building the next generation of health and medical leaders—the potential members of tomorrow. The Emerging Leaders in Health and Medicine Program (ELHMP), established in 2016, engaged "exceptional early- to mid-career professionals in health and medicine, NAM leaders and members, and other experts to promote interdisciplinary collaboration and spark new ways of thinking about shared challenges that could lead to transformative change" (NAM, 2019c). New classes of ELHMP Scholars were appointed annually to 3-year terms by the NAM Council and assigned NAM member mentors. The Scholars also organized an annual Emerging Leaders Forum to discuss priority issues with their peers. The ELHMP complemented the NAM's seven fellowship programs as of 2021 (described in Chapter 2).

BUILDING LEADERSHIP CAPACITY ACROSS DIVERSE DISCIPLINES (STRATEGIC GOAL 3)

The third major goal of the NAM's strategic plan called for it to forge new ground by building leadership capacity in emerging areas—in terms of human capital, policy and infrastructure, and financial investment. Between 2015 and 2021, the NAM established innovative, cross-sectoral programs in developing areas including healthy longevity; climate change, human health, and equity; emerging science and technology; health misinformation; and global mental health.

Healthy Longevity Global Grand Challenge

In the face of rapidly aging populations worldwide, the race to prepare health care and social systems became the subject of the NAM's inaugural Grand Challenge program. When the Healthy Longevity Global Grand Challenge (HLGGC) launched in 2019 (see Figure 7-5), it was projected that by 2030, the population of adults over age 65 would outnumber children under age 18 (U.S. Census Bureau, 2018). This shift presented significant hurdles across health, social, and economic sectors, but also constituted an opportunity to accelerate research, innovation, and entrepreneurism in the new field of healthy longevity.

To tackle this mammoth challenge, the NAM combined the International Commission program model with a novel approach—a global prize competition. An International Commission was appointed to author a Global Roadmap for Healthy Longevity report assessing challenges and opportunities in three domains: social, behavioral, and environmental enablers; health care

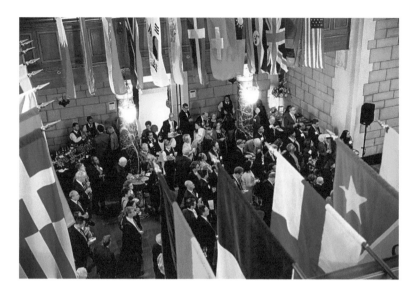

FIGURE 7-5 The launch event for the NAM Healthy Longevity Global Grand Challenge at the National Academy of Sciences Building in Washington, DC.
SOURCE: National Academy of Medicine.

systems and public health; and science and technology. The report, due for publication in early 2022, would also recommend short-term actions for global societies to capitalize on the benefits of a longer health span.

The Healthy Longevity Global Competition was launched to complement the International Commission's work by fomenting worldwide research and innovation through a series of monetary prizes and awards. The competition model was uncharted territory for the NAM—an attempt to jumpstart an under-resourced field. Dzau said,

> The global competition model is uniquely capable of activating innovation and stimulating break-throughs. It can energize thousands of scientists, innovators, and entrepreneurs globally to focus on a challenge in a concentrated timespan and generate a wide variety of bold ideas across many disciplines. This wellspring of activity will build momentum around healthy longevity, create new markets, and ultimately lead to transformative innovations that will impact the lives of generations. (NAM, 2019d)

The competition netted more than $30 million in commitments from sponsors and global collaborators by 2020.

The competition was designed to unfold in three phases. In the first phase (2020 to 2022), Healthy Longevity Catalyst Awards worth $50,000 USD each would be issued in recognition of an innovative idea capable of extending the human health span globally and equitably. Eight international organizations initially joined the NAM in issuing Catalyst Awards for the 2020 cycle: Academia Sinica of Taiwan, the Ministry of Health and National Research Foundation of Singapore, the Chinese Academy of Medical Sciences, UK Research and Innovation, EIT Health of the European Union, the Japan Agency for Medical Research and Development, and the U.S. National Institute on Aging.[18] In 2021, three more organizations joined the competition—Chile Agencia Nacional de Investigación y Desarrollo and the Chinese University of Hong Kong and The University of Hong Kong (acting together)—bringing the total of countries and regions represented to more than 50.

---

[18] The National Institute on Aging participated during only 2020.

In October 2020, the NAM announced more than 150 global Catalyst Award winners, totaling more than $7.7 million in prizes. Twenty-four U.S.-based winners received prizes directly from the NAM for ideas including an app to detect early signs of Parkinson's disease, a deep learning tool to predict biological age from chest radiographs, and software to allow older adults to inhabit avatars of their younger selves (NAM, 2020e).

The second phase of the competition, the Accelerator Phase (which began in 2021), was designed to provide resources, including infrastructure and mentorship, to advance promising ideas that have demonstrated progress and achieved proof of concept. The second cycle of the Catalyst Award competition kicked off in January 2021, and an inaugural Innovator Summit for winners took place in Fall 2021. In the third phase, projected for 2023 or later, one or more grand prizes were projected to be awarded to breakthrough innovations that extend the human healthspan.

Climate Change, Human Health, and Equity

At the NAM's 50th Annual Meeting on October 19, 2020, Dzau announced the NAM's next grand challenge—Climate Change, Human Health, and Equity. At the time, the Intergovernmental Panel on Climate Change predicted that temperatures were on a trajectory to increase from 2.5 to as much as 10 degrees Fahrenheit by the end of the 21st century (NAM, 2020a). In addition to the COVID-19 pandemic, 2020 had been plagued by unusually severe weather events, including a record number of tropical storms making landfall in the United States and devastating wildfires in California and Colorado (NOAA, 2021). However, "extreme events aren't the only threats," Dzau noted in his annual President's Address:

> Climate change will have adverse consequences for livelihoods, public health, food security, and water availability. This in turn will impact human mobility, likely leading to an even greater rise in the scale of migration and displacement. Negative impacts on food production will further contribute to social and political instability. And all of these effects disproportionately fall on the most vulnerable: low-income communities, people of color, young children, and the chronically ill. (NAM, 2020a)

To plan the Grand Challenge on Climate Change, Human Health, and Equity, the NAM assembled a 30-member international, multi-sectoral committee, co-chaired by NAM members Judith Rodin[19] and Philip Pizzo.[20] Modeled in large part on the HLGGC, the Grand Challenge on Climate Change and Human Health was designed around four objectives:

1. Communicate the climate crisis as a public health and equity crisis
2. Develop a roadmap for systems transformation
3. Catalyze the health sector to reduce its climate footprint and ensure its resilience
4. Accelerate research and innovation at the intersection of climate, health, and equity (NAM, n.d.m)

In September 2021, as part of the climate grand challenge, the NAM launched an Action Collaborative on Decarbonizing the U.S. Health Sector. The press release noted that

> the health sector is responsible for approximately 8.5% of U.S. carbon emissions, a leading cause of climate change. The harmful effects of climate change are not distributed equally, but are experienced disproportionally by communities that have been historically and persistently marginalized and disenfranchised—in particular Black, Indigenous, and people of color—who also face the greatest barriers to accessing and receiving quality care. Reducing the carbon footprint of the

---

[19] Judith Rodin was affiliated with the University of Pennsylvania at this time.
[20] Philip Pizzo was affiliated with Stanford University at this time.

entire health care sector will benefit society and the economy, as well as advance health equity. (NAM, 2021m)

The Action Collaborative was co-chaired by Dzau, Rachel Levine (Assistant Secretary for Health, Department of Health and Human Services); George Barrett (former Chair and Chief Executive Officer, Cardinal Health); and Andrew Witty (Chief Executive Officer, UnitedHealth Group). The program had four initial workstreams: (1) health care supply chain and infrastructure; (2) health care delivery; (3) health professional education and communication; and (4) policy, financing, and metrics. A primary goal of the Action Collaborative was to achieve collective commitment to carbon reduction goals consistent with those recommended by the U.S. government (50–52 percent reduction from 2005 levels by 2030 (The White House, 2021b).

Emerging Science and Technology

Building on the global impact of its Human Gene Editing Initiative (described in Chapter 4), the NAM established the Committee on Emerging Science, Technology, and Innovation in Health and Medicine (CESTI) in 2020 to consider not only the positive but also the potentially negative implications of developments in biomedical science and technology. The committee sought to identify emerging developments in biological and medical research and technology and attendant social, ethical, regulatory, and workforce impacts and develop an approach to anticipating the impact of these developments. CESTI undertook case studies on noninvasive neurotechnology, telehealth, and regenerative medicine. To build on this work, the NAM announced the launch of a consensus study, *Creating a Framework for Emerging Science, Technology, and Innovation in Health and Medicine* (chaired by NAM members Keith Wailoo of Princeton University and Keith Yamamoto of the University of California, San Francisco). The study committee, whose report was due to be completed in Spring 2023, set out to "develop a cross-sectoral coordinated governance framework founded upon core ethical principles with a focus on equity, for considering the potential benefits and risks that emerging science, technology, and innovation in health and medicine can bring to society" (NASEM, n.d.b1). Following the release of the study, the NAM planned to launch an Action Collaborative that would facilitate implementation of the framework.

Health Misinformation

As a final example of an area in which greater leadership and focus was needed, the NAM launched an initiative to identify credible sources of health information in social media. False information spread through social media during the COVID-19 pandemic had helped to fuel negative health impacts including hampered uptake of COVID-19 vaccines (Kington et al., 2021). The NAM assembled an advisory committee chaired by NAM member Raynard Kington, former principal deputy director of the NIH. The committee authored a paper that laid out three key principles and associated material attributes that could help to identify credible sources of health information in social and other digital media. In late 2021, the WHO held a meeting of international public health experts to assess the applicability of the principles and attributes to global contexts. As summarized in the meeting report, attendees affirmed the broad applicability of the NAM paper, and the WHO began to promote use of the principles and attributes by members of its "Tech Task Force" (a group of social/digital media companies including Meta, TikTok, YouTube, and Amazon) (WHO, 2022).

CONCLUSION

The NAM's first 6 years became a defining new era for the organization. It successfully defined a unique role and innovative programmatic approach within the National Academies that leveraged public–private partnerships and novel program models such as the International Commission, Action Collaborative, and Grand Challenge. These approaches leveraged the NAM's greater degree of independence and flexibility as an Academy alongside the NAS and the NAE and were quickly adopted by program units across the broader organization. Yet, the NAM remained true to its roots by maintaining a steadfast commitment to scientific rigor and evidence-based advice, drawing often on the resources and time-tested processes of NRC program divisions such as the HMD.

Well before the conclusion of its first decade, the NAM developed a national and international reputation for impact in the areas of pandemic preparedness, clinician well-being, human gene editing, the U.S. opioid epidemic, the learning health system, health equity, healthy longevity, and climate change, among others. Amid its explosive program growth, the NAM also focused on enriching its membership through initiatives to increase its diversity and strengthen its role in governance. By early 2022, as it launched the second phase of its strategic planning, the NAM had come a long way from the uncertainty of the IOM-NAM transition.

8

Conclusion

At the beginning of 2020, just as the National Academy of Medicine (NAM) was preparing for a year-long commemoration of the half-century since its founding as the Institute of Medicine (IOM), a rapidly developing global crisis posed the greatest challenge to the institution in its history. In January, officials in the United States and other countries became aware that a new respiratory virus, SARS-CoV-2, was spreading in China. By the time of the first reported U.S. case, on January 20, and the first reported U.S. death, on February 6, the disease, later named COVID-19, was already spreading rapidly in the United States and many other countries. Over the course of the year, infection rates and fatalities skyrocketed as policy makers struggled to mount effective public health responses and scientists worked to understand how the disease could be treated and prevented. By the end of 2021, more than 5 million people around the world had died as a result of the virus (JHU, n.d.).

The COVID-19 pandemic revealed the flaws in the health system that the IOM/NAM had highlighted throughout its first five decades. The public health response was inadequate in key respects and poorly coordinated. Groups already experiencing health inequities—including Black, Indigenous, and people of color (BIPOC)—suffered much higher levels of infection and death. The U.S. health care system was severely strained in providing critical care for so many desperately ill patients. The global response lacked coordination and failed to adequately protect poorer nations.

The COVID-19 pandemic also revealed the tremendous potential of science and medicine to meet formidable challenges. Researchers from all over the world set aside their individual interests to understand the virus and rapidly develop diagnostics, therapeutics, and vaccines. Better understanding of how the virus was transmitted led to increasingly effective public health measures. Chinese health authorities and the WHO announced the discovery of SARS-CoV-2 on January 9, 2020; just 2 days later, full genomic sequence of the virus was posted online (Institut Pasteur, 2020). Within 69 days of the virus's discovery, the first vaccine candidate entered a clinical trial (Kim et al., 2020). By the end of 2020, two new vaccines, based on revolutionary mRNA technology, had been authorized for emergency use in the United States and other countries. In 2021, death rates in the United States and other countries began to fall, although virus variants and uneven adherence to public health measures led to new spikes in infection. By the end of the year, it was clear that COVID-19 would remain a pressing and uncertain threat indefinitely.

The year 2020 was notable for other reasons. The killing of George Floyd triggered worldwide protests against the centuries of systemic and structural racism experienced by Black Americans and other people of color. At the same time, heatwaves, wildfires, hurricanes, droughts, rising sea levels, floods, and other extreme events highlighted the ongoing crisis of climate change. All three of these global traumas—the COVID-19 pandemic, systemic racism, and climate change—disproportionately affected the most vulnerable people, including low-income communities, BIPOC, children, and the chronically ill. These challenges came at a moment when mistrust in science, fueled by a fraught political environment in the United States, appeared to be at an all-time high.

BOX 8-1
Selected Major Areas of Impact from Institute of Medicine
and National Academy of Medicine Work

Improving safety in health care

Supporting and promoting the role of nurses in health care

Ensuring that medicines are safe, effective, affordable, and accessible

Preventing violence

Providing opportunities for early-career professionals

Advancing embryonic stem cell research

Promoting health equity

Reducing tobacco use

Promoting women's health

Advancing precision medicine

Protecting the health of pregnant people

Advancing healthy longevity

Guiding human genome editing technologies

Mapping the intersection of environment and health

Improving care and coverage for veterans and members of the military

Preventing the spread of infectious disease and responding to infectious disease emergencies

Guiding organ transplantation policy and practice

Advancing care for serious illness

Preventing injury

Advancing cancer biology, prevention, and treatment

Supporting all members of the health care team

Promoting the health of LGBTQIA+ individuals

Advising science policy in the U.S. government

Advancing disaster preparedness and response

Promoting mental health

Protecting the health of children and families

Designing a continuously learning health care system

Building a robust health care workforce

Addressing disability as a public health concern

Promoting U.S. leadership and investment in global health

Advancing vaccine science and policy

Advancing the field of population health

Elevating the challenge of clinician burnout as a patient safety issue

Improving care and policy for substance use disorders

Addressing obesity across the lifespan

Improving the diet and eating habits of Americans

Improving care for older adults

Promoting health literacy

Informing U.S. health care reform movements

Improving end-of-life care

Advancing health information technology

Revealing the scale of waste in U.S. health care spending

Improving education and training for health care providers

Guiding Medicare implementation and expansion

Defining and advancing the field of public health

Advancing understanding of neurobiological development

Catalyzing the public health response to the AIDS epidemic

Facilitating reintegration of veterans into civilian life

Highlighting disparities in health care

Improving the quality of cancer care and treatment

The NAM and its members mounted a broad and aggressive response across all these fronts, leveraging its influence as an impartial, trusted, and authoritative advisor, as well as its ability to convene leading experts and facilitate their implementation of scientific, medical, public health, and policy solutions. Plans for the IOM/NAM anniversary celebration, including this history volume, were largely deferred to 2022 or later. Yet, in many ways, the 50th anniversary year unfolded as a testament to the NAM's historical influence as well as a window into the impact it could have in the future—exactly the themes the Academy had hoped to emphasize in its commemorative activities.

The "tagline" the NAM selected for its anniversary celebrations captured this dual focus: "Celebrating a legacy of impact. Forging a healthier future" (NAM, n.d.j). A survey of the IOM/NAM's major historical impacts (see Box 8-1) showed that it played an influential role in many major U.S. and global health policy developments—from the expansion of Medicare to the quality and patient safety movement to the application of the Patient Protection and Affordable Care Act. As major advances in science and technology led to unimagined progress in understanding and treatment of diseases such as cancer and HIV/AIDS, the IOM/NAM was a steady and trusted advisor to researchers, regulators, and providers—ensuring the safe and appropriate application of breakthroughs. The IOM/NAM advanced the field of population health, building the evidence base for foundational concepts including the social determinants of health, disparities in health and health care, and strategies to advance health equity. And, despite its original mandate as an advisor to the nation, the IOM/NAM built a strong body of work globally, helping to ensure the U.S. government's ongoing investment in global health, securing the future of important international programs such as PEPFAR and leading global efforts in pandemic preparedness and response.

The upheaval of 2020–2021 brought the IOM/NAM's historic mission into sharp relief. The world was confronted with what Dzau described as the triple "existential threats" of pandemics, climate change, and systemic racism. In each of these crises, there was a role for the NAM to advance evidence-based solutions and spur action among stakeholders across sectors. The organization's impact in the future would rely on both its longtime reputation as a trusted, nonpartisan advisor and its innovative and proactive approach as an Academy. In his 2020 annual address to NAM members, Dzau said it best:

> As individuals, and as the NAM, now is the time for us to lead—and to act. Together we can reverse course on decades of woefully insufficient action and investments in our public health systems and national and global emergency preparedness. This year can mark a new beginning in reckoning with our shameful legacy of systemic racism and structural inequality. And this can be the year that we begin to reverse years of neglect and inaction on climate change.
>
> Health and medicine are at the intersection of every one of these crises. I know that you, like me, firmly believe that science and medicine offer solutions that can save lives, reduce inequity, and create a better nation and world for generations to come. (NAM, 2020a)

Epilogue

Although the scope of this volume concludes with 2021, the following year brought ongoing major sociopolitical and health challenges. In February 2022, Russia invaded Ukraine, causing the displacement of millions of people, destruction of health care facilities, and long-term public health consequences for the region. The National Academy of Medicine (NAM) and the National Academies of Sciences, Engineering, and Medicine (the National Academies) rallied to provide support, including public statements (e.g., NAM, 2022a; NASEM, 2022a), programs to relocate Ukrainian scientists and rebuild the Ukrainian research system (NASEM, 2022c,d), and efforts to protect and support health care workers (NAM, 2022d; NASEM, 2022b).

Meanwhile, in the United States, two particularly grievous mass shooting incidents in Buffalo, New York, and Uvalde, Texas, in spring 2022 reinvigorated public health attention to preventing gun violence. NAM President Victor Dzau called for urgent action by the public health and science communities and assembled a Task Force of NAM members to recommend actions for the NAM and the National Academies to undertake (NAM, 2022b).

In June 2022, the U.S. Supreme Court announced its decision to overturn the 1973 *Roe v. Wade* decision, threatening access to safe abortion care for millions of women across the United States, particularly women of color, poor women, and women living in rural areas. Dzau and National Academy of Sciences President Marcia McNutt spoke out against the decision, highlighting its detrimental impact on women's health (NAM, 2022c). The NAM and the National Academies began scoping a research agenda to comprehensively map the health impacts of the reversal as well as other activities to advise health workers, patients, and policy makers in the wake of the decision.

Bibliography

ACEP (American College of Emergency Physicians). 2020. ACEP Applauds Introduction of Dr. Lorna Breen Health Care Provider Protection Act. https://www.emergencyphysicians.org/press-releases/2020/7-29-20-acep-applauds-introduction-of-dr.-lorna-breen-health-care-provider-protection-act (accessed July 5, 2022).

ACGME (Accreditation Council on Graduate Medical Education). 2021. ACGME Common Program Requirements (Residency). https://www.acgme.org/globalassets/PFAssets/ProgramRequirements/CPRResidency2021.pdf (accessed December 30, 2021).

ACP (American College of Physicians). 2008. Internal Medicine Organization Issues Guidelines to Improve Care of 3 Symptoms at End of Life. https://www.eurekalert.org/news-releases/893792 (accessed August 7, 2022).

AHRQ (Agency for Healthcare Research and Quality). 2015. Efforts to Improve Patient Safety Result in 1.3 Million Fewer Patient Harms. Rockville, MD: Agency for Healthcare Research and Quality. https://www.ahrq.gov/hai/pfp/interimhacrate2013.html (accessed July 5, 2021).

AHRQ. n.d. Patient Safety and Quality Improvement Act of 2005. https://www.ahrq.gov/policymakers/psoact.html (accessed July 5, 2021).

Aizenman, N. 2019. How to Demand a Medical Breakthrough: Lessons from the AIDS Fight. *NPR*, February 19. https://www.npr.org/sections/health-shots/2019/02/09/689924838/how-to-demand-a-medical-breakthrough-lessons-from-the-aids-fight (accessed June 29, 2021).

Altman, L. 1992. Surveillance of Diseases Is Deficient, Report Says. *The New York Times*, October 17, 14.

Altman, L. K. 2003. F.C. Robbins, Virus Researcher, Dies at 86. *The New York Times*, August 5. https://www.nytimes.com/2003/08/05/us/f-c-robbins-virus-researcher-dies-at-86.html (accessed July 30, 2021).

Altman, L. K. 2007. John R. Hogness, 85, Dies; Led Institute of Medicine. *The New York Times*, July 10. https://www.nytimes.com/2007/07/10/health/policy/10hogness.html (accessed July 30, 2021).

Angier, N. 1990. Great 15-Year Project to Decipher Genes Stirs Opposition. *The New York Times*, June 5. https://www.nytimes.com/1990/06/05/science/great-15-year-project-to-decipher-genes-stirs-opposition.html (accessed December 29, 2021).

AP (Associated Press). 2020. Members of President-Elect Biden's Coronavirus Task Force. https://apnews.com/article/members-biden-coronavirus-task-force-319dee82242fe00091cdf98b8f5df29a (accessed January 4, 2022).

APHA (American Public Health Association). n.d. Environmental Health. https://www.apha.org/topics-and-issues/environmental-health (accessed July 15, 2021).

APHA and NAM (National Academy of Medicine). n.d. Responding to COVID-19: A Science-Based Approach. https://covid19conversations.org (accessed July 21, 2021).

Applebaum, A. 2005. The Drug Approval Pendulum. *The Washington Post*, April 13, A17.

Bahuguna, K. 2016. World Health Assembly Agrees to New "Health Emergencies Programme." https://www.downtoearth.org.in/news/health/world-health-assembly-agrees-to-new-health-emergencies-programme--54093 (accessed January 4, 2022).

Baumgartner, J. C., and D. C. Radley. 2021. The Spike in Drug Overdose Deaths During the COVID-19 Pandemic and Policy Options to Move Forward. *The Commonwealth Fund*, March 25. https://www.commonwealthfund.org/blog/2021/spike-drug-overdose-deaths-during-covid-19-pandemic-and-policy-options-move-forward (accessed July 21, 2021).

BBC. 2020. Coronavirus: Trump Terminates US Relationship with WHO. https://www.bbc.com/news/world-us-canada-52857413 (accessed July 21, 2021).

Bendix, A. 2022. In a First, Firearms Were Leading Cause of Death for U.S. Children and Teens in 2020. *NBC News*. https://www.nbcnews.com/health/health-news/guns-leading-cause-death-children-teens-rcna25443 (accessed July 11, 2022).

Berkowitz, E., and M. J. Santangelo. 1999. *The Medical Follow-Up Agency: The First 50 Years, 1946–1996*. Washington, DC: National Academy Press.

Blumenthal, D., and M. McGinnis. 2015. Vital Signs: An IOM Report on Core Metrics for Health and Health Care. Draft manuscript prepared for JAMA Viewpoint.

Board on Medicine, National Academy of Sciences. 1968. *Cardiac Transplantation in Man*. Washington, DC: National Academy of Sciences.

Boffey, P. M. 1986. Federal Efforts on AIDS Criticized as Gravely Weak. *The New York Times*, October 30, 1.

Boffey, P. M. 1988. Expert Panel Sees Poor Leadership in U.S. AIDS Battle. *The New York Times*, June 2, 1.

Bond, A. 2017. Medical Student's Death Highlights High Rates of Physician Suicides. *ABC News*, April 25. https://abcnews.go.com/Health/medical-students-death-highlights-high-rates-physician-suicides/story?id=47006198 (accessed July 19, 2021).

Borger, J. 2020. Trump Announces US to Sever All Ties with WHO. *The Guardian*. https://www.theguardian.com/us-news/2020/may/29/trump-who-china-white-house-us (accessed December 22, 2021).

Brennan, T. 2000. The Institute of Medicine Report on Medical Errors—Could It Do Harm? *New England Journal of Medicine* 342:1123–1125. https://doi.org/10.1056/NEJM200004133421510.

Brown University. n.d. About Samuel M. Nabrit. https://www.brown.edu/academics/biomed/molecular-cell-biochemistry/samuel-milton-nabrit (accessed June 21, 2021).

Burstin, H., S. Leatherman, and D. Goldmann. 2016. The evolution of healthcare quality measurement in the United States. *Journal of Internal Medicine* 279(2):154–159. https://doi.org/10.1111/joim.12471.

Butler, D. n.d. Health and Scientific Research on Dioxins and Agent Orange: Past, Present, and Future. Presentation. https://www.vietnam.ttu.edu/events/presentations/3c-Butler.ppt (accessed December 29, 2021).

Carnegie Council for Ethics in International Affairs. 2009. A Conversation with David Hamburg: The Commitment to Prevention, March 4. https://www.carnegiecouncil.org/studio/multimedia/20090323-a-conversation-with-david-hamburg-the-commitment-to-prevention (accessed July 30, 2021).

CASAA (Consumer Advocates for Smoke-Free Alternatives Association). n.d. Historical Timeline of Vaping and Electronic Cigarettes. https://casaa.org/education/vaping/historical-timeline-of-electronic-cigarettes (accessed July 8, 2021).

CBS News. 2013. FDA Handheld Device to Spot Fake Malaria Drugs, April 25. https://www.cbsnews.com/news/fda-develops-handheld-device-to-spot-fake-malaria-drugs (accessed July 23, 2021).

CDC (Centers for Disease Control and Prevention). 1985. Current Trends Education and Foster Care of Children Infected with Human T-Lymphotropic Virus Type III/ Lymphadenopathy-Associated Virus. *Morbidity and Mortality Weekly Report* 34, August 30:517–521. https://www.cdc.gov/mmwr/preview/mmwrhtml/00033069.htm (accessed July 27, 2021).

CDC. 2009. National Health Interview Survey: No. 17. Health Insurance Coverage Trends, 1959–2007: Estimates from the National Health Interview Survey. https://www.cdc.gov/nchs/nhis/nhis_nhsr.htm (accessed July 6, 2021).

CDC. 2017. At a Glance 2017: Epilepsy. https://www.cdc.gov/media/pdf/releases/aag-epilepsy-2017_508c.pdf (accessed July 14, 2021).

CDC. n.d.a. Vaccine Safety. https://www.cdc.gov/vaccinesafety/ensuringsafety/history/index.html (accessed June 24, 2021).

CDC. n.d.b. Institute of Medicine (IOM) Reports. https://www.cdc.gov/vaccinesafety/research/iomreports/index.html (accessed June 24, 2021).

CDC. n.d.c. The National Institute for Occupational Safety and Health (NIOSH). https://www.cdc.gov/niosh/about/default.html (accessed June 30, 2021).

CDC. n.d.d. Tracking the Global Tobacco Epidemic Among Youth. https://www.cdc.gov/globalhealth/stories/global_tobacco_epidemic.html (accessed July 8, 2021).

CDC. n.d.e. Outbreak of Lung Injury Associated with E-Cigarette Use, or Vaping. https://www.cdc.gov/tobacco/basic_information/e-cigarettes/severe-lung-disease.html (accessed July 8, 2021).

CDC. n.d.f. 2014–2016 Ebola Outbreak in West Africa. https://www.cdc.gov/vhf/ebola/history/2014-2016-outbreak/index.html (accessed July 19, 2021).

CDC. n.d.g. Provisional Drug Overdose Death Counts. https://www.cdc.gov/nchs/nvss/vsrr/drug-overdose-data.htm (accessed December 29, 2021).

CDC. n.d.h. History of the 1918 Flu Pandemic. https://www.cdc.gov/flu/pandemic-resources/1918-commemoration/1918-pandemic-history.htm (accessed July 22, 2022).

CEPI (Coalition for Epidemic Preparedness Innovations). n.d.a. https://cepi.net/about/whyweexist (accessed July 21, 2021).

CEPI. n.d.b. A Global Coalition for a Global Problem. https://cepi.net/about/whoweare (accessed January 4, 2022).

Chapin, C. F. 2015. *Ensuring America's Health: The Public Creation of the Corporate Health Care System*. New York: Cambridge University Press.

Chassin, M. R., and J. M. Loeb. 2011. Improvement journey: Next stop, high reliability. *Health Affairs* 30(4). https://doi.org/10.1377/hlthaff.2011.0076.

Choma, N. N., E. E. Vasilevskis, K. C. Sponsler, J. Hathaway, and S. Kripalani. 2013. Effect of the ACGME 16-Hour Rule on Efficiency and Quality of Care: Duty Hours 2.0. *JAMA Internal Medicine* 173(9):819-821. https://doi.org/10.1001/jamainternmed.2013.3014.

Cicerone, R. J., V. J. Dzau, C. Bai, and V. Ramakrishnan. 2015. Statement by the Co-Sponsoring Presidents of the Summit on Human Gene Editing. https://www.nationalacademies.org/news/2015/12/statement-by-the-co-sponsoring-presidents-of-the-summit-on-human-gene-editing (accessed September 7, 2022).

Clark, E. 1967. Medical Board Set Up to Speed Benefits of Research to Public; Doctors to Speed Medical Benefits. *The New York Times*, November 14. https://www.nytimes.com/1967/11/14/archives/medical-board-set-up-to-speed-benefits-of-research-to-public.html (accessed December 23, 2021).

Clark, E. 1968. Guidelines Urged for Transplants: Academy Cautions Doctors on New Heart Operations. *The New York Times*, February 28. https://www.nytimes.com/1968/02/28/archives/guidelines-urged-for-transplants-academy-cautions-doctors-on-new.html (accessed December 23, 2021).

CMS (Centers for Medicare & Medicaid Services). 2005. Medicare "Pay for Performance (P4P) Initiatives." January 31. https://www.cms.gov/newsroom/fact-sheets/medicare-pay-performance-p4p-initiatives (accessed July 5, 2021).

CMS. 2015. Oncology Care Model (OCM) Request for Applications (RFA) February 2015. https://innovation.cms.gov/files/x/ocmrfa.pdf (accessed July 6, 2021).

Coffey, M. J., and C. E. Coffey. 2016. How We Dramatically Reduced Suicide. *NEJM Catalyst*, April 20. https://doi.org/10.1056/CAT.16.0859.

Darrough, C., and D. Adib. 2020. Health Experts on COVID-19 Vaccine: Americans Have "a Lot of Distrust." *ABC News*, December 4. https://abcnews.go.com/Health/health-experts-covid-19-vaccine-americans-lot-distrust/story?id=74519119 (accessed July 19, 2021).

Davis, M. H., and S. T. Burner. 1995. Three decades of Medicare: What the numbers tell us. *Health Affairs* 14(4). https://doi.org/10.1377/hlthaff.14.4.231.

Department of State. 2017. Notice of Information Collection Under OMB Emergency Review: Supplemental Questions for Visa Applicants. https://www.federalregister.gov/documents/2017/05/04/2017-08975/notice-of-information-collection-under-omb-emergency-review-supplemental-questions-for-visa (accessed July 21, 2021).

DeSalvo, K., B. Hughes, M. Bassett, G. Benjamin, M. Fraser, S. Galea, N. Garcia, and J. Howard. 2021. Public Health COVID-19 Impact Assessment: Lessons Learned and Compelling Needs. *NAM Perspectives*. Discussion Paper, National Academy of Medicine, Washington, DC. https://doi.org/10.31478/202104c.

Durch, J., and L. Klerman. 1994. Overcoming immunization barriers. *JAMA* 272(14):1092.

Dzau, V. J. 2015a. The National Academy of Medicine's vision: Leadership, innovation, and impact for a healthier future. *JAMA* 314(20):2127–2128.

Dzau, V. J. 2015b. 2015 President's Address. https://nam.edu/2015-nam-presidents-address (accessed February 18, 2022).

Dzau, V. J. 2020. Statement on Racial Equity and the Adverse Effects of Racism by NAM President Victor J. Dzau. https://nam.edu/statement-on-racial-equity-and-the-adverse-effects-of-racism-by-nam-president-victor-j-dzau (accessed December 22, 2021).

Dzau, V. J. 2021. Op-Ed: We Need a National Strategy to Help Health Workers Recover from the Stress of the Pandemic. *Los Angeles Times*, March 5. https://www.latimes.com/opinion/story/2021-03-05/national-strategy-healthcare-workers-mental-health (accessed July 19, 2021).

Dzau, V. J., D. Kirch, and T. Nasca. 2020. Preventing a Parallel Pandemic — A National Strategy to Protect Clinicians' Well-Being. *New England Journal of Medicine* 383:513–515. https://doi.org/10.1056/NEJMp2011027.

Elders, M. J, C. L. Perry, M. P. Eriksen, and G. A. Giovino. 1994. The report of the Surgeon General: Preventing tobacco use among young people. *American Journal of Public Health* 84(4):543–547. https://doi.org/10.2105/ajph.84.4.543.

Ensign, R. L. 2012. It's Now a Grind for 2-Year-Olds. *The Wall Street Journal*, March 12. https://www.wsj.com/articles/SB10001424052970204603004577271432291154436 (accessed August 7, 2022).

European Commission. 2020. Coronavirus Global Response Pledging Conference. https://ec.europa.eu/international-partnerships/events/coronavirus-global-reponse-pledging-conference_en (accessed December 22, 2021).

European Union and Italian G20 Presidency. 2021. *Science and Innovation for a Safer World: Report of the Global Health Summit Scientific Expert Panel*. https://global-health-summit.europa.eu/panel-scientific-experts_en (accessed December 22, 2021).

Evans, G. 2006. Update on vaccine liability in the United States: Presentation at the National Vaccine Program Office workshop on strengthening the supply of routinely recommended vaccines in the United States, 12 February 2002. *Clinical Infectious Diseases* 42(Issue Supplement 3):S130–S137. https://doi.org/10.1086/499592.

Evelyn, K. 2020. Fauci Accepts Offer of Chief Medical Adviser Role in Biden Administration. *The Guardian*, December 4. https://www.theguardian.com/us-news/2020/dec/04/fauci-accepts-biden-offer-chief-medical-adviser (accessed July 26, 2021).

Fauci, A. 2020. Remarks at the NAM Annual Meeting. Video, October 19. https://youtu.be/q2ZTqj05Btk?list=PLqRL5HO_hA8fYdOdiFTwP5PPe3Zc5e-c8&t=2058 (accessed December 23, 2021).

Faulkner, K. W. 2003. Review of When Children Die. *New England Journal of Medicine*. October 10, 3485.

Feist, J., C. Feist, and P. Cipriano. 2020. Stigma Compounds the Consequences of Clinician Burnout During COVID-19: A Call to Action to Break the Culture of Silence. *NAM Perspectives*. Commentary, National Academy of Medicine, Washington, DC. https://doi.org/10.31478/202008b.

Fineberg, H. 2012. IOM Announces Perspectives. https://nam.edu/perspectives-2012-iom-announces-perspectives (accessed July 21, 2021).

Fineberg, H. 2013. The Institute of Medicine: What Makes It Great? Annual President's Address to the IOM Membership. October 21, Washington, DC. https://nam.edu/the-institute-of-medicine-what-makes-it-great (accessed December 23, 2021).

Fogarty International Center. 2014. Overview of Brain Disorders: Research Across the Lifespan. *Global Health Matters* 13(1). https://www.fic.nih.gov/News/GlobalHealthMatters/january-february-2014/Pages/brain-disorders-overview.aspx (accessed July 15, 2021).

Frueh, S. 2021. Confronting a "Triple Existential Threat"—NAM President Victor Dzau Discusses How Health and Medicine Can Respond to Current Crises. https://www.nationalacademies.org/news/2021/10/confronting-a-triple-existential-threat-nam-president-victor-dzau-discusses-how-health-and-medicine-can-respond-to-current-crises (accessed December 22, 2021).

Fryhofer, S. A. 2012. *Weight of the Nation*: A Review of the HBO Series. *Medscape*, May 15. https://www.medscape.com/viewarticle/763786 (accessed July 15, 2021).

G20 (G20 High Level Independent Panel on Financing the Global Commons for Pandemic Preparedness and Response). 2021a. *A Global Deal for Our Pandemic Age*. https://pandemic-financing.org/wp-content/uploads/2021/07/G20-HLIP-Report.pdf (accessed December 30, 2021).

G20. 2021b. Victor J. Dzau. https://pandemic-financing.org/team/victor-j-dzau (accessed December 30, 2021).

Gatz, M., and D. Butler. 2020. National Academy of Sciences-National Research Council Twin Registry (NAS-NRC Twin Registry), 1958–2013 [RESTRICTED]. Inter-university Consortium for Political and Social Research [distributor], 2020-11-16. https://doi.org/10.3886/ICPSR36234.v6.

Gavi. n.d. What Is COVAX? https://www.gavi.org/covax-facility (accessed December 29, 2021).

Giovino, G. A. 2007. The tobacco epidemic in the United States. *American Journal of Preventive Medicine* 33(6):S318–S326. https://doi.org/10.1016/j.amepre.2007.09.008.

Goldstein, A. 1999. Clinton to Urge Steps to Curb Medical Errors. *The Washington Post*, December 7, A14.

GPMB (Global Preparedness Monitoring Board). n.d.a. Board. https://www.gpmb.org/board (accessed January 4, 2022).

GPMB. n.d.b. Dr. Victor Dzau. https://www.gpmb.org/board/item/dr-victor-dzau (accessed January 4, 2022).

Greene, S. M., M. Ahmed, P. S. Chua, and C. Grossmann (Eds.). 2021. *Sharing Health Data: The Why, the Will, and the Way Forward*. NAM Special Publication. Washington, DC: National Academy of Medicine.

Harris, G. 2011. Vaccine Cleared Again as Autism Culprit. *The New York Times*, August 26, A19.

Harvard T.H. Chan School of Public Health. n.d. A Passion for Justice: Alonzo Yerby. https://www.hsph.harvard.edu/news/centennial-a-passion-for-justice (accessed June 21, 2021).

Health Affairs. 2021. Vital Directions for Health and Health Care: Priorities for 2021. https://www.healthaffairs.org/health-policy-priorities-2021 (accessed July 21, 2021).

Health.mil. n.d. TRICARE Beneficiary. https://health.mil/I-Am-A/TRICARE-Beneficiary (accessed July 15, 2021).

Hill, E., A. Tiefenthäler, C. Triebert, D. Jordan, H. Willis, and R. Stein. 2020. How George Floyd Was Killed in Police Custody. *The New York Times*, May 31. https://www.nytimes.com/2020/05/31/us/george-floyd-investigation.html (accessed July 21, 2021).

HRSA (Health Resources and Services Administration). n.d. Vaccine Injury Table. https://www.hrsa.gov/sites/default/files/hrsa/vaccine-compensation/vaccine-injury-table.pdf (accessed July 21, 2021).

Huebner, G., N. Boothby, J. L. Aber, G. L. Darmstadt, A. Diaz, A. S. Masten, H. Yoshikawa, I. Redlener, A. Emmel, M. Pitt, L. Arnold, B. Barber, B. Berman, R. Blum, M. Canavera, J. Eckerle, N. A. Fox, J. L. Gibbons, S. W. Hargarten, C. Landers, C. A. Nelson III, S. D. Pollak, V. Rauh, M. Samson, F. Ssewamala, N. St Clair, L. Stark, R. Waldman, M. Wessells, S. L. Wilson, and C. H. Zeanah. 2016. Beyond Survival: The Case for Investing in Children Globally. https://nam.edu/beyond-survival-the-case-for-investing-in-young-children-globally (accessed August 4, 2021).

IHI (Institute for Healthcare Improvement). 2018. IHI Timeline. http://www.ihi.org/about/Documents/IHI_Timeline_2018.pdf (accessed July 5, 2021).

Ince, S. 2015. Victor Dzau cardiovascular physician scientist takes helm at IOM. *Circulation Research* 117:13–16.

Infection Control Today. 2010. Walgreens, HHS Partner to Provide $10 Million Worth of Flu Shots to Uninsured and Underserved. December 10. https://www.infectioncontroltoday.com/vaccines-vaccination/walgreens-hhs-partner-provide-10-million-worth-flu-shots-uninsured-and (accessed July 6, 2021).

Institut Pasteur. 2020. Whole Genome of Novel Coronavirus, 2019-nCoV, Sequenced. ScienceDaily, January 31. https://www.sciencedaily.com/releases/2020/01/200131114748.htm (accessed July 5, 2022).

IOM (Institute of Medicine). 1975. *Legalized Abortion and the Public Health: Report of a Study.* Washington, DC: National Academy Press. https://doi.org/10.17226/21527.

IOM. 1978. *Strengthening US Programs to Improve Health in Developing Countries.* Washington, DC: National Academy Press.

IOM. 1982. *Marijuana and Health.* Washington, DC: National Academy Press. https://doi.org/10.17226/18942.

IOM. 1983. *Nursing and Nursing Education: Public Policies and Private Actions.* Washington, DC: National Academy Press. https://doi.org/10.17226/1120.

IOM. 1984a. *Responding to Health Needs and Scientific Opportunity: The Organizational Structure of the National Institutes of Health.* Washington, DC: National Academy Press. https://doi.org/10.17226/762.

IOM. 1984b. *Bereavement: Reactions, Consequences, and Care.* Washington, DC: National Academy Press. https://doi.org/10.17226/8.

IOM. 1985. *Preventing Low Birthweight.* Washington, DC: National Academy Press. https://doi.org/10.17226/511.

IOM. 1987. *Pain and Disability: Clinical, Behavioral, and Public Policy Perspectives.* Washington, DC: National Academy Press. https://doi.org/10.17226/991.

IOM. 1988a. *The Future of Public Health.* Washington, DC: National Academy Press. https://doi.org/10.17226/1091.

IOM. 1988b. *Confronting AIDS: Update 1988.* Washington, DC: National Academy Press. https://doi.org/10.17226/771.

IOM. 1988c. *An Evaluation of Poliomyelitis Vaccine Policy Options.* Washington, DC: National Academy Press. https://doi.org/10.17226/19091.

IOM. 1990a. *Consensus Development at the NIH: Improving the Program.* Washington, DC: National Academy Press. https://doi.org/10.17226/1563.

IOM. 1990b. *Medicare: A Strategy for Quality Assurance, Volume 1.* Washington, DC: National Academy Press. https://doi.org/10.17226/1547.

IOM. 1990c. *Nutrition During Pregnancy: Part I: Weight Gain, Part II: Nutrient Supplements.* Washington, DC: National Academy Press. https://doi.org/10.17226/1451.

IOM. 1990d. *Healthy People 2000: Citizens Chart the Course.* Washington, DC: National Academy Press. https://doi.org/10.17226/1627.

IOM. 1990e. *Treating Drug Problems: Volume 1.* Washington, DC: National Academy Press. https://doi.org/10.17226/1551.

IOM. 1991a. *Oral Contraceptives and Breast Cancer.* Washington, DC: National Academy Press. https://doi.org/10.17226/1814.

IOM. 1991b. *Kidney Failure and the Federal Government.* Washington, DC: National Academy Press. https://doi.org/10.17226/1818.

IOM. 1991c. *Malaria: Obstacles and Opportunities.* Washington, DC: National Academy Press. https://doi.org/10.17226/1812.

IOM. 1991d. *The AIDS Research Program of the National Institutes of Health.* Washington, DC: National Academy Press. https://doi.org/10.17226/1769.

IOM. 1991e. *Nutrition During Lactation.* Washington, DC: National Academy Press. https://doi.org/10.17226/1577.

IOM. 1991f. *Adverse Effects of Pertussis and Rubella Vaccines.* Washington, DC: National Academy Press. https://doi.org/10.17226/1815.

IOM. 1992a. Comprehensive, Systematic Effort Needed to Combat Emerging Infectious Diseases. Press Release, October 15. https://www8.nationalacademies.org/onpinews/newsitem.aspx?RecordID=2008 (accessed December 29, 2021).

IOM. 1992b. *Emerging Infections: Microbial Threats to Health in the United States.* Washington, DC: National Academy Press. https://doi.org/10.17226/2008.

IOM. 1992c. *Treating Drug Problems: Volume 2.* Washington, DC: National Academy Press. https://doi.org/10.17226/1971.

IOM. 1993a. *Veterans at Risk: The Health Effects of Mustard Gas and Lewisite.* Washington, DC: National Academy Press. https://doi.org/10.17226/2058.

IOM. 1993b. *Access to Health Care in America.* Washington, DC: National Academy Press. https://doi.org/10.17226/2009.

IOM. 1994a. *Adverse Events Associated with Childhood Vaccines: Evidence Bearing on Causality.* Washington, DC: National Academy Press. https://doi.org/10.17226/2138.

IOM. 1994b. *Health Data in the Information Age: Use, Disclosure, and Privacy.* Washington, DC: National Academy Press. https://doi.org/10.17226/2312.

IOM. 1994c. *America's Health in Transition: Protecting and Improving Quality.* Washington, DC: National Academy Press. https://doi.org/10.17226/9147.

IOM. 1994d. *Growing Up Tobacco Free: Preventing Nicotine Addiction in Children and Youths.* Washington, DC: National Academy Press. https://doi.org/10.17226/4757.

220

IOM. 1994e. *Committee on Military Nutrition Research: Activity Report 1992–1994*. Washington, DC: National Academy Press. https://doi.org/10.17226/9169

IOM. 1994f. *Reducing Risks for Mental Disorders: Frontiers for Preventive Intervention Research*. Washington, DC: National Academy Press. https://doi.org/10.17226/2139.

IOM. 1995. *Adverse Reproductive Outcomes in Families of Atomic Veterans: The Feasibility of Epidemiologic Studies*. Washington, DC: National Academy Press. https://doi.org/10.17226/4992.

IOM. 1996a. *Veterans and Agent Orange: Update 1996*. Washington, DC: National Academy Press. https://doi.org/10.17226/5203

IOM. 1996b. *Telemedicine: A Guide to Assessing Telecommunications for Health Care*. Washington, DC: National Academy Press. https://doi.org/10.17226/5296.

IOM. 1996c. *Primary Care: America's Health in a New Era*. Washington, DC: National Academy Press. https://doi.org/10.17226/5152.

IOM. 1996d. *WIC Nutrition Risk Criteria: A Scientific Assessment*. Washington, DC: National Academy Press. https://doi.org/10.17226/5071.

IOM. 1996e. *In Her Lifetime: Female Morbidity and Mortality in Sub-Saharan Africa*. Washington, DC: National Academy Press. https://doi.org/10.17226/5112.

IOM. 1996f. *Lead in the Americas: A Call for Action*. Washington, DC: National Academy Press. https://doi.org/10.17226/9168.

IOM. 1996g. *Vaccines Against Malaria*. Washington, DC: National Academy Press. https://doi.org/10.17226/9027.

IOM. 1996h. *Pathways of Addiction: Opportunities in Drug Abuse Research*. Washington, DC: National Academy Press. https://doi.org/10.17226/5297.

IOM. 1997a. *The Computer-Based Patient Record: An Essential Technology for Health Care, Revised Edition*. Washington, DC: National Academy Press. https://doi.org/10.17226/5306.

IOM. 1997b. *Approaching Death: Improving Care at the End of Life*. Washington, DC: National Academy Press. https://doi.org/10.17226/5801.

IOM. 1997c. *America's Vital Interest in Global Health: Protecting Our People, Enhancing Our Economy, and Advancing Our International Interests*. Washington, DC: National Academy Press. https://doi.org/10.17226/5717.

IOM. 1997d. *Dietary Reference Intakes for Calcium, Phosphorus, Magnesium, Vitamin D, and Fluoride*. Washington, DC: National Academy Press. https://doi.org/10.17226/5776.

IOM. 1998a. *To Improve Human Health: A History of the Institute of Medicine*. Washington, DC: National Academy Press. https://doi.org/10.17226/6382.

IOM. 1998b. *Statement on Quality of Care*. Washington, DC: National Academy Press. https://doi.org/10.17226/9439.

IOM. 1998c. *Control of Cardiovascular Diseases in Developing Countries: Research, Development, and Institutional Strengthening*. Washington, DC: National Academy Press. https://doi.org/10.17226/6218.

IOM. 1998d. *Scientific Opportunities and Public Needs: Improving Priority Setting and Public Input at the National Institutes of Health*. Washington, DC: National Academy Press. https://doi.org/10.17226/6225.

IOM. 1999a. *Organ Procurement and Transplantation: Assessing Current Policies and the Potential Impact of the DHHS Final Rule*. Washington, DC: National Academy Press. https://doi.org/10.17226/9628.

IOM. 1999b. *The Unequal Burden of Cancer: An Assessment of NIH Research and Programs for Ethnic Minorities and the Medically Underserved*. Washington, DC: National Academy Press. https://doi.org/10.17226/6377.

IOM. 1999c. *Ensuring Quality Cancer Care*. Washington, DC: National Academy Press. https://doi.org/10.17226/6467.

IOM. 1999d. *Marijuana and Medicine: Assessing the Science Base*. Washington, DC: National Academy Press. https://doi.org/10.17226/6376.

IOM. 1999e. *Leading Health Indicators for Healthy People 2010: Final Report*. Washington, DC: National Academy Press. https://doi.org/10.17226/9436.

IOM. 2000a. *To Err Is Human: Building a Safer Health System*. Washington, DC: National Academy Press. https://doi.org/10.17226/9728.

IOM. 2000b. *Protecting Data Privacy in Health Services Research*. Washington, DC: National Academy Press. https://doi.org/10.17226/9952.

IOM. 2000c. *Promoting Health: Intervention Strategies from Social and Behavioral Research*. Washington, DC: National Academy Press. https://doi.org/10.17226/9939.

IOM. 2000d. *Extending Medicare Reimbursement in Clinical Trials*. Washington, DC: National Academy Press. https://doi.org/10.17226/9742.

IOM. 2000e. *Clearing the Air: Asthma and Indoor Air Exposures*. Washington, DC: National Academy Press. https://doi.org/10.17226/9610.

IOM. 2000f. *State Programs Can Reduce Tobacco Use*. Washington, DC: National Academy Press. https://doi.org/10.17226/9762.

IOM. 2001a. *Immunization Safety Review: Measles-Mumps-Rubella Vaccine and Autism*. Washington, DC: National Academy Press. https://doi.org/10.17226/10101.

IOM. 2001b. *Immunization Safety Review: Thimerosal-Containing Vaccines and Neurodevelopmental Disorders.* Washington, DC: National Academy Press. https://doi.org/10.17226/10208.

IOM. 2001c. *Safe Passage: Astronaut Care for Exploration Missions.* Washington, DC: National Academy Press. https://doi.org/10.17226/10218.

IOM. 2001d. *Crossing the Quality Chasm: A New Health System for the 21st Century.* Washington, DC: National Academy Press. https://doi.org/10.17226/10027.

IOM. 2001e. *Coverage Matters: Insurance and Health Care.* Washington, DC: National Academy Press. https://doi.org/10.17226/10188.

IOM. 2001f. *Clearing the Smoke: Assessing the Science Base for Tobacco Harm Reduction.* Washington, DC: National Academy Press. https://doi.org/10.17226/10029.

IOM. 2001g. *Neurological, Psychiatric, and Developmental Disorders: Meeting the Challenge in the Developing World.* Washington, DC: National Academy Press. https://doi.org/10.17226/10111.

IOM. 2001h. *Perspectives on the Department of Defense Global Emerging Infections Surveillance and Response System: A Program Review.* Washington, DC: National Academy Press. https://doi.org/10.17226/10203.

IOM. 2002a. *Cancer and the Environment: Gene–Environment Interaction.* Washington, DC: National Academy Press. https://doi.org/10.17226/10464.

IOM. 2002b. *Care Without Coverage: Too Little, Too Late.* Washington, DC: National Academy Press. https://doi.org/10.17226/10367.

IOM. 2002c. *Reducing Suicide: A National Imperative.* Washington, DC: The National Academies Press. https://doi.org/10.17226/10398.

IOM. 2002d. *Preparing for Terrorism: Tools for Evaluating the Metropolitan Medical Response System Program.* Washington, DC: National Academy Press. https://doi.org/10.17226/10412.

IOM. 2002e. *The Anthrax Vaccine: Is It Safe? Does It Work?* Washington, DC: The National Academies Press. https://doi.org/10.17226/10310.

IOM. 2002f. *Health Insurance Is a Family Matter.* Washington, DC: The National Academies Press. https://doi.org/10.17226/10503.

IOM. 2002g. *Confronting Chronic Neglect: The Education and Training of Health Professionals on Family Violence.* Washington, DC: The National Academies Press. https://doi.org/10.17226/10127.

IOM. 2002h. *Dietary Risk Assessment in the WIC Program.* Washington, DC: The National Academies Press. https://doi.org/10.17226/10342.

IOM. 2003a. *Responsible Research: A Systems Approach to Protecting Research Participants.* Washington, DC: The National Academies Press. https://doi.org/10.17226/10508.

IOM. 2003b. *Unequal Treatment: Confronting Racial and Ethnic Disparities in Health Care.* Washington, DC: The National Academies Press. https://doi.org/10.17226/12875.

IOM. 2003c. *Health Professions Education: A Bridge to Quality.* Washington, DC: The National Academies Press. https://doi.org/10.17226/10681.

IOM. 2003d. *When Children Die: Improving Palliative and End-of-Life Care for Children and Their Families.* Washington, DC: The National Academies Press. https://doi.org/10.17226/10390.

IOM. 2003e. *Hidden Costs, Value Lost: Uninsurance in America.* Washington, DC: The National Academies Press. https://doi.org/10.17226/10719.

IOM. 2003f. *The Future of the Public's Health in the 21st Century.* Washington, DC: The National Academies Press. https://doi.org/10.17226/10548.

IOM. 2003g. *Who Will Keep the Public Healthy?: Educating Public Health Professionals for the 21st Century.* Washington, DC: The National Academies Press. https://doi.org/10.17226/10542.

IOM. 2003h. *Priority Areas for National Action: Transforming Health Care Quality.* Washington, DC: The National Academies Press. https://doi.org/10.17226/10593.

IOM. 2003i. *Microbial Threats to Health: Emergence, Detection, and Response.* Washington, DC: The National Academies Press. https://doi.org/10.17226/10636.

IOM. 2003j. *Preparing for the Psychological Consequences of Terrorism: A Public Health Strategy.* Washington, DC: The National Academies Press. https://doi.org/10.17226/10717.

IOM. 2003k. *Informing the Future: Critical Issues in Health: Second Edition.* Washington, DC: The National Academies Press. https://doi.org/10.17226/10853.

IOM. 2003l. *A Shared Destiny: Community Effects of Uninsurance.* Washington, DC: The National Academies Press. https://doi.org/10.17226/10602.

IOM. 2004a. *The 1st Annual Crossing the Quality Chasm Summit: A Focus on Communities: Report of a Summit.* Washington, DC: The National Academies Press. https://doi.org/10.17226/11085.

IOM. 2004b. *Health Literacy: A Prescription to End Confusion.* Washington, DC: The National Academies Press. https://doi.org/10.17226/10883.

IOM. 2004c. *Immunization Safety Review: Vaccines and Autism*. Washington, DC: The National Academies Press. https://doi.org/10.17226/10997.

IOM. 2004d. *In the Nation's Compelling Interest: Ensuring Diversity in the Health-Care Workforce*. Washington, DC: The National Academies Press. https://doi.org/10.17226/10885.

IOM. 2004e. *Insuring America's Health: Principles and Recommendations*. Washington, DC: The National Academies Press. https://doi.org/10.17226/10874.

IOM. 2004f. *Damp Indoor Spaces and Health*. Washington, DC: The National Academies Press. https://doi.org/10.17226/11011.

IOM. 2004g. *Saving Lives, Buying Time: Economics of Malaria Drugs in an Age of Resistance*. Washington, DC: The National Academies Press. https://doi.org/10.17226/11017.

IOM. 2004h. *Keeping Patients Safe: Transforming the Work Environment of Nurses*. Washington, DC: The National Academies Press. https://doi.org/10.17226/10851.

IOM. 2005a. *Review of the HIVNET 012 Perinatal HIV Prevention Study*. Washington, DC: The National Academies Press. https://doi.org/10.17226/11264.

IOM. 2005b. *Healers Abroad: Americans Responding to the Human Resource Crisis in HIV/AIDS*. Washington, DC: The National Academies Press. https://doi.org/10.17226/11270.

IOM. 2005c. *Preventing Childhood Obesity: Health in the Balance*. Washington, DC: The National Academies Press. https://doi.org/10.17226/11015.

IOM. 2005d. *The Smallpox Vaccination Program: Public Health in an Age of Terrorism*. Washington, DC: The National Academies Press. https://doi.org/10.17226/11240.

IOM. 2005e. *Dietary Reference Intakes for Energy, Carbohydrate, Fiber, Fat, Fatty Acids, Cholesterol, Protein, and Amino Acids*. Washington, DC: The National Academies Press. https://doi.org/10.17226/10490.

IOM. 2005f. *Dietary Reference Intakes for Water, Potassium, Sodium, Chloride, and Sulfate*. Washington, DC: The National Academies Press. https://doi.org/10.17226/10925.

IOM. 2006a. *Organ Donation: Opportunities for Action*. Washington, DC: The National Academies Press. https://doi.org/10.17226/11643.

IOM. 2006b. *Examining the Health Disparities Research Plan of the National Institutes of Health: Unfinished Business*. Washington, DC: The National Academies Press. https://doi.org/10.17226/11602.

IOM. 2006c. *Plan for a Short-Term Evaluation of PEPFAR Implementation: Letter Report #1*. Washington, DC: The National Academies Press. https://doi.org/10.17226/11472.

IOM. 2006d. *WIC Food Packages: Time for a Change*. Washington, DC: The National Academies Press. https://doi.org/10.17226/11280.

IOM. 2006e. *Food Marketing to Children and Youth: Threat or Opportunity?* Washington, DC: The National Academies Press. https://doi.org/10.17226/11514.

IOM. 2006f. *Posttraumatic Stress Disorder: Diagnosis and Assessment*. Washington, DC: The National Academies Press. https://doi.org/10.17226/11674.

IOM. 2006g. *The Future of Drug Safety: Promoting and Protecting the Health of the Public*. Washington, DC: The National Academies Press. https://doi.org/10.17226/11750.

IOM. 2006h. *Improving the Quality of Health Care for Mental and Substance-Use Conditions*. Washington, DC: The National Academies Press. https://doi.org/10.17226/11470.

IOM. 2007a. *Cancer Biomarkers: The Promises and Challenges of Improving Detection and Treatment*. Washington, DC: The National Academies Press. https://doi.org/10.17226/11892.

IOM. 2007b. *Long-Term Health Effects of Participation in Project SHAD (Shipboard Hazard and Defense)*. Washington, DC: The National Academies Press. https://doi.org/10.17226/11900.

IOM. 2007c. *Challenges for the FDA: The Future of Drug Safety: Workshop Summary*. Washington, DC: The National Academies Press. https://doi.org/10.17226/11969.

IOM. 2007d. *Understanding the Benefits and Risks of Pharmaceuticals: Workshop Summary*. Washington, DC: The National Academies Press. https://doi.org/10.17226/11910.

IOM. 2007e. *Improving the Social Security Disability Decision Process*. Washington, DC: The National Academies Press. https://doi.org/10.17226/11859.

IOM. 2007f. *Preventing Medication Errors*. Washington, DC: The National Academies Press. https://doi.org/10.17226/11623.

IOM. 2007g. *PEPFAR Implementation: Progress and Promise*. Washington, DC: The National Academies Press. https://doi.org/10.17226/11905.

IOM. 2007h. *Ending the Tobacco Problem: A Blueprint for the Nation*. Washington, DC: The National Academies Press. https://doi.org/10.17226/11795.

IOM. 2007i. *Progress in Preventing Childhood Obesity: How Do We Measure Up?* Washington, DC: The National Academies Press. https://doi.org/10.17226/11722.

IOM. 2007j. *Nutrition Standards for Foods in Schools: Leading the Way Toward Healthier Youth*. Washington, DC: The National Academies Press. https://doi.org/10.17226/11899.

IOM. 2007k. *Cancer Control Opportunities in Low- and Middle-Income Countries.* Washington, DC: The National Academies Press. https://doi.org/10.17226/11797.

IOM. 2007l. *Environmental Public Health Impacts of Disasters: Hurricane Katrina: Workshop Summary.* Washington, DC: The National Academies Press. https://doi.org/10.17226/11840.

IOM. 2007m. *Rewarding Provider Performance: Aligning Incentives in Medicare.* Washington, DC: The National Academies Press. https://doi.org/10.17226/11723.

IOM. 2008a. *Review of NASA's Human Research Program Evidence Books: A Letter Report.* Washington, DC: The National Academies Press. https://doi.org/10.17226/12261.

IOM. 2008b. *Retooling for an Aging America: Building the Health Care Workforce.* Washington, DC: The National Academies Press. https://doi.org/10.17226/12089.

IOM. 2008c. *Cancer Care for the Whole Patient: Meeting Psychosocial Health Needs.* Washington, DC: The National Academies Press. https://doi.org/10.17226/11993.

IOM. 2008d. *Treatment of Posttraumatic Stress Disorder: An Assessment of the Evidence.* Washington, DC: The National Academies Press. https://doi.org/10.17226/11955.

IOM. 2008e. Roundtable on Translating Genomic-Based Research for Health: 2008–2009 Annual Report. https://www.nationalacademies.org/our-work/roundtable-on-genomics-and-precision-health/publications (Annual Reports tab) (accessed July 27, 2021).

IOM. 2009a. *Resident Duty Hours: Enhancing Sleep, Supervision, and Safety.* Washington, DC: The National Academies Press. https://doi.org/10.17226/12508.

IOM. 2009b. *America's Uninsured Crisis: Consequences for Health and Health Care.* Washington, DC: The National Academies Press. https://doi.org/10.17226/12511.

IOM. 2009c. *Combating Tobacco Use in Military and Veteran Populations.* Washington, DC: The National Academies Press. https://doi.org/10.17226/12632.

IOM. 2009d. *Addressing the Threat of Drug-Resistant Tuberculosis: A Realistic Assessment of the Challenge: Workshop Summary.* Washington, DC: The National Academies Press. https://doi.org/10.17226/12570.

IOM. 2009e. *Guidance for Establishing Crisis Standards of Care for Use in Disaster Situations: A Letter Report.* Washington, DC: The National Academies Press. https://doi.org/10.17226/12749.

IOM. 2009f. *The U.S. Commitment to Global Health: Recommendations for the New Administration.* Washington, DC: The National Academies Press. https://doi.org/10.17226/12506.

IOM. 2010a. *A National Cancer Clinical Trials System for the 21st Century: Reinvigorating the NCI Cooperative Group Program.* Washington, DC: The National Academies Press. https://doi.org/10.17226/12879.

IOM. 2010b. *Hepatitis and Liver Cancer: A National Strategy for Prevention and Control of Hepatitis B and C.* Washington, DC: The National Academies Press. https://doi.org/10.17226/12793.

IOM. 2010c. *Redesigning Continuing Education in the Health Professions.* Washington, DC: The National Academies Press. https://doi.org/10.17226/12704.

IOM. 2010d. *Promoting Cardiovascular Health in the Developing World: A Critical Challenge to Achieve Global Health.* Washington, DC: The National Academies Press. https://doi.org/10.17226/12815.

IOM. 2010e. *School Meals: Building Blocks for Healthy Children.* Washington, DC: The National Academies Press. https://doi.org/10.17226/12751.

IOM. 2010f. *Provision of Mental Health Counseling Services Under TRICARE.* Washington, DC: The National Academies Press. https://doi.org/10.17226/12813.

IOM. 2010g. *Forum on Drug Discovery, Development, and Translation: Annual Report 2009.* Washington, DC: The National Academies Press. https://doi.org/10.17226/26110.

IOM. 2010h. *Secondhand Smoke Exposure and Cardiovascular Effects: Making Sense of the Evidence.* Washington, DC: The National Academies Press. https://doi.org/10.17226/12649.

IOM. 2010i. *Strategies to Reduce Sodium Intake in the United States.* Washington, DC: The National Academies Press. https://doi.org/10.17226/12818.

IOM. 2011a. Adverse Effects of Vaccines: Evidence and Causality, Report Brief. https://www.nap.edu/resource/13164/adverseeffectsofvaccinesreportbrief.pdf (accessed July 30, 2021).

IOM. 2011b. *Implementing a National Cancer Clinical Trials System for the 21st Century: Workshop Summary.* Washington, DC: The National Academies Press. https://doi.org/10.17226/13154.

IOM. 2011c. *Long-Term Health Consequences of Exposure to Burn Pits in Iraq and Afghanistan.* Washington, DC: The National Academies Press. https://doi.org/10.17226/13209.

IOM. 2011d. *Learning What Works: Infrastructure Required for Comparative Effectiveness Research: Workshop Summary.* Washington, DC: The National Academies Press. https://doi.org/10.17226/12214.

IOM. 2011e. The Health of Lesbian, Gay, Bisexual, and Transgender People: Building a Foundation for Better Understanding, Report Brief. https://www.nap.edu/resource/13128/LGBT-Health-2011-Report-Brief.pdf (accessed July 6, 2021).

IOM. 2011f. *The Health of Lesbian, Gay, Bisexual, and Transgender People: Building a Foundation for Better Understanding.* Washington, DC: The National Academies Press. https://doi.org/10.17226/13128.

IOM. 2011g. *The Future of Nursing: Leading Change, Advancing Health*. Washington, DC: The National Academies Press. https://doi.org/10.17226/12956.

IOM. 2011h. *Clinical Preventive Services for Women: Closing the Gaps*. Washington, DC: The National Academies Press. https://doi.org/10.17226/13181.

IOM. 2011i. *Climate Change, the Indoor Environment, and Health*. Washington, DC: The National Academies Press. https://doi.org/10.17226/13115.

IOM. 2011j. *Digital Infrastructure for the Learning Health System: The Foundation for Continuous Improvement in Health and Health Care: Workshop Series Summary*. Washington, DC: The National Academies Press. https://doi.org/10.17226/12912.

IOM. 2011k. *Future Opportunities to Leverage the Alzheimer's Disease Neuroimaging Initiative: Workshop Summary*. Washington, DC: The National Academies Press. https://doi.org/10.17226/13017.

IOM. 2011l. *Leading Health Indicators for Healthy People 2020: Letter Report*. Washington, DC: The National Academies Press. https://doi.org/10.17226/13088.

IOM. 2011m. *Advancing Oral Health in America*. Washington, DC: The National Academies Press. https://doi.org/10.17226/13086.

IOM. 2011n. *Dietary Reference Intakes for Calcium and Vitamin D*. Washington, DC: The National Academies Press. https://doi.org/10.17226/13050.

IOM. 2011o. *Dietary Reference Intakes for Calcium and Vitamin D*. Washington, DC: The National Academies Press. https://doi.org/10.17226/13050.

IOM. 2011p. *Early Childhood Obesity Prevention Policies*. Washington, DC: The National Academies Press. https://doi.org/10.17226/13124.

IOM. 2012a. *Evolution of Translational Omics: Lessons Learned and the Path Forward*. Washington, DC: The National Academies Press. https://doi.org/10.17226/13297.

IOM. 2012b. *Breast Cancer and the Environment: A Life Course Approach*. Washington, DC: The National Academies Press. https://doi.org/10.17226/13263.

IOM. 2012c. *Ethical and Scientific Issues in Studying the Safety of Approved Drugs*. Washington, DC: The National Academies Press. https://doi.org/10.17226/13219.

IOM. 2012d. *Health IT and Patient Safety: Building Safer Systems for Better Care*. Washington, DC: The National Academies Press. https://doi.org/10.17226/13269.

IOM. 2012e. *The Mental Health and Substance Use Workforce for Older Adults: In Whose Hands?* Washington, DC: The National Academies Press. https://doi.org/10.17226/13400.

IOM. 2012f. *Essential Health Benefits: Balancing Coverage and Cost*. Washington, DC: The National Academies Press. https://doi.org/10.17226/13234.

IOM. 2012g. *Primary Care and Public Health: Exploring Integration to Improve Population Health*. Washington, DC: The National Academies Press. https://doi.org/10.17226/13381.

IOM. 2012h. *Scientific Standards for Studies on Modified Risk Tobacco Products*. Washington, DC: The National Academies Press. https://doi.org/10.17226/13294.

IOM. 2012i. *Living Well with Chronic Illness: A Call for Public Health Action*. Washington, DC: The National Academies Press. https://doi.org/10.17226/13272.

IOM. 2012j. *Epilepsy Across the Spectrum: Promoting Health and Understanding*. Washington, DC: The National Academies Press. https://doi.org/10.17226/13379.

IOM. 2012k. *Accelerating Progress in Obesity Prevention: Solving the Weight of the Nation*. Washington, DC: The National Academies Press. https://doi.org/10.17226/13275.

IOM. 2012l. *Ensuring Safe Foods and Medical Products Through Stronger Regulatory Systems Abroad*. Washington, DC: The National Academies Press. https://doi.org/10.17226/13296.

IOM. 2012m. *Prepositioning Antibiotics for Anthrax*. Washington, DC: The National Academies Press. https://doi.org/10.17226/13218.

IOM. 2012n. *Crisis Standards of Care: A Systems Framework for Catastrophic Disaster Response: Volume 1: Introduction and CSC Framework*. Washington, DC: The National Academies Press. https://doi.org/10.17226/13351.

IOM. 2012o. Essential Health Benefits: Balancing Coverage and Cost: Report Brief. Washington, DC: The National Academies Press. https://nap.nationalacademies.org/resource/13234/essentialhealthbenefitsreportbrief.pdf.

IOM. 2012p. *Facing the Reality of Drug-Resistant Tuberculosis in India: Challenges and Potential Solutions: Summary of a Joint Workshop by the Institute of Medicine, the Indian National Science Academy, and the Indian Council of Medical Research*. Washington, DC: The National Academies Press. https://doi.org/10.17226/13243.

IOM. 2012q. *Alzheimer's Diagnostic Guideline Validation: Exploration of Next Steps: Workshop Summary*. Washington, DC: The National Academies Press. https://doi.org/10.17226/13312.

IOM. 2013a. *The Childhood Immunization Schedule and Safety: Stakeholder Concerns, Scientific Evidence, and Future Studies*. Washington, DC: The National Academies Press. https://doi.org/10.17226/13563.

IOM. 2013b. *Implementing a National Cancer Clinical Trials System for the 21st Century: Second Workshop Summary.* Washington, DC: The National Academies Press. https://doi.org/10.17226/18362.

IOM. 2013c. *The CTSA Program at NIH: Opportunities for Advancing Clinical and Translational Research.* Washington, DC: The National Academies Press. https://doi.org/10.17226/18323.

IOM. 2013d. *Gulf War and Health: Treatment for Chronic Multisymptom Illness.* Washington, DC: The National Academies Press. https://doi.org/10.17226/13539.

IOM. 2013e. *Best Care at Lower Cost: The Path to Continuously Learning Health Care in America.* Washington, DC: The National Academies Press. https://doi.org/10.17226/13444.

IOM. 2013f. *International Regulatory Harmonization Amid Globalization of Drug Development: Workshop Summary.* Washington, DC: The National Academies Press. https://doi.org/10.17226/18324.

IOM. 2013g. *Delivering High-Quality Cancer Care: Charting a New Course for a System in Crisis.* Washington, DC: The National Academies Press. https://doi.org/10.17226/18359.

IOM. 2013h. Delivering High-Quality Cancer Care: Charting a New Course for a System in Crisis: Presentation Slides. Washington, DC: The National Academies Press. https://doi.org/10.17226/18359.

IOM. 2013i. *Evaluation of PEPFAR.* Washington, DC: The National Academies Press. https://doi.org/10.17226/18256.

IOM. 2013j. *Sodium Intake in Populations: Assessment of Evidence.* Washington, DC: The National Academies Press. https://doi.org/10.17226/18311.

IOM. 2013k. *Educating the Student Body: Taking Physical Activity and Physical Education to School.* Washington, DC: The National Academies Press. https://doi.org/10.17226/18314.

IOM. 2013l. *Substance Use Disorders in the U.S. Armed Forces.* Washington, DC: The National Academies Press. https://doi.org/10.17226/13441.

IOM. 2013m. *Crisis Standards of Care: A Toolkit for Indicators and Triggers.* Washington, DC: The National Academies Press. https://doi.org/10.17226/18338.

IOM. 2013n. *Neurodegeneration: Exploring Commonalities Across Diseases: Workshop Summary.* Washington, DC: The National Academies Press. https://doi.org/10.17226/18341.

IOM. 2013o. *Toward Quality Measures for Population Health and the Leading Health Indicators.* Washington, DC: The National Academies Press. https://doi.org/10.17226/18339.

IOM. 2013p. *Returning Home from Iraq and Afghanistan: Assessment of Readjustment Needs of Veterans, Service Members, and Their Families.* Washington, DC: The National Academies Press. https://doi.org/10.17226/13499.

IOM. 2013q. *Countering the Problem of Falsified and Substandard Drugs.* Washington, DC: The National Academies Press. https://doi.org/10.17226/18272.

IOM. 2014a. *Veterans and Agent Orange: Update 2012.* Washington, DC: The National Academies Press. https://doi.org/10.17226/18395.

IOM. 2014b. *Graduate Medical Education That Meets the Nation's Health Needs.* Washington, DC: The National Academies Press. https://doi.org/10.17226/18754.

IOM. 2014c. *Preventing Psychological Disorders in Service Members and Their Families: An Assessment of Programs.* Washington, DC: The National Academies Press. https://doi.org/10.17226/18597.

IOM. 2014d. Preventing Psychological Disorders in Service Members and Their Families: An Assessment of Programs, Report Brief. Washington, DC: The National Academies Press. https://doi.org/10.17226/18597.

IOM. 2014e. Investing in Global Health Systems. https://www.nap.edu/resource/18940/IGHS-keyfindings.pdf (accessed July 15, 2021).

IOM. 2014f. *Treatment for Posttraumatic Stress Disorder in Military and Veteran Populations: Final Assessment.* Washington, DC: The National Academies Press. https://doi.org/10.17226/18724.

IOM. 2015a. *Vital Signs: Core Metrics for Health and Health Care Progress.* Washington, DC: The National Academies Press. https://doi.org/10.17226/19402.

IOM. 2015b. Vital Signs: Core Metrics for Health and Health Care Progress. Report Brief. Washington, DC: The National Academies Press. https://nap.nationalacademies.org/resource/19402/VitalSigns_RB.pdf.

IOM. 2015c. *Measuring the Impact of Interprofessional Education on Collaborative Practice and Patient Outcomes.* Washington, DC: The National Academies Press. https://doi.org/10.17226/21726.

IOM. 2015d. *Dying in America: Improving Quality and Honoring Individual Preferences Near the End of Life.* Washington, DC: The National Academies Press. https://doi.org/10.17226/18748.

IOM. 2015e. Public Health Implications of Raising the Minimum Age of Legal Access to Tobacco Products, Report Brief. Washington, DC: The National Academies Press. https://nap.nationalacademies.org/resource/18997/tobacco_minimum_age_report_brief.pdf.

IOM. 2015f. *Psychosocial Interventions for Mental and Substance Use Disorders: A Framework for Establishing Evidence-Based Standards.* Washington, DC: The National Academies Press. https://doi.org/10.17226/19013.

IOM. 2015g. *Transforming Health Care Scheduling and Access: Getting to Now.* Washington, DC: The National Academies Press. https://doi.org/10.17226/20220.

IOM. 2015h. *Healthy, Resilient, and Sustainable Communities After Disasters: Strategies, Opportunities, and Planning for Recovery.* Washington, DC: The National Academies Press. https://doi.org/10.17226/18996.

IOM. 2015i. *Cognitive Aging: Progress in Understanding and Opportunities for Action.* Washington, DC: The National Academies Press. https://doi.org/10.17226/21693.

IOM. 2015j. *Strategies to Improve Cardiac Arrest Survival: A Time to Act.* Washington, DC: The National Academies Press. https://doi.org/10.17226/21723.

IOM and NAS (National Academy of Sciences). 1977. *Evaluation of Poliomyelitis Vaccines: Report of the Committee for the Study of Poliomyelitis Vaccines.* Washington, DC: National Academy of Sciences.

IOM and NAS. 1986. *Confronting AIDS: Directions for Public Health, Health Care, and Research.* Washington, DC: National Academy Press. https://doi.org/10.17226/938.

IOM and NRC (National Research Council). 1998a. *Taking Action to Reduce Tobacco Use.* Washington, DC: National Academy Press. https://doi.org/10.17226/6060.

IOM and NRC. 1998b. *Violence in Families: Assessing Prevention and Treatment Programs.* Washington, DC: National Academy Press. https://doi.org/10.17226/5285.

IOM and NRC. 2000. *From Neurons to Neighborhoods: The Science of Early Childhood Development.* Washington, DC: National Academy Press. https://doi.org/10.17226/9824.

IOM and NRC. 2001. *Improving Palliative Care for Cancer.* Washington, DC: National Academy Press. https://doi.org/10.17226/10149.

IOM and NRC. 2003a. *Large-Scale Biomedical Science: Exploring Strategies for Future Research.* Washington, DC: The National Academies Press. https://doi.org/10.17226/10718.

IOM and NRC. 2003b. *Fulfilling the Potential of Cancer Prevention and Early Detection.* Washington, DC: The National Academies Press. https://doi.org/10.17226/10263.

IOM and NRC. 2004. *Meeting Psychosocial Needs of Women with Breast Cancer.* Washington, DC: The National Academies Press. https://doi.org/10.17226/10909.

IOM and NRC. 2005. *Guidelines for Human Embryonic Stem Cell Research.* Washington, DC: The National Academies Press. https://doi.org/10.17226/11278.

IOM and NRC. 2006. *From Cancer Patient to Cancer Survivor: Lost in Transition.* Washington, DC: The National Academies Press. https://doi.org/10.17226/11468.

IOM and NRC. 2007a. *2007 Amendments to the National Academies' Guidelines for Human Embryonic Stem Cell Research.* Washington, DC: The National Academies Press. https://doi.org/10.17226/11871.

IOM and NRC. 2007b. *PTSD Compensation and Military Service.* Washington, DC: The National Academies Press. https://doi.org/10.17226/11870.

IOM and NRC. 2008a. *2008 Amendments to the National Academies' Guidelines for Human Embryonic Stem Cell Research.* Washington, DC: The National Academies Press. https://doi.org/10.17226/12260.

IOM and NRC. 2008b. *The National Children's Study Research Plan: A Review.* Washington, DC: The National Academies Press. https://doi.org/10.17226/12211.

IOM and NRC. 2009a. *Evaluating Occupational Health and Safety Research Programs: Framework and Next Steps.* Washington, DC: The National Academies Press. https://doi.org/10.17226/12639.

IOM and NRC. 2009b. *Sustaining Global Surveillance and Response to Emerging Zoonotic Diseases.* Washington, DC: The National Academies Press. https://doi.org/10.17226/12625.

IOM and NRC. 2009c. *Weight Gain During Pregnancy: Reexamining the Guidelines.* Washington, DC: The National Academies Press. https://doi.org/10.17226/12584.

IOM and NRC. 2011a. *Chimpanzees in Biomedical and Behavioral Research: Assessing the Necessity.* Washington, DC: The National Academies Press. https://doi.org/10.17226/13257.

IOM and NRC. 2011b. *Improving Access to Oral Health Care for Vulnerable and Underserved Populations.* Washington, DC: The National Academies Press. https://doi.org/10.17226/13116.

IOM and NRC. 2012. *From Neurons to Neighborhoods: An Update: Workshop Summary.* Washington, DC: The National Academies Press. https://doi.org/10.17226/13119.

IOM and NRC. 2013a. *Priorities for Research to Reduce the Threat of Firearm-Related Violence.* Washington, DC: The National Academies Press. https://doi.org/10.17226/18319.

IOM and NRC. 2013b. *Leveraging Action to Support Dissemination of the Pregnancy Weight Gain Guidelines: Workshop Summary.* Washington, DC: The National Academies Press. https://doi.org/10.17226/18410.

IOM and NRC. 2013c. *Guidelines on Weight Gain and Pregnancy.* Washington, DC: The National Academies Press. https://doi.org/10.17226/18291.

IOM and NRC. 2013d. *Implementing Guidelines on Weight Gain and Pregnancy.* Washington, DC: The National Academies Press. https://doi.org/10.17226/18292.

IOM and NRC. 2014a. *New Directions in Child Abuse and Neglect Research.* Washington, DC: The National Academies Press. https://doi.org/10.17226/18331.

IOM and NRC. 2014b. *The National Children's Study Research Plan: A Review.* Washington, DC: The National Academies Press. https://doi.org/10.17226/18826.

JHU (Johns Hopkins University). n.d. Coronavirus Resource Center. https://coronavirus.jhu.edu/map.html (accessed February 18, 2022)

Kaplan, S. 2018. Congress Quashed Research into Gun Violence. Since Then, 600,000 People Have Been Shot. *The New York Times,* March 12. https://www.nytimes.com/2018/03/12/health/gun-violence-research-cdc.html (accessed July 14, 2021).

KFF (Kaiser Family Foundation). 2021. Tracking U.S. COVID-19 Vaccine Donations. https://www.kff.org/coronavirus-covid-19/issue-brief/tracking-u-s-covid-19-vaccine-donations (accessed July 6, 2022).

Kim, Y. C., B. Dema, and A. Reyes-Sandoval. 2020. COVID-19 Vaccines: Breaking Record Times to First-in-Human Trials. *npj Vaccines* 5(34). https://www.nature.com/articles/s41541-020-0188-3 (accessed July 5, 2022).

Kington, R., S. Arnesen, W.-Y. S. Chou, S. Curry, D. Lazer, and A. Villarruel. 2021. Identifying Credible Sources of Health Information in Social Media: Principles and Attributes. *NAM Perspectives.* Discussion Paper, National Academy of Medicine, Washington, DC. https://doi.org/10.31478/202107a.

Klein, B., and J. Hansler. 2020. Trump Halts World Health Organization Funding Over Handling of Coronavirus Outbreak. CNN, April 15. https://www.cnn.com/2020/04/14/politics/donald-trump-world-health-organization-funding-coronavirus/index.html (accessed July 21, 2021).

Knoll, C., A. Watkins, and M. Rothfeld. 2020. "I Couldn't Do Anything": The Virus and an E.R. Doctor's Suicide. *The New York Times,* July 11. https://www.nytimes.com/2020/07/11/nyregion/lorna-breen-suicide-coronavirus.html (accessed July 19, 2021).

Kodjak. A. 2019. Prescription Drug Costs Driven by Manufacturer Price Hikes, Not Innovation. NPR, January 7. https://www.npr.org/sections/health-shots/2019/01/07/682986630/prescription-drug-costs-driven-by-manufacturer-price-hikes-not-innovation (accessed July 6, 2021).

Langer, E. 2021. Richard Lewontin, a Preeminent Geneticist of His Era, Dies at 92. *The Washington Post,* July 8. https://www.washingtonpost.com/local/obituaries/richard-lewontin-dead/2021/07/08/5aaf3c58-dfe9-11eb-b507-697762d090dd_story.html (accessed December 29, 2021).

LaVeist, T., and G. Benjamin. 2021. 60 Black Health Experts Urge Black Americans to Get Vaccinated. *The New York Times,* February 7. https://www.nytimes.com/2021/02/07/opinion/covid-black-americans.html (accessed July 19, 2021).

Leape, L. L. 2000. Institute of Medicine medical error figures are not exaggerated. *JAMA* (284):95–97.

Lohr, K. N., and J. Harris-Wehling. 1991. Medicare: A strategy for quality assurance I: A recapitulation of the study and a definition of the quality of care. *QRB Quality Review Bulletin* 17(1):6–9. https://10.1016/s0097-5990(16)30413-4.

Long, P., M. Abrams, A. Milstein, G. Anderson, K. Lewis Apton, M. Lund Dahlberg, and D. Whicher (Eds.). 2017. *Effective Care for High-Need Patients: Opportunities for Improving Outcomes, Value, and Health.* Washington, DC: National Academy of Medicine.

Lopez, G. 2019. Marijuana Has Been Legalized in 11 States and Washington, DC. *Vox,* June 19. https://www.vox.com/identities/2018/8/20/17938336/marijuana-legalization-states-map (accessed July 14, 2021).

Lowry, B. 2012. The Weight of the Nation. *Variety,* May 13. https://variety.com/2012/tv/reviews/the-weight-of-the-nation-1117947544 (accessed July 15, 2021).

Matheny, M., S. Thadaney Israni, M. Ahmed, and D. Whicher (Eds.). 2022. *Artificial Intelligence in Health Care: The Hope, the Hype, the Promise, the Peril.* NAM Special Publication. Washington, DC: National Academy of Medicine.

McFeatters, A. 2002. Seriously Ill Children and Their Families Overlooked, Study Says. *Pittsburgh Post Gazette,* July 31, A-3.

Miller, R. 1995. Looking for Adverse Reproductive Outcomes in "Atomic Veterans": Are Such Studies Feasible? *JAMA* 274(11):865. https://doi.org/10.1001/jama.1995.03530110021007.

NAE (National Academy of Engineering). n.d. About the National Academy of Engineering. https://www.nae.edu/19580/About (accessed December 23, 2021).

NAM. 2015. Annual Report 2015. https://nam.edu/wp-content/uploads/2016/06/NAM-Annual-Report-2015.pdf (accessed December 29, 2021).

NAM. 2016a. *The Neglected Dimension of Global Security: A Framework to Counter Infectious Disease Crises.* Washington, DC: The National Academies Press. https://doi.org/10.17226/21891.

NAM. 2016b. National Academy of Medicine Launches "Action Collaborative" to Promote Clinician Well-Being and Combat Burnout, Depression, and Suicide Among Health Care Workers. https://nam.edu/national-academy-of-medicine-launches-action-collaborative-to-promote-clinician-well-being-and-combat-burnout-depression-and-suicide-among-health-care-workers (accessed July 19, 2021).

NAM. 2016c. 2016 President's Address. https://nam.edu/2016-presidents-address (accessed July 28, 2021).

NAM. 2017a. The Leadership Consortium for a Value & Science-Driven Health System. https://nam.edu/wp-content/uploads/2017/01/Updated2pager.07.28.17.pdf (accessed July 5, 2021).

NAM. 2017b. *First, Do No Harm: Marshaling Clinician Leadership to Counter the Opioid Epidemic*. NAM Special Publication. https://nam.edu/wp-content/uploads/2017/09/First-Do-No-Harm-Marshaling-Clinician-Leadership-to-Counter-the-Opioid-Epidemic.pdf (accessed July 19, 2021).

NAM. 2017c. *Vital Directions for Health & Health Care: A Special Publication of the National Academy of Medicine*. https://nam.edu/initiatives/vital-directions-for-health-and-health-care/vital-directions-for-health-health-care-special-publication (accessed July 21, 2021).

NAM. 2017d. Strategic Plan 2018–2023: Goalposts for a Healthier Future. https://nam.edu/wp-content/uploads/2017/10/National-Academy-of-Medicine-2018-2023-Strategic-Plan.pdf (accessed July 16, 2021).

NAM. 2018a. More Than 130 Organizations Join the National Academy of Medicine in Committing to Clinician Well-Being. https://nam.edu/130-organizations-join-national-academy-medicine-committing-clinician-well (accessed July 19, 2021).

NAM. 2018b. National Academy of Medicine Launches Action Collaborative to Counter Opioid Epidemic; Public–Private Partnership Will Coordinate Initiatives Across Sectors to Drive Collective Solutions. https://nam.edu/national-academy-of-medicine-launches-action-collaborative-to-counter-opioid-epidemic-public-private-partnership-will-coordinate-initiatives-across-sectors-to-drive-collective-solutions (accessed July 19, 2021).

NAM. 2018c. 2018 Annual Report. https://nam.edu/wp-content/uploads/2019/05/National-Academy-of-Medicine-2018-Annual-Report.pdf (accessed July 21, 2021).

NAM. 2018d. National Academy of Medicine Code of Conduct. https://nam.edu/national-academy-of-medicine-code-of-conduct (accessed July 21, 2021).

NAM. 2019a. To Ensure High Quality Patient Care, the Health Care System Must Address Clinician Burnout Tied to Work and Learning Environments, Administrative Requirements, October 23. https://nam.edu/to-ensure-high-quality-patient-care-the-health-care-system-must-address-clinician-burnout-tied-to-work-and-learning-environments-administrative-requirements (accessed July 19, 2021).

NAM. 2019b. More Than 100 Organizations Join the National Academy of Medicine in Countering the Opioid Epidemic. https://nam.edu/more-than-100-organizations-join-the-national-academy-of-medicine-in-countering-the-opioid-epidemic (accessed July 19, 2021).

NAM. 2019c. Engaging the Next Generation of Leaders in Health and Medicine: Summary of the 2019 NAM Emerging Leaders Forum. https://nam.edu/programs/emerging-leaders-forum/2019-emerging-leaders-forum-summary (accessed July 27, 2021).

NAM. 2019d. National Academy of Medicine Launches Global Competition Seeking Solutions for Improving Healthy Longevity, October 21. https://nam.edu/national-academy-of-medicine-launches-global-competition-seeking-solutions-for-improving-healthy-longevity (accessed July 28, 2021).

NAM. 2020a. 2020 President's Address to the NAM Membership. October 19, 2020. https://nam.edu/2020-annual-presidents-address-to-the-nam-membership (accessed June 24, 2020).

NAM. 2020b. National Organizations Call for Action to Implement Crisis Standards of Care During COVID-19 Surge, December 18. https://nam.edu/national-organizations-call-for-action-to-implement-crisis-standards-of-care-during-covid-19-surge (accessed July 19, 2021).

NAM. 2020c. Statement on Political Interference in Peer-Reviewed Federal Research Grants. https://nam.edu/statement-on-political-interference-in-peer-reviewed-federal-research-grants (accessed July 21, 2021).

NAM. 2020d. Statement on Racial Equity and the Adverse Effects of Racism by NAM President Victor J. Dzau. https://nam.edu/statement-on-racial-equity-and-the-adverse-effects-of-racism-by-nam-president-victor-j-dzau (accessed July 21, 2021).

NAM. 2020e. More Than 150 Innovators Awarded in Inaugural Round of Global Competition Seeking Solutions to Improve Healthy Longevity. https://nam.edu/more-than-150-innovators-awarded-in-inaugural-round-of-global-competition-seeking-solutions-to-improve-healthy-longevity (accessed July 201, 2021).

NAM. 2020f. Leading the Way: Transforming Global Brain Health with a Bold and Radical Approach. https://nam.edu/leading-the-way-transforming-global-brain-health-with-a-bold-and-radical-approach (accessed July 21, 2021).

NAM. 2020g. NAM Elects Dzau for Second Term as President, Elects Del Rio as Foreign Secretary. https://nam.edu/nam-elects-dzau-for-second-term-as-president-elects-del-rio-as-foreign-secretary (accessed July 21, 2021).

NAM. 2020h. NAM Awards First-Ever Presidential Citation for Exemplary Leadership to Anthony Fauci. https://nam.edu/nam-awards-first-ever-presidential-citation-for-exemplary-leadership-to-anthony-fauci (accessed July 26, 2021).

NAM. 2020i. NAM President Victor J. Dzau Joins Fellow Members of Global Preparedness Monitoring Board in Issuing Statement on Outbreak of 2019-Novel Coronavirus. News Release, January 30. https://nam.edu/nam-president-victor-dzau-joins-fellow-members-of-global-preparedness-monitoring-board-in-issuing-statement-on-outbreak-of-2019-novel-coronavirus (accessed December 30, 2021).

NAM. 2020j. Victor Dzau Speaks at Coronavirus Global Response International Pledging Event. News Release, May 8. https://nam.edu/victor-dzau-speaks-at-coronavirus-global-response-international-pledging-event (accessed December 30, 2021).

NAM. 2020k. *NAM President Victor Dzau Speaks at Coronavirus Global Response International Pledging Event.* Video. https://youtu.be/Gv-mZUgih3M (accessed December 30, 2021).

NAM. 2021a. *National Academy of Medicine Extends Action Collaborative on Clinician Well-Being and Resilience until 2022.* https://nam.edu/national-academy-of-medicine-extends-action-collaborative-on-clinician-well-being-and-resilience-until-2022 (accessed July 19, 2021).

NAM. 2021b. *National Academy of Medicine Extends Action Collaborative on Countering the U.S. Opioid Epidemic Through 2022,* March 25. https://nam.edu/national-academy-of-medicine-extends-action-collaborative-on-countering-the-u-s-opioid-epidemic-through-2022 (accessed July 21, 2021).

NAM. 2021c. *National Academy of Medicine Extends Culture of Health Program until 2024.* https://nam.edu/national-academy-of-medicine-extends-culture-of-health-program-until-2024 (accessed July 21, 2021).

NAM. 2021d. *Letter from Victor Dzau, William Foege, and Helene Gayle to Xavier Becerra and Jeffrey Zients.* March 26. https://nam.edu/wp-content/uploads/2021/04/NAM-letter-to-Becerra-Zients-Global-COVID-19-vaccine-allocation-%E2%80%93-a-critical-opportunity-for-the-U.S.-to-reclaim-global-health-leadership.pdf (accessed December 29, 2021).

NAM. 2021e. *G20 High Level Independent Panel Releases Report on Financing the Global Commons for Pandemic Preparedness and Response.* News Release, July 9. https://nam.edu/g20-high-level-independent-panel-releases-report-on-financing-the-global-commons-for-pandemic-preparedness-and-response (accessed December 30, 2021).

NAM. 2021f. *Advancing Pandemic and Seasonal Influenza Vaccine Preparedness and Response: Harnessing Lessons from the Efforts Mitigating the COVID-19 Pandemic—Overview of the Four Consensus Studies.* https://nam.edu/wp-content/uploads/2021/11/Flu-Studies-Overview-FINAL.pdf (accessed December 30, 2021).

NAM. 2021g. *Emerging Stronger After COVID-19: Priorities for Health System Transformation.* https://nam.edu/programs/value-science-driven-health-care/emerging-stronger-after-covid-19-priorities-for-health-system-transformation (accessed December 30, 2021).

NAM. 2021h. *National Academy of Medicine Releases Video Encouraging Latinx/Latino(a)/Hispanic Americans to Accept the COVID-19 Vaccine.* News Release, September 28. https://nam.edu/national-academy-of-medicine-releases-video-encouraging-latinx-latinoa-hispanic-americans-to-accept-the-covid-19-vaccine (accessed December 30, 2021).

NAM. 2021i. *Letter from Latinx/Latino(a)/Hispanic Members of the National Academy of Medicine Urging Latinx/Latino(a)/Hispanic Americans to Get the COVID-19 Vaccine.* https://nam.edu/wp-content/uploads/2021/10/Latinx-Member-Letter_FINAL-10.25_w-citations.pdf (accessed December 30, 2021).

NAM. 2021j. *Promoting Vaccine Uptake in Communities of Color.* https://nam.edu/promoting-vaccination-uptake-english (accessed December 30, 2021).

NAM. 2021k. *National Academy of Medicine Members Urge Latinx/Latino(a)/Hispanic Americans to Get Vaccinated.* Video. https://youtu.be/0T38-d45Ok4 (accessed December 30, 2021).

NAM. 2021l. *Working Group on Urgent Priorities for Science, Medicine, & Public Health After COVID-19.* https://nam.edu/programs/working-group-on-urgent-priorities-for-science-medicine-public-health-based-on-lessons-learned-from-covid-19 (accessed December 30, 2021).

NAM. 2021m. *National Academy of Medicine Launches Action Collaborative on Decarbonizing the U.S. Health Sector.* https://nam.edu/national-academy-of-medicine-launches-action-collaborative-on-decarbonizing-the-u-s-health-sector (accessed January 4, 2022).

NAM. 2021n. *21st Surgeon General Joins National Academy of Medicine Action Collaborative on Clinician Well-Being and Resilience as Co-Chair.* https://nam.edu/21st-surgeon-general-vivek-murthy-named-as-co-chair-of-national-academy-of-medicine-action-collaborative-on-clinician-well-being-and-resilience (accessed February 18, 2022).

NAM. 2021o. *National Academy of Medicine Announces Creation of David and Beatrix Hamburg Award for Advances in Biomedical Research and Clinical Medicine.* https://nam.edu/national-academy-of-medicine-announces-creation-of-david-and-beatrix-hamburg-award-for-advances-in-biomedical-research-and-clinical-medicine (accessed July 8, 2022).

NAM. 2022a. *Statement by NAM President Victor Dzau on Responding to the Health Crisis in and Around Ukraine.* https://nam.edu/statement-by-nam-president-victor-dzau-on-responding-to-the-health-crisis-in-and-around-ukraine (accessed July 5, 2022).

NAM. 2022b. *Statement by NAM President Victor J. Dzau in Response to Multiple Mass Shootings in May 2022.* https://nam.edu/statement-by-nam-president-victor-j-dzau-in-response-to-multiple-mass-shootings-in-may-2022 (accessed July 5, 2022).

NAM. 2022c. *Statement from NAM President Victor Dzau and NAS President Marcia McNutt on the Decision to Overturn* Roe v. Wade. https://nam.edu/statement-from-nam-president-victor-dzau-and-nas-president-marcia-mcnutt-on-the-decision-to-overturn-roe-v-wade (accessed July 5, 2022).

NAM. 2022d. *Violent Conflict: The Challenges of Protecting Public Health & Health Care.* https://nam.edu/event/violent-conflict-the-challenges-of-protecting-public-health-health-care (accessed July 22, 2022).

NAM. n.d.a. *Publications of the NAM Leadership Consortium: The Learning Health System Series.* https://nam.edu/publications-of-the-leadership-consortium (accessed July 5, 2021).

NAM. n.d.b. Action Collaborative on Clinician Well-Being and Resilience. https://nam.edu/initiatives/clinician-resilience-and-well-being (accessed July 5, 2021).

NAM. n.d.c. NAM Leadership Consortium: Collaboration for a Value & Science-Driven Health System. https://nam.edu/programs/value-science-driven-health-care (accessed July 6, 2021).

NAM. n.d.d. Global Health Risk Framework. https://nam.edu/initiatives/global-health-risk-framework (accessed July 19, 2021).

NAM. n.d.e. Resources from the NAM's Action Collaborative on Countering the U.S. Opioid Epidemic. https://nam.edu/programs/action-collaborative-on-countering-the-u-s-opioid-epidemic/resources-on-addiction-and-pain-management-services-during-covid-19 (accessed July 19, 2021).

NAM. n.d.f. Resources on Health Equity in the Context of COVID-19 and Disproportionate Outcomes for Marginalized Groups. https://nam.edu/programs/culture-of-health/resources-on-health-equity-in-the-context-of-covid-19-and-disproportionate-outcomes-for-marginalized-groups (accessed July 19, 2021).

NAM. n.d.g. Advancing Pandemic and Seasonal Influenza Vaccine Preparedness and Response. https://nam.edu/programs/advancing-pandemic-and-seasonal-influenza-vaccine-preparedness-and-response-a-global-initiative (accessed July 19, 2021).

NAM. n.d.h. Sharing Knowledge to Combat Clinician Burnout. https://nam.edu/clinicianwellbeing (accessed July 19, 2021).

NAM. n.d.i. Culture of Health: Community-Driven Health Equity Action Plans. https://nam.edu/programs/culture-of-health/community-driven-health-equity-action-plans (accessed July 21, 2021).

NAM. n.d.j. The IOM/NAM 50th Anniversary. https://nam.edu/celebrating-50-years-since-the-founding-of-the-institute-of-medicine (accessed July 27, 2021).

NAM. n.d.k. Culture of Health Program. https://nam.edu/programs/culture-of-health (accessed December 30, 2021).

NAM. n.d.l. About the National Academy of Medicine. https://nam.edu/about-the-nam (accessed January 3, 2022).

NAM, n.d.m. Grand Challenge on Climate Change, Human Health, and Equity. https://nam.edu/programs/climate-change-and-human-health (accessed July 22, 2022).

NAP (National Academies Press). 2014. The National Children's Study 2014. "Description." https://www.nap.edu/catalog/18826/the-national-childrens-study-2014-an-assessment (accessed December 29, 2021).

NAS (National Academy of Sciences). 1947. *Report of the National Academy of Sciences, National Research Council, Fiscal Year 1945–46*. Washington, DC: U.S. Government Printing Office.

NASEM (National Academies of Sciences, Engineering, and Medicine). 1967a. Minutes of Organizational Meeting for a National Academy of Medicine, January 7. Board on Medicine Files, NAS-NRC Archives, Washington DC.

NASEM. 1967b. Minutes of Second Organizational Meeting for a National Academy of Medicine. March 7, Board on Medicine Files, NAS-NRC Archives.

NASEM. 2002a. *The Anthrax Vaccine: Is It Safe? Does It Work?*. Washington, DC: The National Academies Press. https://doi.org/10.17226/10310.

NASEM. 2002b. Report Offers New Eating and Physical Activity Targets to Reduce Chronic Disease Risk. http://www8.nationalacademies.org/onpinews/newsitem.aspx?RecordID=10490 (accessed July 14, 2021).

NASEM. 2004. Indoor Mold, Building Dampness Linked to Respiratory Problems and Require Better Prevention; Evidence Does Not Support Links to Wider Array of Illnesses, May 25. https://www.nationalacademies.org/news/2004/05/indoor-mold-building-dampness-linked-to-respiratory-problems-and-require-better-prevention-evidence-does-not-support-links-to-wider-array-of-illnesses (accessed July 15, 2021).

NASEM. 2006. Fixing Drug Safety System Will Require "New Drug" Symbols on Labels, Major Boost in FDA Staffing and Funding, and Increased Access to Information. News Release, September 22.

NASEM. 2009. *Ensuring the Integrity, Accessibility, and Stewardship of Research Data in the Digital Age*. Washington, DC: The National Academies Press. https://doi.org/10.17226/12615.

NASEM. 2010. Health Care Reform and Increased Patient Needs Require Transformation of Nursing Profession. News Release. https://www.nationalacademies.org/news/2010/10/health-care-reform-and-increased-patient-needs-require-transformation-of-nursing-profession (accessed July 8, 2021).

NASEM. 2013. New IOM Report Highlights PEPFAR's Successes, Calls on Initiative to Intensify Efforts to Enhance Partner Countries' Management of Programs and to Improve Prevention. News from the National Academies, February 20. https://www8.nationalacademies.org/onpinews/newsitem.aspx?RecordID=18256 (accessed July 8, 2021).

NASEM. 2015. Roundtable on Genomics and Precision Health: 2015 Annual Report. https://www.nationalacademies.org/our-work/roundtable-on-genomics-and-precision-health/publications (Annual Reports tab) (accessed July 27, 2021).

NASEM. 2016a. *Advancing the Discipline of Regulatory Science for Medical Product Development: An Update on Progress and a Forward-Looking Agenda: Workshop Summary*. Washington, DC: The National Academies Press. https://doi.org/10.17226/23438.

NASEM. 2016b. *Veterans and Agent Orange: Update 2014*. Washington, DC: The National Academies Press. https://doi.org/10.17226/21845.

NASEM. 2016c. *Assessing Health Outcomes Among Veterans of Project SHAD (Shipboard Hazard and Defense)*. Washington, DC: The National Academies Press. https://doi.org/10.17226/21846.

NASEM. 2016d. Report Release Slides: Assessing Progress on the Institute of Medicine Report: The Future of Nursing. Washington, DC: The National Academies Press. https://doi.org/10.17226/21838.

NASEM. 2016e. *Assessing Progress on the Institute of Medicine Report* The Future of Nursing. Washington, DC: The National Academies Press. https://doi.org/10.17226/21838.

NASEM. 2016f. Families Caring for an Aging America: Report in Brief. Washington, DC: The National Academies Press. https://nap.nationalacademies.org/resource/23606/Caregiving-RiB.pdf.

NASEM. 2016g. *Families Caring for an Aging America.* Washington, DC: The National Academies Press. https://doi.org/10.17226/23606.

NASEM. 2016h. *Hearing Health Care for Adults: Priorities for Improving Access and Affordability.* Washington, DC: The National Academies Press. https://doi.org/10.17226/23446.

NASEM. 2016i. Hearing Health Care for Adults: Priorities for Improving Access and Affordability: Report in Brief. Washington, DC: The National Academies Press. https://nap.nationalacademies.org/resource/23446/Hearing-RiB.pdf.

NASEM. 2016j. *Potential Research Priorities to Inform Public Health and Medical Practice for Domestic Zika Virus: Workshop in Brief.* Washington, DC: The National Academies Press. https://doi.org/10.17226/23404.

NASEM. 2016k. Potential Research Priorities to Inform Public Health and Medical Practice for Domestic Zika Virus. Workshop in Brief, February 29. https://www.nap.edu/resource/23404/interactive (accessed July 19, 2021).

NASEM. 2016l. *Global Health Risk Framework: Resilient and Sustainable Health Systems to Respond to Global Infectious Disease Outbreaks: Workshop Summary.* Washington, DC: The National Academies Press. https://doi.org/10.17226/21856.

NASEM. 2016m. Roundtable on Genomics and Precision Health: 2016 Annual Report. https://www.nationalacademies.org/our-work/roundtable-on-genomics-and-precision-health/publications (Annual Reports tab) (accessed July 27, 2021).

NASEM. 2016n. International Summit on Human Gene Editing: A Global Discussion, Meeting in Brief, Dec 1–3, 2015. https://www.ncbi.nlm.nih.gov/books/NBK343651 (accessed June 24, 2021).

NASEM. 2017a. *Opportunities for Organ Donor Intervention Research: Saving Lives by Improving the Quality and Quantity of Organs for Transplantation.* Washington, DC: The National Academies Press. https://doi.org/10.17226/24884.

NASEM. 2017b. *Human Genome Editing: Science, Ethics, and Governance.* Washington, DC: The National Academies Press. https://doi.org/10.17226/24623.

NASEM. 2017c. *Assessment of the Department of Veterans Affairs Airborne Hazards and Open Burn Pit Registry.* Washington, DC: The National Academies Press. https://doi.org/10.17226/23677.

NASEM. 2017d. *Review of NASA's Evidence Reports on Human Health Risks: 2016 Letter Report.* Washington, DC: The National Academies Press. https://doi.org/10.17226/23678.

NASEM. 2017e. Accounting for Social Risk Factors in Medicare Payment. http://nationalacademies.org/hmd/Activities/Quality/Accounting-SES-in-Medicare-Payment-Programs/Medicare-Social-Risk-Factors-Overview (accessed July 6, 2021).

NASEM. 2017f. *The Health Effects of Cannabis and Cannabinoids: The Current State of Evidence and Recommendations for Research.* Washington, DC: The National Academies Press. https://doi.org/10.17226/24625.

NASEM. 2017g. *Preventing Cognitive Decline and Dementia: A Way Forward.* Washington, DC: The National Academies Press. https://doi.org/10.17226/24782.

NASEM. 2017h. *Guiding Principles for Developing Dietary Reference Intakes Based on Chronic Disease.* Washington, DC: The National Academies Press. https://doi.org/10.17226/24828.

NASEM. 2017i. Report Highlights: Review of WIC Food Packages. https://www.nap.edu/resource/23655/WIC-highlights.pdf (accessed July 14, 2021).

NASEM. 2017j. *Review of WIC Food Packages: Improving Balance and Choice: Final Report.* Washington, DC: The National Academies Press. https://doi.org/10.17226/23655.

NASEM. 2017k. *Microbiomes of the Built Environment: A Research Agenda for Indoor Microbiology, Human Health, and Buildings.* Washington, DC: The National Academies Press. https://doi.org/10.17226/23647.

NASEM. 2017l. Microbiomes of the Built Environment: A Research Agenda for Indoor Microbiology, Human Health, and Buildings, Report Brief. Washington, DC: The National Academies Press. https://nap.nationalacademies.org/resource/23647/Microbiomes_of_Built_Envt_Highlights.pdf.

NASEM. 2017m. National Academies' Presidents Comment on Proposal for New Questions for Visa Applicants. https://www.nationalacademies.org/news/2017/05/national-academies-presidents-comment-on-proposal-for-new-questions-for-visa-applicants (accessed July 21, 2021).

NASEM. 2017n. Global Health and the Future Role of the United States, Report Brief. Washington, DC: The National Academies Press. https://nap.nationalacademies.org/resource/24737/Global_health_report_highlights.pdf.

NASEM. 2017o. *Communities in Action: Pathways to Health Equity.* Washington, DC: The National Academies Press. https://doi.org/10.17226/24624.

NASEM. 2018a. *Veterans and Agent Orange: Update 11.* Washington, DC: The National Academies Press. https://doi.org/10.17226/25137.

NASEM. 2018b. *Crossing the Global Quality Chasm: Improving Health Care Worldwide.* Washington, DC: The National Academies Press. https://doi.org/10.17226/25152.

NASEM. 2018c. *People Living with Disabilities: Health Equity, Health Disparities, and Health Literacy: Proceedings of a Workshop.* Washington, DC: The National Academies Press. https://doi.org/10.17226/24741.

NASEM. 2018d. *Making Medicines Affordable: A National Imperative.* Washington, DC: The National Academies Press. https://doi.org/10.17226/24946.

NASEM. 2018e. *Considerations for the Design of a Systematic Review of Care Interventions for Individuals with Dementia and Their Caregivers: Letter Report.* Washington, DC: The National Academies Press. https://doi.org/10.17226/25326.

NASEM. 2018f. Public Health Consequences of E-Cigarettes: Consensus Study Report, Highlights. https://www.nap.edu/resource/24952/012318ecigaretteHighlights.pdf (accessed July 8, 2021).

NASEM. 2018g. *Getting to Zero Alcohol-Impaired Driving Fatalities: A Comprehensive Approach to a Persistent Problem.* Washington, DC: The National Academies Press. https://doi.org/10.17226/24951.

NASEM. 2018h. *Evaluation of the Department of Veterans Affairs Mental Health Services.* Washington, DC: The National Academies Press. https://doi.org/10.17226/24915.

NASEM. 2018i. Statement by NAS, NAE, and NAM Presidents on the Political Review of Scientific Proposals. https://www.nationalacademies.org/news/2018/01/statement-by-nas-nae-and-nam-presidents-on-the-political-review-of-scientific-proposals (accessed July 21, 2021).

NASEM. 2018j. *The Safety and Quality of Abortion Care in the United States.* Washington, DC: The National Academies Press. https://doi.org/10.17226/24950.

NASEM. 2019a. 2019 President's Address to the NAM Membership. October 21, 2019. https://nam.edu/2019-nam-annual-meeting-information/2019-presidents-address (accessed June 24, 2021).

NASEM. 2019b. New International Commission Launched on Clinical Use of Heritable Human Genome Editing. http://www8.nationalacademies.org/onpinews/newsitem.aspx?RecordID=5222019 (accessed June 24, 2021).

NASEM. 2019c. *Vibrant and Healthy Kids: Aligning Science, Practice, and Policy to Advance Health Equity.* Washington, DC: The National Academies Press. https://doi.org/10.17226/25466.

NASEM. 2019d. Vibrant and Healthy Kids: Aligning Science, Practice, and Policy to Advance Health Equity: Consensus Study Report, Roadmap to Apply the Science of Early Development. https://www.nap.edu/resource/25466/072519_VibrantandHealthyKids_roadmap.pdf (accessed June 24, 2021).

NASEM. 2019e. The Promise of Adolescence: Realizing Opportunity for All Youth: Consensus Study Report, Highlights. https://www.nap.edu/resource/25388/Adolescent%20Development.pdf (accessed June 24, 2021).

NASEM. 2019f. *The Promise of Adolescence: Realizing Opportunity for All Youth.* Washington, DC: The National Academies Press. https://doi.org/10.17226/25388.

NASEM. 2019g. *Guiding Cancer Control: A Path to Transformation.* Washington, DC: The National Academies Press. https://doi.org/10.17226/25438.

NASEM. 2019h. *Reusable Elastomeric Respirators in Health Care: Considerations for Routine and Surge Use.* Washington, DC: The National Academies Press. https://doi.org/10.17226/25275.

NASEM. 2019i. *Taking Action Against Clinician Burnout: A Systems Approach to Professional Well-Being.* Washington, DC: The National Academies Press. https://doi.org/10.17226/25521.

NASEM. 2019j. *Health Systems Interventions to Prevent Firearm Injuries and Death: Proceedings of a Workshop.* Washington, DC: The National Academies Press. https://doi.org/10.17226/25354.

NASEM. 2019k. *Criteria for Selecting the Leading Health Indicators for Healthy People 2030.* Washington, DC: The National Academies Press. https://doi.org/10.17226/25531.

NASEM. 2019l. *Dietary Reference Intakes for Sodium and Potassium.* Washington, DC: The National Academies Press. https://doi.org/10.17226/25353.

NASEM. 2019m. *Integrating Social Care into the Delivery of Health Care: Moving Upstream to Improve the Nation's Health.* Washington, DC: The National Academies Press. https://doi.org/10.17226/25467.

NASEM. 2020a. Discussion Draft of the Preliminary Framework for Equitable Allocation of COVID-19 Vaccine. https://www.nap.edu/resource/25917/25914.pdf (accessed August 24, 2021).

NASEM. 2020b. *Framework for Equitable Allocation of COVID-19 Vaccine.* Washington, DC: The National Academies Press. https://doi.org/10.17226/25917.

NASEM. 2020c. Workshop on Allocation of COVID-19 Monoclonal Antibody Therapies and Other Novel Therapeutics. https://www.nationalacademies.org/event/12-16-2020/workshop-on-allocation-of-covid-19-monoclonal-antibody-therapies-and-other-novel-therapeutics (accessed July 19, 2021).

NASEM. 2020d. U.S. Funding for World Health Organization Should Not Be Interrupted During COVID-19 Pandemic, Say Presidents of the NAS, NAE, and NAM. https://www.nationalacademies.org/news/2020/04/us-funding-for-world-health-organization-should-not-be-interrupted-during-covid-19-pandemic-say-presidents-of-the-nas-nae-and-nam (accessed July 21, 2021).

NASEM. 2020e. NAS and NAM Presidents Alarmed by Political Interference in Science Amid Pandemic. https://www. nationalacademies.org/news/2020/09/nas-and-nam-presidents-alarmed-by-political-interference-in-science-amid-pandemic (accessed July 21, 2021).

NASEM. 2021a. National Academy of Medicine Names 10 Inaugural Scholars in Diagnostic Excellence for 2021. https://www. nationalacademies.org/news/2021/05/national-academy-of-medicine-names-10-inaugural-scholars-in-diagnostic-excellence-for-2021 (accessed July 5, 2021).

NASEM. 2021b. To Achieve Health Equity, Leverage Nurses and Increase Funding for School and Public Health Nursing, Says New Report. https://www.nationalacademies.org/news/2021/05/to-achieve-health-equity-leverage-nurses-and-increase-funding-for-school-and-public-health-nursing-says-new-report (accessed July 6, 2021).

NASEM. 2021c. National Cancer Policy Forum: About the Forum. https://www.nationalacademies.org/our-work/national-cancer-policy-forum (Resources – Forum Overview) (accessed July 27, 2021).

NASEM. 2021d. National Cancer Policy Forum: Workshop Proceedings and Related Publications. https://www.national academies.org/our-work/national-cancer-policy-forum (Resources – Publications) (accessed July 27, 2021).

NASEM. 2021e. *The Future of Nursing 2020–2030: Charting a Path to Achieve Health Equity.* Washington, DC: The National Academies Press. https://doi.org/10.17226/25982.

NASEM. 2022a. "We Stand with Our Colleagues in Ukraine," Say U.S. National Academies Presidents. https://www. nationalacademies.org/news/2022/03/we-stand-with-our-colleagues-in-ukraine-say-u-s-national-academies-presidents (accessed July 22, 2022).

NASEM. 2022b. CHR Statement Regarding Attacks on Health Care in Ukraine. https://www.nationalacademies.org/ news/2022/03/chr-statement-regarding-attacks-on-health-care-in-ukraine (accessed July 22, 2022).

NASEM. 2022c. NAS Launches Effort to Help Support Ukrainian Researchers as They Relocate to Poland. https://www. nationalacademies.org/news/2022/03/nas-launches-effort-to-help-support-ukrainian-researchers-as-they-resettle-in-poland (accessed July 22, 2022).

NASEM. 2022d. International Science Academies Meet in Poland to Explore How to Support Ukrainian Science and Researchers. https://www.nationalacademies.org/news/2022/06/international-science-academies-meet-in-poland-to-explore-how-to-support-ukrainian-science-and-researchers (accessed July 22, 2022).

NASEM. n.d.a. Roundtable on Genomics and Precision Health. http://www.nationalacademies.org/hmd/Activities/Research/ GenomicBasedResearch.aspx (accessed June 24, 2021).

NASEM. n.d.a1. Forum on Regenerative Medicine. http://www.nationalacademies.org/hmd/Activities/Research/Regenerative Medicine.aspx (accessed June 24, 2021).

NASEM. n.d.b. Immunization Safety Review. http://www.nationalacademies.org/hmd/Activities/PublicHealth/Immunization Safety.aspx (accessed July 24, 2021).

NASEM. n.d.b1. Creating a Framework for Emerging Science, Technology, and Innovation in Health and Medicine. https://www.nationalacademies.org/our-work/creating-a-framework-for-emerging-science-technology-and-innovation-in-health-and-medicine (accessed February 18, 2022).

NASEM. n.d.c. Board on Children, Youth, and Families. https://sites.nationalacademies.org/dbasse/bcyf (accessed June 24, 2021).

NASEM. n.d.c1. Review of Omics-Based Tests for Predicting Patient Outcomes in Clinical Trials. https://www.national academies.org/our-work/review-of-omics-based-tests-for-predicting-patient-outcomes-in-clinical-trials (accessed September 7, 2022).

NASEM. n.d.d. Forum for Children's Well-Being: Promoting Cognitive, Affective, and Behavioral Health for Children and Youth. http://www.nationalacademies.org/hmd/Activities/Children/ChildrensHealthForum.aspx (accessed June 24, 2021).

NASEM. n.d.d1. Accelerating Progress in Obesity Prevention. https://www.nationalacademies.org/our-work/accelerating-progress-in-obesity-prevention (accessed September 8, 2022).

NASEM. n.d.e. Standing Committee on Personal Protective Equipment for Workplace Safety and Health. http://www. nationalacademies.org/hmd/Activities/PublicHealth/PPEinWorkplace.aspx (accessed July 5, 2021).

NASEM. n.d.e1. Reducing Risks for Mental Disorders. https://nap.nationalacademies.org/catalog/2139/reducing-risks-for-mental-disorders-frontiers-for-preventive-intervention-research (accessed September 8, 2022).

NASEM. n.d.f. Standing Committee on Aerospace Medicine and the Medicine of Extreme Environments. http://www. nationalacademies.org/hmd/Activities/Research/AerospaceMedicine.aspx (accessed June 30, 2021).

NASEM. n.d.f1. Emerging Infections. https://nap.nationalacademies.org/catalog/2008/emerging-infections-microbial-threats-to-health-in-the-united-states (accessed September 8, 2022).

NASEM. n.d.g. Standing Committee of Medical and Vocational Experts for the Social Security Administration's Disability Programs. http://www.nationalacademies.org/hmd/Activities/HealthServices/SSAStandingCmte.aspx (accessed July 5, 2021).

NASEM. n.d.h. African Science Academy Development Initiative. https://www.nationalacademies.org/our-work/african-science-academy-development-initiative (accessed June 30, 2021).

NASEM. n.d.i. The Quality of Health Care in America. https://www.nationalacademies.org/our-work/the-quality-of-health-care-in-america (accessed July 5, 2021).

NASEM. n.d.j. Committee on Core Metrics for Better Health at Lower Cost. https://www.nationalacademies.org/our-work/committee-on-core-metrics-for-better-health-at-lower-cost (accessed July 6, 2021).

NASEM. n.d.k. Roundtable on Health Literacy. https://www.nationalacademies.org/our-work/roundtable-on-health-literacy (accessed July 6, 2021).

NASEM. n.d.l. Health Literacy and Communication Strategies in Oncology: A Workshop. https://www.nationalacademies.org/our-work/health-literacy-and-communication-strategies-in-oncology-a-workshop (accessed July 6, 2021).

NASEM. n.d.m. The Future of Nursing 2020–2030. http://www.nationalacademies.org/hmd/Activities/Workforce/futureofnursing2030.aspx (accessed July 6, 2021).

NASEM. n.d.n. National Cancer Policy Forum. https://www.nationalacademies.org/our-work/national-cancer-policy-forum (accessed July 6, 2021).

NASEM. n.d.o. Forum on Neuroscience and Nervous System Disorders. https://www.nationalacademies.org/our-work/forum-on-neuroscience-and-nervous-system-disorders (accessed July 6, 2021).

NASEM. n.d.p. Consequences of Uninsurance. https://www.nationalacademies.org/our-work/consequences-of-uninsurance (accessed July 6, 2021).

NASEM. n.d.q. Vital Directions for Health and Health Care. https://nam.edu/initiatives/vital-directions-for-health-and-health-care (accessed July 6, 2021).

NASEM. n.d.r. Roundtable on Population Health Improvement. https://www.nationalacademies.org/our-work/roundtable-on-population-health-improvement (accessed July 7, 2021).

NASEM. n.d.s. Forum on Global Violence Prevention. https://www.nationalacademies.org/our-work/forum-on-global-violence-prevention (accessed September 8, 2022).

NASEM. n.d.t. Food Forum. https://www.nationalacademies.org/our-work/food-forum/about (accessed July 14, 2021).

NASEM. n.d.u. Summary Report of the Dietary Reference Intakes. http://www.nationalacademies.org/hmd/Activities/Nutrition/SummaryDRIs/DRI-Tables.aspx (accessed July 14, 2021).

NASEM. n.d.v. Roundtable on Obesity Solutions. https://www.nationalacademies.org/our-work/roundtable-on-obesity-solutions (accessed July 15, 2021).

NASEM. n.d.w. Key Policy Challenges to Improve Care for People with Mental Health and Substance Use Disorders. http://www.nationalacademies.org/hmd/Activities/MentalHealth/MentalHealthSubstanceUseDisorderForum/2019-OCT-15.aspx (accessed July 15, 2021).

NASEM. n.d.x. Roundtable on Environmental Health Sciences, Research, and Medicine. https://www.nationalacademies.org/our-work/roundtable-on-environmental-health-sciences-research-and-medicine (accessed July 15, 2021).

NASEM. n.d.y. Action Collaborative on Preventing Sexual Harassment in Higher Education. https://www.nationalacademies.org/our-work/action-collaborative-on-preventing-sexual-harassment-in-higher-education (accessed July 19, 2021).

NASEM. n.d.z. About: Forum on Medical and Public Health Preparedness for Disasters and Emergencies. https://www.nationalacademies.org/our-work/forum-on-medical-and-public-health-preparedness-for-disasters-and-emergencies/about (accessed July 26, 2021).

NCATS (National Center for Advancing Translational Sciences). 2014. NCATS Advisory Council Working Group on the IOM Report: The CTSA Program at NIH, Draft Report. https://ncats.nih.gov/files/CTSA-IOM-WG-report-5-2014.pdf (accessed June 29, 2021).

NCHS (National Center for Health Statistics). 2020. NCHS Data Brief 394. https://www.cdc.gov/nchs/data/databriefs/db394-tables-508.pdf#page=1 (accessed July 21, 2021).

NCMJ (*North Carolina Medical Journal*). 2020. Vital Directions for Health and Health Care in North Carolina. https://www.ncmedicaljournal.com/content/81/3 (accessed July 21, 2021).

NEJM (*New England Journal of Medicine*). n.d. Progress in Health: The NAM at 50. https://www.nejm.org/nam-health-progress (accessed July 27, 2021).

Network Television Evening News. 1986. Abstracts for October 29, 1986, Vanderbilt Television News Archives, Vanderbilt University.

Neustadt, R. E., and H. V. Fineberg. 1978. *The Swine Flu Affair*. Washington, DC: Department of Health, Education, and Welfare. https://www.nap.edu/catalog/12660/the-swine-flu-affair-decision-making-on-a-slippery-disease.

Newcott, B. 2021. Fauci Recalls the Terrifying Early Days of the AIDS Epidemic. *National Geographic,* June 3. https://www.nationalgeographic.com/history/article/fauci-recalls-the-terrifying-early-days-of-the-aids-epidemic (accessed July 7, 2021).

NHGRI (National Human Genome Research Institute). n.d. Human Genome Project Timeline of Events. https://www.genome.gov/human-genome-project/Timeline-of-Events (accessed June 24, 2021).

Nichols, E. K. 1986. *Mobilizing Against AIDS*. Cambridge, MA: Harvard University Press, 1989.

NIH (National Institutes of Health). 2014. Statement on the National Children's Study, December 11. https://www.nih.gov/about-nih/who-we-are/nih-director/statements/statement-national-childrens-study (accessed June 24, 2021).

NIH. n.d.a. James A. Shannon, M.D. The NIH Almanac. https://www.nih.gov/about-nih/what-we-do/nih-almanac/james-shannon-md (accessed June 21, 2021).

NIH. n.d.b. An Overview of NCI's National Clinical Trials Network. https://ctep.cancer.gov/initiativesPrograms/nctn.htm (accessed June 24, 2021).

NIH. n.d.c. Retirement of the National Institutes of Health Consensus Development Program. https://consensus.nih.gov (accessed June 29, 2021).

NIH. n.d.d. NIH Plan to Retire All NIH-Owned and -Supported Chimpanzees. https://orip.nih.gov/comparative-medicine/programs/nih-plan-retire-all-nih-owned-and-supported-chimpanzees (accessed June 29, 2021).

NLM (National Library of Medicine). n.d. What Is the Precision Medicine Initiative? https://ghr.nlm.nih.gov/primer/precision medicine/initiative (accessed June 24, 2021).

NOAA (National Oceanic and Atmospheric Administration). 2021. Record Number of Billion-Dollar Disasters Struck U.S. in 2020. https://www.noaa.gov/stories/record-number-of-billion-dollar-disasters-struck-us-in-2020 (accessed July 21, 2021).

NRC (National Research Council). 1977. *Computed Tomographic Scanning: A Policy Statement*. Washington, DC: National Academy Press. https://doi.org/10.17226/19927.

NRC. 1989a. *Diet and Health: Implications for Reducing Chronic Disease Risk: Executive Summary*. Washington, DC: National Academy Press. https://doi.org/10.17226/19023.

NRC. 1989b. *AIDS, Sexual Behavior, and Intravenous Drug Use*. Washington, DC: National Academy Press. https://doi.org/10.17226/1195.

NRC. 1990. *AIDS: The Second Decade*. Washington, DC: National Academy Press. https://doi.org/10.17226/1534.

NRC. 1993. *Understanding Child Abuse and Neglect*. Washington, DC: National Academy Press. https://doi.org/10.17226/2117.

NRC and IOM (Institute of Medicine). 2004. *Reducing Underage Drinking: A Collective Responsibility*. Washington, DC: The National Academies Press. https://doi.org/10.17226/10729.

NRC and IOM. 2010. *Final Report of the National Academies' Human Embryonic Stem Cell Research Advisory Committee and 2010 Amendments to the National Academies' Guidelines for Human Embryonic Stem Cell Research*. Washington, DC: The National Academies Press. https://doi.org/10.17226/12923.

Oak Ridge National Laboratory. n.d. Human Genome Project Information Archive. https://web.ornl.gov/sci/techresources/Human_Genome/index.shtml (accessed June 24, 2021).

ONC (Office of the National Coordinator for Health Information Technology). 2013. Health Information Technology Patient Safety Action & Surveillance Plan. https://www.healthit.gov/sites/default/files/safety_plan_master.pdf (accessed July 5, 2021)

Page, I. 1964. Needed—A National Academy of Medicine. *Modern Medicine,* July 20, 77–79.

Page, I. 1965. More on a National Academy of Medicine. *Modern Medicine,* March 15, 189–90.

Panangala, S. V., D. T. Shedd, and U. Moulta-Ali. 2014. Veterans Affairs: Presumptive Service Connection and Disability Compensation. Congressional Research Service Report R41405. https://fas.org/sgp/crs/misc/R41405.pdf (accessed June 30, 2021).

Panchal, N., R. Kamal, C. Cox, and R. Garfield. 2021. The Implications of COVID-19 for Mental Health and Substance Use. Kaiser Family Foundation. https://www.kff.org/coronavirus-covid-19/issue-brief/the-implications-of-covid-19-for-mental-health-and-substance-use (accessed December 29, 2021).

Pariseault, A. B. 2021. Current Status of COVID-19 Vaccines Rollout Nationwide. https://www.naag.org/attorney-general-journal/current-status-of-covid-19-vaccines-rollout-nationwide-december-2021-update-for-the-attorney-general-community (accessed July 6, 2022).

Pear, R. 1999. A Clinton Order Seeks to Reduce Medical Errors. *The New York Times,* December 7, A1.

Pear, R. 2000. Clinton to Order Steps to Reduce Medical Mistakes. *The New York Times,* February 22, A1.

Pear, R. 2018. Trump Rule Would Compel Drug Makers to Disclose Prices in TV Commercials. *The New York Times,* October 15.

Pechura, M. 1993. *From the Institute of Medicine. JAMA* 269(4):453. https://doi.org/10.1001/jama.1993.03500040015008.

Philadelphia Inquirer. 1999. Put Patient Safety First. Editorial, December 1.

Preston, R. 1992. Crisis in the Hot Zone: Lessons from an Outbreak of Ebola. *The New Yorker.* https://www.newyorker.com/magazine/1992/10/26/crisis-in-the-hot-zone (accessed December 29, 2021).

Pronovost, P., M. M. E. Johns, S. Palmer, R. C. Bono, D. B. Fridsma, A. Gettinger, J. Goldman, W. Johnson, M. Karney, C. Samitt, R. D. Sriram, A. Zenooz, and Y. C. Wang (Eds.). 2018. *Procuring Interoperability: Achieving High-Quality, Connected, and Person-Centered Care.* Washington, DC: National Academy of Medicine.

Rakoczy, K. L. 2001. Ex-Provost Will Head Institute of Medicine. *The Harvard Crimson,* November 9. https://www.thecrimson.com/article/2001/11/9/ex-provost-will-head-institute-of-medicine/?page=1 (accessed July 30, 2021).

Rapaport, L. 2017. Another Look at the Surge in EpiPen Costs. *Reuters,* March 17. https://www.reuters.com/article/us-health-epipen-costs/another-look-at-the-surge-in-epipen-costs-idUSKBN16Y24O (accessed July 6, 2021).

Ratzan, S. C., and R. M. Parker. 2000. Introduction. In *National Library of Medicine Current Bibliographies in Medicine: Health Literacy.* NLM Pub. No. CBM 2000-1. C. R. Selden, M. Zorn, S. C. Ratzan, and R. M. Parker (Eds.). Bethesda, MD: National Institutes of Health, Department of Health and Human Services.

Robernicks, A. 2002. Pediatric End-of-Life Care Found Lacking. *amnednews.com*, August 19.

Roberts, S. 2019. David Hamburg, Leader in Conflict Resolution, Dies at 93. *The New York Times,* April 23. https://www.nytimes.com/2019/04/23/obituaries/dr-david-hamburg-dead.html (accessed August 24, 2021).

Russell, C. 1986. Escalate AIDS Fight, Scientists Urge. *The Washington Post*, October 30, A-1.

RWJF (Robert Wood Johnson Foundation). 2010. Pursuing Perfection: Raising the Bar for Health Care Performance. https://www.rwjf.org/content/dam/farm/reports/program_results_reports/2011/rwjf69593 (accessed July 5, 2021).

Sack, K. 2008. Medicare Won't Pay for Medical Errors. *The New York Times,* September 30. https://www.nytimes.com/2008/10/01/us/01mistakes.html (accessed July 5, 2021).

Science History Institute. n.d. Jonas Salk and Albert Bruce Sabin. https://www.sciencehistory.org/historical-profile/jonas-salk-and-albert-bruce-sabin (accessed June 24, 2021).

Seitz, F. 2007. *A Selection of Highlights from the History of the National Academy of Sciences, 1863–2005.* Lanham, MD: University Press of America.

Shear, M. D. 2017. Trump Administration Orders Tougher Screening of Visa Applicants. *The New York Times,* March 23. https://www.nytimes.com/2017/03/23/us/politics/visa-extreme-vetting-rex-tillerson.html (accessed July 21, 2021).

Siddiqui, S., L. Gambino and O. Laughland. 2017. Trump Travel Ban: New Order Targeting Six Muslim-Majority Countries Signed. *The Guardian*, March 6. https://www.theguardian.com/us-news/2017/mar/06/new-trump-travel-ban-muslim-majority-countries-refugees (accessed July 21, 2021).

Sklar, D. P. 2014. Graduate education and the Institute of Medicine report. *Academic Medicine* 89(12):1575–1577. https://doi.org/10.1097/ACM.0000000000000532.

Slade, J. 1992. The tobacco epidemic: Lessons from history. *Journal of Psychoactive Drugs* 24(2):99–109. https://doi.org/10.1080/02791072.1992.10471631.

STAT. n.d. The COVID-19 Tracker. https://www.statnews.com/feature/coronavirus/covid-19-tracker (accessed July 26, 2021).

Stolberg, S. G., M. Haberman and N. Weiland. 2020. Trump Calls Fauci "a Disaster" and Shrugs Off Virus as Infections Soar. *The New York Times*, October 19. https://www.nytimes.com/2020/10/19/us/politics/trump-fauci-covid.html (accessed July 21, 2021).

Tavernise, S. 2021. An Arms Race in America: Gun Buying Spiked During the Pandemic. It's Still Up. *The New York Times*, May 29. https://www.nytimes.com/2021/05/29/us/gun-purchases-ownership-pandemic.html (accessed July 14, 2021).

The Joint Commission. n.d. The Joint Commission: Over a Century of Quality and Safety. https://www.jointcommission.org/-/media/tjc/documents/about-us/tjc-history-timeline-through-2019-pdf.pdf (accessed July 5, 2021).

The Skin You're In. 2021. National Academy of Medicine Members Urge Black Americans to Get Vaccinated. Video. https://www.youtube.com/watch?v=_2qQxFrdNSw (accessed December 30, 2021).

The Washington Post. 2011. Obituaries. https://www.washingtonpost.com/local/obituaries/2011/09/07/gIQAzN2AAK_story.html?_=ddid-6-1574447700 (accessed July 30, 2021).

The White House. 2000. President Clinton Takes New Action to Encourage Participation in Clinical Trials. June 7. https://clintonwhitehouse3.archives.gov/WH/New/html/20000607.html (accessed July 6, 2021).

The White House. 2021a. FACT SHEET: Biden-Harris Administration Unveils Strategy for Global Vaccine Sharing, Announcing Allocation Plan for the First 25 Million Doses to Be Shared Globally. https://www.whitehouse.gov/briefing-room/statements-releases/2021/06/03/fact-sheet-biden-harris-administration-unveils-strategy-for-global-vaccine-sharing-announcing-allocation-plan-for-the-first-25-million-doses-to-be-shared-globally (accessed December 29, 2021).

The White House. 2021b. FACT SHEET: President Biden Sets 2030 Greenhouse Gas Pollution Reduction Target Aimed at Creating Good-Paying Union Jobs and Securing U.S. Leadership on Clean Energy Technologies. https://www.whitehouse.gov/briefing-room/statements-releases/2021/04/22/fact-sheet-president-biden-sets-2030-greenhouse-gas-pollution-reduction-target-aimed-at-creating-good-paying-union-jobs-and-securing-u-s-leadership-on-clean-energy-technologies (accessed July 22, 2022).

Thurber, J. 2000. Lucile Petry Leone; Led U.S. Cadet Nurse Corps. *Los Angeles Times*, January 3. https://www.latimes.com/archives/la-xpm-2000-jan-03-mn-50357-story.html (accessed June 21, 2021).

Tolbert, J., K. Orgera, and A. Damico. 2020. Key Facts About the Uninsured Population. Kaiser Family Foundation. https://www.kff.org/uninsured/issue-brief/key-facts-about-the-uninsured-population (accessed July 6, 2021).

TRB, IOM, and NRC (Transportation Research Board, Institute of Medicine, and National Research Council). 2009. *Local Government Actions to Prevent Childhood Obesity.* Washington, DC: The National Academies Press.

Umstead, R. T. 2012. Review: HBO's "The Weight of the Nation." *Next TV*, May 13. https://www.multichannel.com/news/review-hbos-weight-nation-360575 (accessed July 15, 2021).

UN (United Nations). 2018. New Health Board Aims to Break "Cycle of Panic and Neglect" on Pandemics." https://news.un.org/en/story/2018/05/1010641 (accessed January 4, 2022).

U.S. Census Bureau. 2018. Older People Projected to Outnumber Children for First Time in U.S. History. https://www. census.gov/newsroom/press-releases/2018/cb18-41-population-projections.html (accessed July 21, 2021).

U.S. Census Bureau. 2019. 2020 Census Will Help Policymakers Prepare for the Incoming Wave of Aging Boomers. https:// www.census.gov/library/stories/2019/12/by-2030-all-baby-boomers-will-be-age-65-or-older.html (accessed July 6, 2021).

U.S. Congress, Senate. 2009. S. 717 (111th): 21st Century Cancer ALERT (Access to Life-Saving Early detection, Research and Treatment) Act. Washington, DC: Government Printing Office. https://www.govtrack.us/congress/bills/111/s717/text (accessed June 24, 2021).

U.S. Congress, Senate Committee on Appropriations. 2020. Subcommittee Hearing: Review of Operation Warp Speed: Researching, Manufacturing, & Distributing a Safe & Effective Coronavirus Vaccine. Video, July 2. https://www. appropriations.senate.gov/hearings/review-of-operation-warp-speed-researching-manufacturing-and-distributing-a-safe_effective-coronavirus-vaccine (accessed July 6, 2022).

VA (Department of Veterans Affairs). 2016. Gulf War Newsletter. https://www.publichealth.va.gov/exposures/publications/gulf-war/gulf-war-winter-2016/gulf-war-presumptives.asp (accessed June 30, 2021).

VA. n.d.a. Veterans Health Administration. https://www.va.gov/health (accessed June 30, 2021).

VA. n.d.b. Public Health: Gulf War Health and Medicine Division Reports. https://www.publichealth.va.gov/exposures/gulfwar/reports/health-and-medicine-division.asp (accessed June 30, 2021).

Wadman, M. 2005. Strong medicine. *Nature Medicine* 11(4):465–466.

Wakefield, A. J., S. H. Murch, A. Anthony, J. Linnell, D. M. Casson, M. Malik, M. Berelowitz, A. P. Dhillon, M. A. Thomson, P. Harvey, A. Valentine, S. E. Davies, and J. A. Walker-Smith. 1998. RETRACTED: Ileal-lymphoid-nodular hyperplasia, non-specific colitis, and pervasive developmental disorder in children. *The Lancet* 351(9103):P637–P641.

Wan, W. 2019. Health-Care System Causing Rampant Burnout Among Doctors, Nurses. *The Washington Post*, October 23. https://www.washingtonpost.com/health/2019/10/23/broken-health-care-system-is-causing-rampant-burnout-among-doctors-nurses (accessed July 19, 2021).

Weir, K. 2021. A Thaw in the Freeze on Federal Funding for Gun Violence and Injury Prevention Research. *Monitor on Psychology* 52(3). https://www.apa.org/monitor/2021/04/news-funding-gun-research (accessed July 14, 2021).

WHO (World Health Organization). 2004. WHO Guidelines for Indoor Air Quality: Dampness and Mould. https://www. who.int/airpollution/guidelines/dampness-mould/en (accessed July 15, 2021).

WHO. 2019. WHO Report on the Global Tobacco Epidemic 2019: Offer Help to Quit Tobacco Use. https://www.who.int/teams/health-promotion/tobacco-control/who-report-on-the-global-tobacco-epidemic-2019 (accessed July 8, 2021).

WHO. 2022. WHO and NAM Encourage Digital Platforms to Apply Global Principles for Identifying Credible Sources of Health Information. https://www.who.int/news/item/24-02-2022-who-and-nam-encourage-digital-platforms-to-apply-global-principles-for-identifying-credible-sources-of-health-information (accessed July 5, 2022).

Yaktine, A., and A. C. Ross. 2019. Milestones in DRI Development: What Does the Future Hold?" *Advances in Nutrition* 10(3):537–545.

Editor and Author Biographies

EDITORS

The editors of this volume are members of the National Academy of Medicine (NAM) who contributed their time and expertise to the organization, review, and revision of this book. Final responsibility for the content rests with the authors and the NAM.

Evelynn Hammonds, SM, PhD, is the Barbara Gutmann Rosenkrantz Professor of the History of Science, a Professor of African and African American Studies, Harvard University, and a Professor of the Social and Behavioral Sciences, Harvard T.H. Chan School of Public Health. Dr. Hammonds is the author of *Childhood's Deadly Scourge: The Campaign to Control Diphtheria in New York City, 1880–1930* (Johns Hopkins University Press, 1999). She co-edited *Gender and Scientific Authority* (University of Chicago Press, 1996). She has published articles on the history of disease, race, and science; African American feminism; African American women and the epidemic of HIV/AIDS; and analyses of gender and race in science and medicine. She is also the author of the article "Gendering the Epidemic: Feminism and the Epidemic of HIV/AIDS in the United States, 1981–1999," which appeared in *Science, Medicine, and Technology in the 20th Century: What Difference Has Feminism Made?* (University of Chicago Press, 2000). Dr. Hammonds's current work focuses on the intersection of scientific, medical, and socio-political concepts of race in the United States. Her most recent article, co-authored with S. Reverby, is "Toward a Historically Informed Analysis of Racial Health Disparities Since 1619" *(American Journal of Public Health* 108[10]).

Howard Markel, MD, PhD, is the George E. Wantz Distinguished Professor of the History of Medicine and the Director of the Center for the History of Medicine at the University of Michigan. He is also a Professor of Psychiatry, Public Health, History, English Literature and Language, and Pediatrics and Communicable Diseases. An acclaimed social and cultural historian of medicine, Dr. Markel is the author, co-author, or co-editor of 10 books, including the award-winning *Quarantine!: East European Jewish Immigrants and the New York City Epidemics of 1892* (Johns Hopkins University Press, 1997) and *When Germs Travel: Six Major Epidemics That Have Invaded America*

Since 1900 and the Fears They Have Unleashed (Pantheon Books/Alfred A. Knopf, 2004). His national best-selling book *An Anatomy of Addiction: Sigmund Freud, William Halsted, and the Miracle Drug Cocaine* (Pantheon Books/Alfred A. Knopf, 2011) garnered wide critical praise and was a *New York Times* best-seller. From 2005 to 2006, Dr. Markel served as a historical consultant on pandemic influenza preparedness planning for the Department of Defense.

David Rosner, PhD, MPH, is the Ronald H. Lauterstein Professor, Sociomedical Sciences, and the Co-Director, Center for the History & Ethics of Public Health, at Columbia University. Dr. Rosner focuses on research at the intersection of public health and social history and the politics of occupational disease and industrial pollution. He has been actively involved in lawsuits on behalf of cities, states, and communities around the nation who are trying to hold the lead, asbestos, and chemical industry accountable for past acts that have resulted in tremendous damage to America's children. Cases aimed at removing lead from children's environments, removing PCBs from state waterways, and asbestos lawsuits aimed at providing funds for remediation and compensation for victims of environmental and occupational disease have grown out of his academic work. His work on the history of industry understanding the harms done by their industrial toxins has been part of lawsuits on behalf of asbestos workers and silicosis victims as well. Dr. Rosner is the author and editor of 12 books, including, with NAM member Gerald Markowitz, the forthcoming *Building the Worlds That Kill Us: Disease, Death, and American History* (Columbia University Press).

Rosemary Stevens, PhD, MPH, is a DeWitt Wallace Distinguished Scholar in Social Medicine and Public Policy in the Department of Psychiatry at Weill Cornell Medical College. She is also the Stanley I. Sheerr Professor Emeritus in Arts and Sciences at the University of Pennsylvania, where she was a member (and sometime chair) of the Department of History and Sociology of Science and a Senior Fellow at the Leonard Davis Institute of Health Economics. Between 1968 and 1976, she held subsequent Assistant, Associate, and full Professor positions at the Yale Medical School in the Department of Epidemiology and Public Health, and was also a Fellow at Yale's Institute for Social and Policy Studies. In 1976 she moved to Tulane University, serving as the Chair of the Department of Health Systems Management. She moved to the University of Pennsylvania in 1979 and joined the emeritus faculty in 2002. Stevens's publications include books on the history of medical practice in England, the history of specialization in American medicine, the early implementation of Medicaid, physician migration policy and its implications, and the history of American hospitals. Her current research focuses on the formal organization of specialization in American medicine today, and the public roles and self-regulatory structures of the medical profession.

AUTHORS

Laura Harbold DeStefano is the Director of Strategic Communications & Engagement at the National Academy of Medicine, where she has served in various editing and communications roles since 2011. Previously, she was the manager of the AEI Press, the book publisher for the American Enterprise Institute. She has a B.A. in English from Dickinson College and resides in Takoma Park, Maryland, with her husband, two sons, and two dogs.

Andrea Schultz, MPH, is the Technical Program Manager at Cleerly Health, a digital health care company dedicated to promoting cardiovascular health. Previously, she held research and project management positions at LGS Innovations, PCM TRIALS, and the Department of State. From 2004 until 2013, Schultz held roles at the Institute of Medicine (IOM), including a position supporting research and organizational change initiatives for IOM President Harvey Fineberg. She served as the Co-Director of five IOM consensus studies and three standing committees.

Edward Berkowitz, PhD, is a Professor Emeritus of History and Public Policy at The George Washington University. He is the author of *To Improve Human Health: A History of the Institute of Medicine* (Washington, DC: National Academy Press, 1998). His most recent book is *Making Social Welfare Policy: Three Case Studies Since 1959* (Chicago: University of Chicago Press, 2020).